CONTROL OF HOSPITAL INFECTION

CONTROL OF HOSPITAL INFECTION
A practical handbook

Third edition
Edited by

G. A. J. Ayliffe

Emeritus Professor of Medical Microbiology,
University of Birmingham and formerly Hon. Director, Hospital Infection
Research Laboratory, Dudley Road Hospital, Birmingham

E. J. L. Lowbury

Formerly Hon. Visiting Professor of Medical Microbiology, Aston University
and formerly Hon. Director of Hospital Infection Research Laboratory
and Bacteriologist MRC Burns Unit, Birmingham Accident Hospital

A. M. Geddes

Professor of Infection, University of Birmingham,
Consultant Physician, South Birmingham Health Authority and
Consultant Adviser in Infectious Diseases, Department of Health

J. D. Williams

Professor of Medical Microbiology, London Hospital Medical College
and Consultant Microbiologist, The Royal London Hospital

CHAPMAN & HALL MEDICAL
London · Glasgow · New York · Tokyo · Melbourne · Madras

Published by Chapman & Hall, 2-6 Boundary Row, London SE1 8HN

Chapman & Hall, 2-6 Boundary Row, London SE1 8HN, UK

Blackie Academic & Professional, Wester Cleddens Road, Bishopbriggs, Glasgow G64 2NZ, UK

Chapman & Hall, 29 West 35th Street, New York NY10001, USA

Chapman & Hall Japan, Thomson Publishing Japan, Hirakawacho Nemoto Building, 6F, 1-7-11 Hirakawa-cho, Chiyoda-ku, Tokyo 102, Japan

Chapman & Hall Australia, Thomas Nelson Australia, 102 Dodds Street, South Melbourne, Victoria 3205, Australia

Chapman & Hall India, R. Seshadri, 32 Second Main Road, CIT East, Madras 600 035, India

First edition 1975
Second edition 1981
Reprinted 1982, 1988
Third edition 1992
Reprinted 1993

© 1975, 1981, 1992 Chapman & Hall

Typeset in 10/12pt Palatino by Intype, London
Printed in Great Britain by TJ Press (Padstow) Ltd, Padstow, Cornwall

ISBN 0 412 28440 5   0 442 31669 0(USA)

A catalogue record for this book is available from the British Library
Library of Congress Cataloging-in-Publication Data available

Contents

Editors

G.A.J. Ayliffe Emeritus Professor of Medical Microbiology, University of Birmingham; formerly Hon. Director, Hospital Infection Research Laboratory, Dudley Road Hospital, Birmingham

E.J.L. Lowbury formerly Hon. Visiting Professor of Medical Microbiology (Aston University); formerly Hon. Director of Hospital Infection Research Laboratory and Bacteriologist MRC Burns Unit, Birmingham Accident Hospital

A.M. Geddes Professor of Infection, University of Birmingham. Consultant Physician, South Birmingham Health Authority. Consultant Adviser in Infectious Diseases, Department of Health

J.D. Williams Professor of Medical Microbiology, Royal London Hospital Medical College. Consultant Microbiologist, The Royal London Hospital

Other contributors

J.R. Babb Hospital Infection Research Laboratory
The late **B.J. Collins** Hospital Infection Research Laboratory
N. Cripps Principal Assistant Engineer, West Midlands Regional Health Authority
J.G.P. Hutchison formerly Director Public Health Laboratory, East Birmingham Hospital
R.H. George Consultant Microbiologist Children's Hospital Birmingham
C.E.A. Deverill Manager, Sterile Services Department, Central District Birmingham
B.H.B. Robinson Consultant Physician, Renal Unit, East Birmingham Hospital
T.H. Flewett formerly Director Regional Virus Unit, East Birmingham Hospital
M.J. Roper-Hall formerly Consultant Ophthalmologist, Eye Hospital, Birmingham

Acknowledgements

We should also like to thank the staff of the Hospital Infection Research Laboratory: Christina Bradley, Jean Davies, Lynda Taylor (now at the Division of Hospital Infection, Colindale), Elaine Josse, Katherine Mitchell and the other infection control nurses in Dudley Road Hospital for present and past contributions, also Dr J. Harry, Consultant Pathologist, Eye Hospital, Dr P. Brown, formerly Consultant Microbiologist Central District Birmingham, Dr J. C. Lawrence, Burns Research Group, Birmingham Accident Hospital, Mr T.H. Waterhouse formerly legal adviser to West Midlands Regional Health Authority, and the other members of the original working party who are listed in the previous edition of this book. We are grateful to Pauline Surman and Ruth Jones for typing the script.

Acknowledgement

Preface to the third edition

Since the publication of the second edition 10 years ago a number of new problems of hospital infection have emerged. Epidemics of methicillin-resistant *Staphylococcus aureus* have been reported in many hospitals and methods for the control of staphylococcal infection have required re-evaluation. These epidemics which sometimes have had severe clinical effects have often been costly and have demonstrated the need for isolation units and effective hygienic practices in general hospitals.

The emergence of human immunodeficiency virus (HIV) infection has probably had the greatest impact on control of infection procedures. Although transmission in hospitals has been rare, except through transfused blood in the early days, HIV infection has caused considerable anxiety among hospital staff. Numerous guidelines have been produced often providing contradictory and sometimes unnecessary recommendations, particularly for hospitals where the incidence of HIV infection is low. Nevertheless, attention focused on the disease has revealed deficiencies in routine control of infection practices in the community as well as in hospital.

The increased usage of expensive heat-labile equipment, such as flexible fibreoptic endoscopes, has required further research into effective decontamination procedures. This has highlighted problems of toxicity of disinfectants such as glutaraldehyde, and has demonstrated a need for the development of non-toxic, non-corrosive antiviral disinfectants.

Outbreaks of food poisoning and Legionnaire's disease in hospitals in the UK were responsible for official recommendations on the administrative aspects of control of infection both in hospitals and the community. The large US project on 'The study on the Efficacy of Nosocomial Infection Control' (SENIC) demonstrated the importance of the surveillance and effective control measures and of an infection control doctor (Officer) or hospital epidemiologist and an infection control nurse in reducing infection rates. High costs of hospital care have had an increasing influence on hospital practice and infection control staff have had to justify their policies and provide evidence of improved quality of care by audit of infection control practices. Increased computerization of data has been associated with new methods of identifying patients at high risk of infection, so that specific control measures can be targeted at these patients.

The increasing involvement of hospital managers and outside agencies in control of infection has led to a tendency for a return of rituals which previously had been eliminated from most hospitals. These are often associated with increased costs without benefit to patients or staff. Examples are microbiological sampling of the environment, increased use of disinfectants in the environment and of expensive single-use products. We hope that control procedures will continue to be based on valid microbiological or clinical evidence rather than on risks assumed groundlessly by inexperienced personnel or by the lay public.

The basic principles of infection control have not changed and spread of infection can still be minimized by simple procedures, such as hand-washing and good aseptic techniques.

A recent document published by the Department of Health titled Health of the Nation includes an objective to reduce as far as possible the incidence of hospital-acquired infection.

This book is intended to be a practical guide and is not a comprehensive textbook. Only a limited number of references have been included with each chapter, but a more general bibliography has been provided at the end of the book. Readers are also referred to specialist journals on hospital infection, for example the *Journal of Hospital Infection*, *Infection Control and Hospital Epidemiology*, and the *American Journal of Infection Control*.

Although many of the references are official guidelines or codes of practice from the UK, the recommendations in the book do not necessarily follow these where they are considered to be inappropriate, and it is hoped that the book will be of interest and useful to infection control workers in all countries.

Preface to the first edition

This *Handbook* has been prepared as a guide for use by the staffs of hospitals. It is addressed to doctors, nurses, physiotherapists, radiographers and others who are involved in the treatment and care of patients, and in part also to administrators, architects, engineers, domestic superintendents and others whose work may influence the chances of infection among patients and staff.

Before the introduction of antiseptic and aseptic methods by Lister and others in the last century, major surgical infection ('hospital gangrene') was an overwhelming hazard and a common cause of death in hospitals. Although fulminating infection of this type was eliminated by the new measures, a residue of less dangerous infection persisted, and the development of new fields of surgery and therapy, including methods which interfere with the patients' immunity, has introduced new hazards of infection. Antibiotic treatment has brought relief against some of these infections, but it has often been frustrated by the emergence of antibiotic resistant bacteria. In addition to the hardship that it causes to patients (and sometimes to members of staff), hospital infection has, in the words of Sir Wilson Jameson, been 'a steady drain on the hospital purse and efficiency'. Abundant research in the past 25 years has shown that hospital infection can be greatly reduced by the correct application of a number of improved methods of asepsis and hygiene; but it is also a familiar experience that hospital infection is still common and that recommendations are often unknown or unobserved. The purpose of this *Handbook* is to offer the guidance and information needed for a more effective use of current knowledge on ways of controlling infection.

To be effective such a handbook must be understood clearly by all who wish to use it, and we have therefore tried to express, in as simple terms as we can, the elaborate and ever-developing strategy and tactics used in the control of hospital infection. This has involved calling many products by the proprietary names which are commonly used rather than (or as well as) by their official or chemical names; in many cases (e.g. the clear soluble phenolic compounds) no other names are available. When we refer to a disinfectant or antiseptic for a particular purpose, it must be regarded as an example, and one which we have examined; other products of which we have no information or personal experience may well be as effective – perhaps even more effective. Where our studies and those of others have shown one product or group of products to be more effective than others, we have naturally chosen that product or group of products; and occasionally where a commonly used product has been found, in careful studies, to fall short of expectation or to be ineffective, it has been necessary to mention this fact so that hospitals should choose a more effective product. The recommendations which we have made refer only to hospital practice and it must not be inferred that methods judged unsuitable for hospital use are not suitable for domestic and other purposes.

Cost as well as effectiveness must be considered, and we have therefore appended some information about retail prices at the time this *Handbook* was prepared, relating to a number of alternative products which we have found to be effective. Of course, prices will change frequently. Furthermore, it has not been possible to include the price structures which might apply to alternatives that we did not have the opportunity to assess, or to take account of special terms which might be available through contracting or bulk purchasing. Because such special terms may affect different materials to a different degree, we have presented some examples of the relative costs to hospitals of different compounds or mixtures which have been used for the same purpose. We feel that the information we have provided will be of some value to Health Authorities.

Hospital hygiene and aseptic practices have changed repeatedly with the arrival of new knowledge and the assessment of new materials. It is expected that many of the recommendations presented here will, in the course of time, be – and some may already have been – superseded by new and improved methods, which will call for a revision of the *Handbook*. Many alternative procedures are equally effective, and there should be no conflict in the choice between such alternatives. Sometimes the most effective method cannot be applied (e.g. because the equipment required is not available); under these circumstances a less desirable alternative must be recommended. It is important that the Bacteriologist, the Infection Control Officer and the Infection Control Nurse should be consulted on questions of uncertainty about procedures or principles; the Area Supplies Officer and the Area Pharmaceutical Officer should be consulted, and other officers as appropriate, in respect of costs. The *Handbook*, supplemented by more recent information, will be used by the Infection Control Team in its handling of current infection problems.

1 *Introduction*

1.1 Definitions

The term **infection** is generally used to mean the deposition and multi-plication of bacteria and other microorganisms in tissues or on surfaces of the body where they can cause adverse effects; such adverse effects are often assumed in the definition. If the response of the host is slight or absent, it is usually termed **colonization**. **Sepsis** means the presence of inflammation, pus formation and other signs of illness in wounds colonized by micro-organisms, and in tissues to which such infection has spread. Other types of infective illness are described by terms which refer to the site of infection (e.g. tonsillitis, peritonitis, pyelitis, gastroenteritis, pneumonia) or to the specific disease, when this is distinctive (e.g. tuberculosis, measles, tetanus). The term **contamination** refers to the soiling of inanimate objects or living material with harmful, potentially infectious or unwanted matter.

✗**Hospital** (or **'nosocomial'***) **infection** means infection acquired by patients while they are in hospital, or by members of hospital staff; the term **hospital-acquired infection** is sometimes used. This may be associated with sepsis or other forms of infective illness, either in hospi-tal or after the patient returns home. **Cross-infection** means infection acquired in hospital from other people, either patients or staff. **Self–** (or **endogenous**) **infection** means infection caused by microbes which the patient carries on normal or septic areas of his own body, including organisms which these areas have acquired in hospital (eg. self-infection supervening on cross-infection or on infection from the environment).

All infections of operation wounds are, for obvious reasons, hospital infections. In other sites, however, it is often impossible to say whether an infection was acquired by the patient in hospital or before he came into hospital. The term **hospital-associated infection** has been used to cover such infections, as well as those acquired in hospital.

A **source** of hospital infection may be defined as a place where **patho-genic** (i.e. potentially disease-producing) microorganisms are growing or have grown and from which they are transmitted to patients (e.g.

---

* νοσοκομεῖον is the Greek (and nosocomium the Latin) word for hospital.

an infected wound, the nose or faeces of a carrier, contaminated food, contaminated solutions). A **reservoir** is a place where pathogens can survive outside the body and from which they could be transferred, directly or indirectly, to patients (e.g. static equipment, furniture, floors). Although the term is sometimes used interchangeably with the term **source**, it is usually accepted that the source is the part of the reservoir which provides organisms that infect or colonize one or more patients. A **vehicle** is a mobile object which can carry pathogenic organisms to a patient (e.g. dust particles, bedpans, blankets, toys etc.). The word **vector** is commonly used interchangeably with **vehicle**, but it is sometimes used in the specialized sense of an insect which carries pathogenic micro-organisms (i.e. an **insect-vector**), and should probably be restricted to this use. These categories overlap: e.g. a fluid in which bacteria multiply may be a 'vehicle' as well as a 'source' of infection, and will have acquired the organism from some antecedent 'source' (e.g. a patient with pseudomonas infection).

1.2   The importance of hospital infection

Prevalence surveys of hospital infection in many countries have shown that about one in ten patients in hospital have acquired an infection and a similar number of infections are community acquired (Meers *et al*. 1981; Mayon White *et al*. 1988). The main acquired infections are of the urinary tract, of surgical wounds, lower respiratory tract and skin. The frequency and severity varies with the age of the patient, type of operation in surgical cases, length of time of catheterization (urinary and vascular), immunosuppressive treatment and other factors. It is necessary to take these 'risk' factors into account when comparing the incidence or prevalence of infection in different hospitals, and in the prediction of expected infection in individual patients or wards in hospitals.

The prevalence rate is the proportion of a defined group having an infection at one point in time. The incidence rate is the proportion of a defined group developing an infection within a stated period and is lower than the prevalence rate. The incidence of hospital-acquired infection is about 5%. This continuous and apparently universal, though variable, incidence is described as **endemic** infection. But sometimes there is a large increase in the commonly occurring types of infection (e.g. postoperative wound sepsis) or the appearance of infection of a type not normally present in the hospital (e.g. salmonella infections in babies, or pseudomonas infections after eye surgery); this is called **epidemic** infection. Typing by serological, bacteriophage or bacteriocine methods shows epidemic infection is usually due to single type, which can often be traced to a source (e.g. a carrier of a virulent strain of *Staphylococcus aureus*, or a solution contaminated with *Pseudomonas aeruginosa*). If aseptic and hygienic measures in a hospital break down, the frequency of infection caused by multiple types of bacteria (i.e. **endemic** infection as defined above) may be increased to epidemic proportions.

The importance of hospital infection can be considered both in terms of the patients' illness, and of the prolonged occupancy of hospital beds. Illness due to hospital infection is today rarely a cause of death, though this may occur in patients with poor resistance (e.g. those with extensive burns) or from highly pathogenic organisms (e.g. some strains of hepatitis B virus). The cost of a prolonged stay is a convenient measure of the cost of infection, although it represents a reduction in the number of beds available from the waiting list rather than an actual increased cost to the hospital. This estimated cost on the basis of an average additional stay of four days was about 120 million pounds per year in England and Wales in 1987 and would now be higher (DHSS 1988). Even this is a considerable underestimate, as an additional stay of eight or more days is more likely. The cost of an outbreak can be very high, e.g. £250 000 for a large outbreak of methicillin-resistant *Staph. aureus* infection (North Thames Microbiology Subcommittee MRSA Working Party 1987).

1.3   Factors involved in hospital infection

The occurrence and the effects of hospital infection depend basically on:

1. the microorganisms;
2. the host (patients and staff);
3. the environment;
4. treatment.

1.3.1   THE MICROORGANISMS

Though virtually any infection may be acquired by patients or staff in hospital, there are certain pathogenic organisms which are particularly associated with hospital infection and some which rarely cause infection in other environments. Their role as a cause of hospital infection depends both on their pathogenicity or virulence (ability of the species or strain to cause disease) and on their numbers; it depends also on the patient's defences, and since many patients in hospital have diminished resistance because of their disease or treatment, organisms which are relatively harmless to healthy people may cause disease in hospital;

such 'opportunistic' organisms (e.g. *Pseudomonas aeruginosa*) are usually
resistant to many antibiotics and able to flourish under conditions in
which most disease-producing organisms cannot multiply. In surgical
wound infection Gram-negative bacilli, particularly *Escherichia coli*, play
a predominant role, but *Staphylococcus aureus* is still of major importance
in clean surgery. *Staph.epidermidis* infections have been increasing, particularly in prosthetic implant surgery, vascular catheterisation, leukaemia and premature neonates. Haemolytic streptococci of Group A
(*Streptococcus pyogenes*), which were formerly a much feared cause of
invasive and rapidly fatal wound infection, are today a relatively
infrequent cause of wound or burn infection and have remained fully
sensitive to penicillin. In spite of its apparently diminished invasive-
ness, however, *Strep.pyogenes* is more likely to cause the complete failure
of skin grafts than other bacteria if it gains access to full skin thickness
burns and is still an occasional cause of septicaemia and death. Tetanus
and gas gangrene are dangerous infections, which are very rare in spite
of the fact that the bacteria that cause them are commonly found in
dust and in human faeces. Their anaerobic growth requirements make
it difficult or impossible for these organisms to colonize tissues with a
good blood supply or exposed to the air. A group of anaerobes more
commonly responsible for clinical infection in hospital is the family of
non-sporing anaerobic bacilli, including *Bacteroides spp*. These organisms
are normal inhabitants of the large intestine, where they greatly
outnumber *E. coli* and other aerobes. In lower intestinal operations
Bacteroides fragilis has recently been recognized as a major pathogen,
often causing peritonitis and wound infection together with aerobic
organisms. Concurrent growth of aerobic organisms in the wound
may enhance the risks of anaerobic infection by reducing the oxygen
content of the tissues. In highly susceptible patients – those
who have had transplants, those infected with the human immunodeficiency virus (HIV) and those requiring prolonged chemotherapy –
certain mycobacteria, fungi (e.g. *Candida albicans*, aspergilli and *Cryptoc-
occus neoformans*), viruses (e.g. herpes simplex and cytomegalovirus),
and protozoa (e.g. *Pneumocystis carinii*), are a cause of severe and often
fatal infections. Cryptosporidia are a cause of severe diarrhoea in
patients with HIV infection. Arthropod parasites (e.g. itch mites and
lice) may be transmitted in hospital.

Outbreaks of infection (**epidemic** infection) may be caused by the
agents of specific infectious diseases, usually due to the admission of
an infected patient or the presence of a carrier in the ward. They may
also occur through exceptional errors in asepsis or sterile supply (e.g.
contamination of eye-drops or infusion fluids).

1.3.2 THE HOST (PATIENT OR MEMBER OF STAFF)

The susceptibility of the host and the virulence of the microorganisms are independent variables which have the same relevance to infection as the qualities of soil and seed have in agriculture.

A patient may have poor general resistance, for example in infancy, before antibodies have been formed and when the tissues that produce antibodies are imperfectly developed; or poor resistance may be associated with disease (such as uncontrolled diabetes, leukaemia or severe burns), or with poor nutrition, or with certain forms of treatment such as the use of immunosuppressive drugs given to prevent the rejection of transplanted organs or in the chemotherapy of cancer. General resistance may also be reduced by infection; the extreme example of this is HIV infection.

The patient may also have poor local resistance because of imperfect blood supply to the tissues, or because of the presence of dead tissue or blood clot in which bacteria can grow without interference from the natural defences; foreign bodies including sutures and prostheses also increase the susceptibility of the tissues to local sepsis. Surgical operations and instrumentation (e.g. catheterization) allow access of bacteria to tissues which are normally protected against contamination. Some of these, in particular the chambers of the eye, the meninges, the joints, the endocardium and the urinary tract, have very low resistance to bacterial invasion and are, therefore, peculiarly susceptible to infection with 'opportunistic' organisms.

Not only the patients, but the staff (including laboratory staff) are exposed to special hazards of infection with virulent organisms. The risk of infection among members of staff through contamination with blood and exudates of patients with hepatitis B (HBV) or HIV has received much attention in recent years. The risk in most hospitals is extremely low, but fear of AIDS has been associated with an excessive response.

1.3.3 THE ENVIRONMENT

The place where the patient is treated has an important influence on the likelihood of his acquiring infection and on the nature of such infection. A wide variety of microorganisms, including virulent strains, is likely to be found in hospitals where many people, including some with infection, are aggregated; these organisms are likely to include a large proportion of antibiotic-resistant bacteria, which can flourish where antibiotic usage has led to the suppression of sensitive bacteria.

Different areas of the hospital have individual infection hazards. In the operating theatre there is a special hazard of wound infection because of the exposure, often for several hours, of susceptible tissues, and the presence of a number of potential human and inanimate sources. In wards the patients may be exposed for many weeks to contaminants from which open surgical wounds will usually be protected by some form of cover – though this is imperfect in many patients, especially those with drains. Special hazards exist in neonatal wards through possible contamination of feeds, suction and resuscitation equipment etc., and because of the frequent handling of infants; and similar problems exist in intensive care units and burns wards. In Infectious Diseases Hospitals there is a special hazard of infection with the agents of acute communicable diseases. There is a risk of Legionnaire's disease through airborne contamination of aerosols containing *Legionella pneumophila* from cooling towers, humidifiers or water supply systems colonized by the organism.

An objective in control of hospital infection is to expose patients to an environment at least as free from microbial hazard as that which they would find outside hospital.

1.3.4   TREATMENT

The clinical results of microbial contamination are influenced by details of treatment – favourably by correct surgical or medical procedures and antimicrobial chemotherapy, but adversely (as mentioned above) by treatment with immunosuppressive drugs or steroids.

1.4   Sources and routes of infection (Fig. 1.1)

Self-infection of an operation wound may be due to bacteria transferred from an area where they are causing infection (e.g. boils), or by bacteria carried by the patient without symptoms on his skin or in his nose (mostly staphylococci), but occasionally in his mouth (especially streptococci), in his intestines (especially coliform bacilli, *Bacteroides spp.* and gas gangrene bacilli). Endogenous infection with *Bacteroides spp.* and coliform bacilli is especially important in the lower intestinal tract, but the upper intestine and stomach may be heavily colonized by these bacteria in patients with gastric carcinoma, other pathological states and during treatment with H_2 receptor blockers.

Cross-infection with some of these organisms may occur from other patients or members of staff by contact or by airborne routes. Infection may be transferred on hands or clothing of staff, visitors or ambulant patients, on unsterile objects or in fluids used in treatment, in food etc. Members of staff (nurses, physiotherapists, doctors) who attend to many patients are likely to transfer infective organisms from one patient

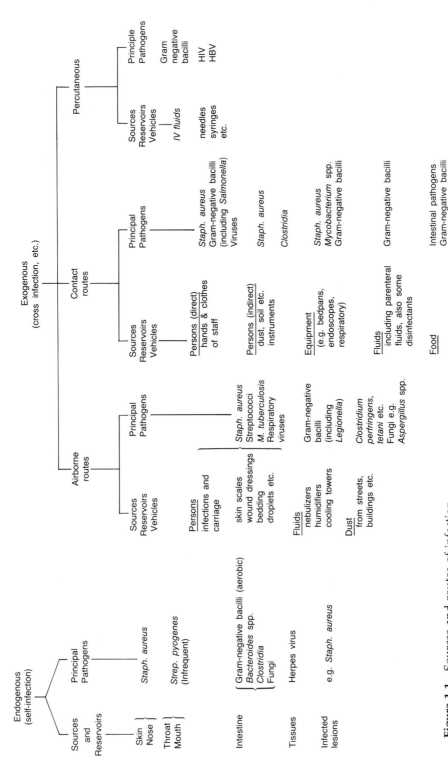

Figure 1.1 Sources and routes of infection.

to another. Visitors who attend one patient present a smaller hazard, though they may transfer their own microorganisms. A fetus may be infected from the mother (e.g. with cytomegalovirus) *in utero* or on delivery (e.g. with *Neisseria gonorrheae*). Airborne transfer may occur through the dispersal of skin scales that are shed continuously from the surface of the body and often carry staphylococci, or on minute dròplets dispersed from the potential source of airborne infection, especially from a patient with respiratory tract infection. Epidemic infections arise through the presence of a case of an infectious disease or of a carrier of the causal organism in the ward, theatre or other place in the hospital where a number of patients may be exposed to contamination; the route or routes of transfer vary, depending on the survival of the organisms outside the body and other factors. Infection may occur also through contamination with organisms acquired from inanimate sources, such as Gram-negative bacilli on inadequately sterilized equipment. Insect vectors (e.g. cockroaches, ants, flies) may convey infective organisms to patients or to sterilized equipment. Legionnaire's disease appears to be acquired from the inanimate environment only; though rare, it is potentially dangerous. Hepatitis B and HIV infections are spread in hospitals and from blood of infected persons or carriers, usually from a needle-stick or other injury or in the past from transfused blood or blood products.

Though the relative importance of different sources and routes can rarely be stated with any precision, there are certain patterns which are relevant to the choice of methods for controlling hospital infection. Of the sources, those in which bacteria are multiplying (e.g. patients with infectious disease and septic wounds, but also healthy surfaces of the body and contaminated solutions) are, in general, more important than dry objects or surfaces on which organisms may survive but cannot multiply (described above as 'reservoirs'). Infected patients and septic wounds are more likely to be a dangerous source than healthy surfaces of the body, because the bacteria in the former can be assumed to be virulent, while those on healthy surfaces may often be avirulent. Vehicles which can convey the pathogenic organisms directly to the patient's susceptible sites (e.g. fluids used for aseptic procedures, surgical instruments, food, the hands of nurses handling newborn babies) are more likely to cause infection than sources or reservoirs which do not come in contact with such sites or with the patient. Some of the latter (e.g. floors, walls, furniture) are of very little importance unless incorrect procedures (e.g. sweeping with a brush) are used. The larger the number of stages of contact transfer from a source or reservoir, the smaller the numbers of bacteria that will reach the patients. Contact transfer is more important than airborne transfer for organisms that do not survive well under dry conditions outside the body. Gram-negative bacilli (e.g. typhoid and dysentery bacilli and *Ps. aeruginosa*), which have this characteristic because they are highly sensitive to drying, are more capable than Gram-positive cocci of survival in water, and are, therefore, more likely to be transferred in a fluid vector. A sufficient number, however, survive the effects of drying for them to be transmissible on the hands of nurses, doctors and other human contacts.

1.5   Principles of control of infection

Patients are protected against infection in hospital by a system of methods, including surgical asepsis and hospital hygiene, the purpose of which can be summarized under three headings:

1. to remove the sources or potential sources of infection (or, more usually, to remove disease-producing microbes from potential sources of infection) – this includes treatment of infected patients as well as sterilizing, disinfection and cleaning of contaminated materials and surfaces;
2. to block the routes of transfer of bacteria from those potential sources and reservoirs to uninfected patients, which include isolation of infected or susceptible patients, barrier nursing, aseptic operations, 'no touch' dressing techniques and particularly handwashing;
3. to enhance the patient's resistance to infection (e.g. during operations by careful handling of tissues and removal of slough and foreign bodies, also by enhancing the general defences, as by control of diabetes, reinforcement of immunity to tetanus, and the use of antibiotic prophylaxis if and when this is indicated).

Methods advocated for the control of surgical infection can be classified under four headings:

1. established methods, for which good evidence is available;
2. provisionally established methods, for which there is some evidence;
3. rational methods, which are consistent with our knowledge of bacteria but which cannot be evaluated by experiments (e.g. avoidance of 'clutter' in operating rooms);
4. 'rituals' – methods which have been shown by experiment or observation to have no value or even to be harmful (Daschner 1989).

From a large amount of research carried out in recent years we know that much infection can be prevented and some lives can be saved by applying certain methods of controlling infection. At the same time there is, in many hospitals, a continuing incidence of endemic infection at levels which are similar to those reported many years ago. This may be due, in part, to more adventurous surgery and medicine, and to the presence of more patients who are highly susceptible to infection; but there is evidence, too, of erratic and unstandardized aseptic methods which probably contribute a large share to the incidence of cross-infection.

In a number of British hospitals there has been a decline since the early 1970s in the incidence of staphylococcal cross-infection and of antibiotic-resistant *Staph. aureus*, but cross-infection still occurs. Methicillin-resistant *Staph. aureus* (MRSA) has been causing problems in many countries. These epidemic strains are now causing major problems in some UK hospitals, particularly in the London area (Duckworth *et al.* 1988) and exemplify the need for continuing effective surveillance and hygienic techniques and the provision of adequate isolation facilities (Report 1990). *Ps. aeruginosa* is still a common cause of death in patients with burns in developing countries. Outbreaks of infection with other antibiotic-resistant Gram-negative bacilli (e.g. *Klebsiella spp, Enterobacter spp, Serratia* and *Acinetobacter spp*) are commonly reported, particularly in intensive care units and urological wards. These infections can be prevented by good aseptic and hygienic techniques and avoiding excessive use of antibiotics. However, there has been a general reduction in cross-infection and the focus of attention is shifting, to some extent, from general problems of cross-infection to the control of endogenous infection in colorectal surgery and in patients with diminished antimicrobial resistance, to problems of sterilization of difficult pieces of equipment and to containment of dangerous communicable disease. The spread of HBV and HIV is prevented by care in taking blood from infected persons, safe disposal of needles, screening of blood and blood products and reliable processing of equipment (ACDP 1990).

The *Study on the Efficacy of Nosocomial Infection Control* (SENIC) carried out by the Centres of Disease Control in the United States has demonstrated the importance of infection control personnel in the prevention of infection (Haley *et al.* 1985). The administrative aspects of infection control have been formalized in the United Kingdom (DHSS 1988).

The increased use of computers has enabled statistical techniques, such as multivariate analysis, to be introduced as a routine into control of infection departments. Formulae for assessing risk of infection assessment have been developed which should enable high risk patients to be more accurately targetted and will improve comparability of infection rates between different units or hospitals (Bibby *et al.* 1986).

A large outbreak of salmonella food-poisoning in a geriatric hospital (DHSS 1986a) and another large outbreak, of Legionnaire's disease in Staffordshire (DHSS 1986b), demonstrated the necessity for effective coordination of effort and communication in the management of large outbreaks.

There is an increasing awareness of the importance of the personal factor in preventing hospital infection, and of the need of a proper understanding of the facts by all members of the hospital staff. Although the subject is complex and involves many disciplines, the basic ideas are simple, and many of the details of asepsis can be made easier by forms of standardization based on evidence of effectiveness and practicability.

References

Advisory Committee on Dangerous Pathogens (ACDP) (1990) *HIV – the Causative Agent of AIDS and Related Conditions*. 2nd revision of guidelines. HMSO, London.

Bibby, B.A., Collins, B.J., and Ayliffe, G.A.J. (1986) A mathematical model for assessing risk of postoperative wound infection. *Journal of Hospital Infection*, **8**, 31.

Daschner, F. (1989) Cost-effectiveness in hospital infection control – lessons for the 1990s. *Journal of Hospital Infection*, **13**, 325.

Department of Health and Social Security (1986a). *The Report of the Committee of Inquiry into an Outbreak of Food-Poisoning at Stanley Royd Hospital*. HMSO, London.

Department of Health and Social Security (1986b). *Public Inquiry into the Cause of the Outbreak of Legionnaires Disease in Staffordshire*. HMSO, London.

Department of Health and Social Security (1988) *Hospital Infection Control: Guidance on the Control of Infection in Hospitals*. Prepared by the DHSS/PHLS Hospital Infection Working Group. HMSO, London.

Duckworth, G.J., Lothian, J.L.E., and Williams, J.D. (1988) Methicillin-resistant *Staphylococcus aureus*: report of an outbreak in a London Teaching Hospital. *Journal of Hospital Infection*, **11**, 1–15.

Haley, R., Culver, D.H., White, J.W., *et al*. (1985) The efficacy of infection surveillance and control programmes in preventing nosocomial infection in US hospitals. *American Journal of Epidemiology*, **121**, 182.

Mayon-White, R.J., Ducel, G.I., Kereselidze, T. and Tikhomirov, E. (1988) An international survey of the prevalence of hospital acquired infection. *Journal of Hospital Infection*, **II** (Supplement A), 43.

Meers, P.D., Ayliffe, G.A.J., Emmerson, A.M., *et al*. (1981) Report on the national survey of infection in hospitals 1980. *Journal of Hospital Infection*, **2**, Supplement.

Report of a combined working party of the Hospital Infection Society and British Society for Antimicrobial Chemotherapy. Revised guidelines for the control of epidemic methicillin-resistant *Staphylococcus aureus* (1990). *Journal of Hospital Infection*, **16**, 351.

2 *Administration and responsibility*

The administrative arrangements for infection control will vary in different countries but most will include an infection control doctor (officer), an infection control nurse and a committee. England and Wales is divided into District Health Authorities, each responsible for a population of about 200 000 and containing at least one general hospital of about 600 beds for the acutely ill patient. A health district may contain chronic care establishments, specialist-hospitals and is also responsible for community health. It is subdivided into Units, (e.g. acute, long-term and community care etc.). Each district has a medical officer (Director of Public Health) responsible to the District General Manager for coordination of public health services, and it is recommended that a medical officer with responsibility for control of communicable disease, particularly in the community, is also appointed (DHSS 1988a). The Director of Public Health and the Public Health Medical Officer for communicable diseases (Consultant in Communicable Disease Control – CCDC) will be responsible for coordination of infection control activities between the hospital and the community and between adjacent hospitals and districts. The infection control doctor (officer) will retain responsibility for hospital infection control and is directly accountable to the District General Manager through the Unit General Manager and will collaborate with the CCDC (DHSS 1988b; Casewell 1989).

The administration of control of hospital infection in the UK is now more complicated following the recent reorganization. District Health Authorities now have two major but clearly separate functions and their organizations should clearly reflect this split. First, they retain responsibility for managing the provision of health care services historically associated with their district through their Directly Managed Units (DMUs). This responsibility is only relinquished when a unit assumes NHS Trust status. Second, District Health Authorities are now the purchasers of health care for their resident population and in discharging this responsibility they should assess the need for health care for their population and should arrange through contracts and other financial links, provision of health care to meet those needs.

Within this structure, the infection control team will be part of the provider arm of the organization and the costs associated with it would normally be recouped by the provider via the prices it charges to purchasers, either through contracts or on an extra contractual referral basis. Purchasers will enforce reasonable infection control standards through explicit clauses in contracts.

Where a District Health Authority has more than one provider unit which is directly managed, the infection control team will normally be managerially responsible to one of those provider units but will provide services to other units, usually on some 'internal trading' basis, with the prices of all provider units reflecting these costs.

The infection control team will advise the Health Authority (as a purchaser) on the measures required for effective infection control.

The infection control team would also be responsible for investigating outbreaks of infection or infection problems either on behalf of the Health Authority as manager of the provider units or for one or more of the provider units directly.

The cost of providing an infection control service must be considered an essential part of the budget of a District, Trust or Unit. In addition to the annual allocation to the infection control doctor for routine control purposes, costs of an outbreak should be borne by a contingency fund.

It is the responsibility of the hospital administration (e.g. District General Manager on behalf of the Health Authority) to ensure that adequate arrangements are made to control hospital infection (DHSS 1988b). These arrangements should include the setting up of a control of infection committee and the appointment of an infection control doctor and an infection control nurse in every district. The Health Authority should be responsible for implementing recommendations of the doctor or committee. It is the responsibility of all members of staff to inform the infection control doctor or nurse of potential hazards of infection. Without this information the infection control team cannot be fully effective. In addition to the official responsibilities of the Health Authority and the infection control team is the personal care and responsibility of the clinician in charge.

2.1 Infection control team

The team consists of members of staff with special interest and knowledge of infection control in hospital. The head of the team will be the infection control doctor; it will include the microbiologist (who will usually also be the infection control doctor), infection control nurses, and where available a member of the scientific or technical staff with responsibilities in infection control. More than one infection control doctor or nurse may be appointed in a large District. The District or

Unit General Manager or representative (e.g. Director of Public Health) could be a member of the team, attending meetings when a major problem arises. If not a member of the team, he or his representative should always be available to the infection control doctor for discussion of problems. Although most of the problems occur within hospital, the present administrative structure also involves the community. A public health medical officer – or Consultant in Communicable Disease Control (CCDC) – should be co-opted on the team if community problems are being considered or an outbreak of a particularly dangerous infection, such as Lassa fever, has occurred for which he has legal responsibilities.

The team is responsible for:

1. monitoring of infections and methods of control, rapid identification and investigation of outbreaks or potentially hazardous procedures;
2. providing advice on isolation of infected patients and on hazardous or ineffective procedures;
3. giving advice, making day-to-day decisions and liaising with staff in all areas in the District where potential risks of infection occur;
4. providing, monitoring and evaluating policies for the prevention of infection and its spread;
5. communication and provision of readily available information to staff on measures of infection control.

The particular duties of the infection control doctor and nurse are described below. The team should meet at least weekly but the infection control doctor and nurse will usually meet more frequently, often daily.

2.1.1   INFECTION CONTROL DOCTOR

The individual holding this appointment should be a senior member of the medical staff with ready access to committees and sufficient authority to command respect with all categories of staff. He or she should have a special interest and training in hospital infection and should be aware of recent developments in the subject. He or she should be appointed by the Health Authority in consultation with the medical staff. The microbiologist is usually the logical choice, being suitably qualified and in an ideal position to keep the record system under constant scrutiny. A survey in 1987 showed that 81% of infection control doctors were microbiologists, 8% pathologists and the remainder were infectious diseases physicians, District community physicians, surgeons and others (Howard 1988). The functions of the infection control doctor in conjunction with other members of the team are to assess risks of infection, to advise on preventive measures and to check their efficacy in all parts of the hospital, including catering, laundry, sterile service departments (SSD), domestic, pharmaceutical and engineering departments, as well as clinical and other areas. Inspection of kitchens and other catering establishments should be regularly carried out (every 6–12 months) by the infection control doctor or his representative. Information and advice may be given by the infection control doctor informally or at meetings of the medical staff committee, control of infection committee or District or Unit teams. However, if any immediate action is required, the infection control doctor or Chairman of the control of infection committee (see below) should be empowered to take whatever steps may be necessary without prior reference to the control of infection committee. He or she should have ready access to the District Manager and laboratory facilities, and work closely with the infection control nurse and the CCDC especially on notifiable infectious diseases. Some of the duties may be delegated to other staff (e.g. senior registrar, infection control nurse or a medical laboratory scientific officer as appropriate).

2.1.2 INFECTION CONTROL NURSE   Role.

The infection control doctor usually has commitments which prevent regular visits to wards and theatres and do not allow him or her personally to carry out many of the day-to-day duties of the team, such as recording of infections and ensuring that procedures are satisfactorily performed. In every large hospital (or District) at least one infection control nurse should be appointed to collaborate with the doctor in these duties. The nurse should be registered, preferably with surgical, paediatric or infectious diseases experience. Experience as a ward or theatre sister or as nurse tutor would be an advantage, but is not essential. Of much greater importance is an agreeable personality and an ability to deal tactfully with all grades of staff.

It is recommended that newly appointed nurses attend, for a short period, a centre in which there is a suitably experienced nurse and microbiologist. The principles of hospital microbiology and methods of collection of specimens should be taught in the microbiology laboratory of her or his own hospital. The acquisition of laboratory skills is not required. It is expected that all nurses will complete the English National Board (ENB) Foundation Course (329) or a course of similar or higher standard. This will take one year, but during most of that time the nurses will continue to work in their own hospital. The attendance of such nurses at the annual conference of the Infection Control Nurses' Association should be considered as part of their training.

The nurse responsible for a district should be graded as a clinical nurse specialist. Grading should depend on area of responsibility and should be reviewed at appropriate intervals. Failure to provide a career structure leads to a wastage of trained experienced nurses.

The infection control nurse is administratively responsible to the District Nursing Officer or nurse manager and technically responsible to the infection control doctor or microbiologist who controls her or his day-to-day activities. The infection control doctor should be responsible for advising on attendance by the nurse at conferences, courses and other relevant meetings. If a person other than a nurse is appointed to take on some of these duties, he or she should be on the laboratory staff and may be described, for example, as 'infection control microbiologist' or 'infection control scientific officer'. The appointment should be in addition to that of a nurse.

The functions of the infection control nurse are described below. These cover the whole field of infection control and involve co-operation with all the departments mentioned in the section on the control of infection committee, and also with the occupational health medical officer; the nurse is a member of, and shares responsibility with, the infection control team. The nurse should visit all wards regularly and discuss problems with staff. The laboratory should be visited every morning. Keeping records should not be the main part of her/his duties. Instruction of nurses and other grades of staff in the practice of infection control is an important function.

The day-to-day tasks of an infection control nurse might include:

1. identifying as promptly as possible potential infection hazards in patients, staff or equipment;
2. compiling records of infected patients from ward notifications, case notes, laboratory reports and information collected in routine visits and discussions;
3. arranging prompt isolation of infected patients (in co-operation with the ward sister and consultant who have initial responsibility) in accordance with hospital policy and ensuring that there are adequate facilities for isolating patients; introducing other measures as necessary to prevent the spread of infection or organisms highly resistant to antibiotics;
4. checking by inspection that infection control and aseptic procedures are being carried out in accordance with hospital policy;
5. liaison between laboratory and ward staff; informing heads of departments and giving advice on infection control problems;
6. collaboration with occupational health staff in maintaining records of infection in medical, nursing, catering, domestic and other grades of staff; ensuring clearance specimens are taken before infected staff return to duty;
7. collaboration with and advising community nurses on problems of infection;

8. prompt information by telephone of notifiable diseases to the public health medical officer (CCDC);
9. informing other hospitals, general practitioners, and others concerned when infected patients are discharged from hospital or transferred elsewhere, and receiving relevant information from other hospitals or from the community where appropriate;
10. participation in teaching and practical demonstrations of control of infection techniques to medical, nursing, auxiliary, domestic, catering, and other staff;
11. informing the District Nursing Manager of practical problems and difficulties in carrying out routine procedures related to nursing aspects of infection control;
12. attending relevant committees, which are usually control of infection and nursing procedures committees;
13. conferring with the sterile services manager about certain infections in hospital (e.g. HBV)

The nurse will collaborate with other members of the team investigating outbreaks, carrying out surveys, visiting kitchen and catering establishments, monitoring special units, collecting microbiological samples, preparing reports for the control of infection committee, clinicians and administrators, and assisting in research projects.

2.2 Control of infection committee

The committee of a large general hospital or District should have representatives from all the major departments which may be concerned with control of infection, i.e. medical, nursing, occupational health, engineering, pharmacy, supplies, domestic, SSD, catering, microbiology, administration and community health, as well as the infection control team. The chairman of the committee may also be the infection control officer, but can be a clinician with an interest in infection control. Some Districts or smaller hospitals may prefer to appoint a small committee, consisting of the infection control team, the CCDC, a senior nurse, clinician and senior manager and to co-opt others as necessary. The main advantages of a large committee are educational and to ensure adequate communication between the different departments. However, major decisions will be made by the Infection Control Team on hospital problems and possibly by a small executive committee as described above for the District.

Meetings should be held 1–12 times a year, but three to four meetings should be adequate for most Districts and yearly for small hospitals where problems tend to arise sporadically. The committee should:

1. discuss any problems brought to them by the infection control doctor, nurse or other members of the committee;
2. take responsibility for major decisions;
3. be given reports on current problems and on the incidence of infection and evaluate other reports involving infection risk (e.g. kitchen inspections);
4. arrange interdepartmental co-ordination and education in control of infection (it is therefore advantageous to have a representation of members with various interests);
5. introduce, maintain and, when necessary, modify policies (e.g. disinfectant, antibiotic, isolation);
6. advise on the selection of equipment for the prevention of infection (e.g. sharps disposal boxes, etc);
7. make recommendations to other committees and departments on infection control techniques;
8. advise Health Authorities on all aspects of infection control and make recommendations for use of resources.

2.2.1   IMPLEMENTATION OF COMMITTEE RECOMMENDATIONS

If the committee or team is to be effective, the results of the investigations and records of infection must be sent to the relevant authorities and recommendations rapidly implemented, especially when the safety of patients or staff is involved.

Although the infection control doctor has an overall advisory responsibility in the hospital, other members of the committee should ensure that recommendations within their own areas of responsibility are carried out as considered necessary by the committee. Heads of departments (e.g. catering, laundry) should be invited to attend committee meetings when problems concerning their own departments are discussed.

The control of infection committee is a sub-committee of the District health services team or equivalent. The Chairman and the infection control doctor should have direct access to the District or Unit General Manager who may also be a member of the committee or team. All recommendations, instructions or procedures involving any aspect of infection in the hospital issued by the administration, other committees, health and safety executive (HSE), or public health medical officer should be referred for approval to the control of infection committee.

2.3   Objectives of the infection control department and implementation of policies

The main objective of the infection control team is to reduce preventable infection to the lowest practical level at acceptable cost, and Health Authorities increasingly require evidence that infection control techniques are cost effective. Although costs can be measured, effectiveness is more difficult to assess since patients vary in age and in other characteristics as well as having different treatments, and units vary in design. Comparisons between infection rates in different hospitals or during different periods in the same hospital are of doubtful validity and require a considerable amount of time collecting data. Even if the data can be collected, the numbers of infections over a year in a single hospital are not usually sufficient to provide statistical evidence of efficacy of measures. In addition, it is not possible to estimate the infections that might have occurred if early preventative measures had not been implemented.

It is difficult, therefore, to assess the infection control measures in terms of outcome (e.g. reduced infection rates) but it may be possible to infer the outcome from process measurements. The 'SENIC' (Study of Efficacy of Nosocomial Infection Control) project carried out in the US showed that 'reduction in infection rates of about one third could be obtained by intensive surveillance and control methods, the appointment of a physician with expertise in infection control and one infection control nurse to 250 beds.' (Haley *et al*. 1985). It is inferred that if the SENIC criteria are met, a reduction in infection rate will be achieved. However, it is unlikely that the appointment of more infection control nurses will be possible in most hospitals in the foreseeable future around the world and maintaining a comprehensive clinical surveillance system will not represent optimal use of the nurse's time. However, the infection control staff should be able to demonstrate to the administration that certain objectives have been achieved. Essential surveillance reports could be presented to the infection control committee as well as evidence of implementation of policies and appropriate infection control techniques which have proven value. Priorities can be defined and unnecessary rituals eliminated, e.g. wearing of caps and overshoes in intensive care units and unnecessary washing of operating theatre walls.

2.3.1   ACTION AT TIME OF AN OUTBREAK OF INFECTION (see Wenzel 1987)

When an outbreak occurs, for example from the sudden appearance of increasing incidence of one type of infection in a ward, immediate action is needed to prevent the further spread to patients and staff. This action will vary with the nature and severity of the infection, but certain general principles apply. The infection control doctor must be notified, and should take immediate steps (e.g. isolation of suspected cases), in consultation with the microbiologist (if not the same person), the infection control nurse and clinicians whose patients are involved. The public health medical officer (CCDC) responsible for communicable diseases should be informed if the outbreak is of a notifiable disease or involves the community. If a major outbreak occurs, a meeting of the 'emergencies' or 'outbreak' committee should be immediately arranged by the chairman of the control of infection committee or infection control doctor and the District Manager or his deputy. Other members of this committee are the infection control team, clinician responsible for affected patients, senior nurse, occupational health team and the public health medical officer (CCDC) responsible for communicable diseases.

A major outbreak is difficult to define in terms of numbers of patients and staff involved. Numbers of cases (e.g. 20) have been suggested, but two cases of diphtheria might be considered a major outbreak. The decision should be made by the infection control doctor, based on factors such as the necessity to close the ward, the need to prevent transfer of staff, provide additional staff, provide additional supplies, linen etc. or open an isolation ward.

The infection control doctor (or chairman of the control of infection committee) will usually be responsible for co-ordinating infection control arrangements in the hospital. The following steps are appropriate.

1. arrangements for the clinical care of patients;
2. adequate channels for communication should be set up and a decision made as to who will be responsible for communication with the media;
3. assessment of the situation should be made; details of patients with infection, including date of admission and first symptoms, and nature of disease are noted; bacteriological samples are examined and pathogens are, when possible, typed (or kept on suitable medium for typing) in the hospital or the Public Health Laboratory;
4. isolation of infected patients – for appropriate methods see Chapter 9;
5. introduction of additional control of infection techniques in affected wards (e.g. alcoholic hand disinfection), closure of ward or wards (which is rarely required, but may be necessary if the outbreak is extensive and particularly if the infection involves a hazard of severe illness or even death in some patients); the ward should be closed to further admissions, and thoroughly cleaned after discharge of

the last patient before re-opening; such a procedure may also apply to a theatre or other affected area;

6. the allocation of beds, e.g. the entire isolation unit, side wards, or possibly a larger ward, for treatment of infected patients may be required;

7. an epidemiological survey should be undertaken to provide evidence of time and place where infection was acquired, including enquiry for possible admission of patients incubating infection.

8. surveillance of contacts – who may be incubating the disease, surveillance is sometimes necessary; this includes clinical surveillance and laboratory screening;

9. bacteriological search for source of infection; examination of all staff and patients for carriage to see whether, for example, the same phage type of *Staph. aureus* is isolated from all infections; search for the infecting strain in the inanimate environment (e.g. fluids if the organism is *Ps. aeruginosa* or other Gram-negative bacilli; food, if the illness is gastroenteritis;

10. survey of methods, equipment, buildings – such a survey would include dressing technique, theatre discipline, kitchen hygiene, for evidence of lapses and the 'personal factor'; also for effectiveness of sterilizers, ventilation systems, disinfection, and protection against recontamination of sterilized objects and solutions;

11. the infection control or occupational health nurse will discuss the situation with heads of departments – e.g. catering, SSD, laundry and domestic – to relieve anxieties and indicate any necessary procedures;

12. the requirement for assistance should be assessed at each meeting and advice sought as necessary (e.g. from a Public Health Laboratory, Division of Hospital Infection, Colindale, other specialist laboratory or physician, e.g. Hospital Infection Research Laboratory, Birmingham or Communicable Disease Surveillance Centre, Colindale).

Check lists of practices should be prepared for investigation of infection arising in surgical, maternity, and general medical wards and in special departments, e.g. operating suites, kitchens, laundries, SSD (Williams *et al.* 1966).

2.4 Visits to patients

Infection may be brought into hospital by visitors, or transferred by them from one patient to another, or acquired by them from infected patients. Though visitors do not appear to play an important role in hospital infection, some precautions are required to meet recognized hazards.

Prospective visitors should be shown a notice warning them not to enter a ward if they have a bad cold, a sore throat, diarrhoea, boils or other communicable diseases. Special precautions (gowns, restricted movement, no touch) should be used if visitors must be admitted to patients with enhanced susceptibility to infection.

The notice should instruct the visitor to confine his visit to one patient. If this instruction is observed, visits by healthy people (e.g. mothers of children) do not present any special hazard of cross-infection. It may be necessary for the ward sister or manager to evict or exclude visitors from a ward if they disregard these instructions or are violent.

Visits by non-immune persons (especially children) to patients in isolation with highly communicable diseases should be prohibited. Where visits must be allowed, the visitors to such patients should be instructed to take self-protective measures, such as wearing a gown, and they should refrain from touching the patient, the patient's bed and his/her belongings. When contact is unavoidable (e.g. in mothers' visits to small children), it may be advisable for the visitor to wear gloves. Intimate contact should be avoided. Hands should be thoroughly washed on leaving the patient.

2.5   Legal responsibility of patients, staff, visitors and hospital authorities in the control of hospital infection

The legal responsibilities of hospital authorities and staff, visitors and patients depend upon the application of general common law principles and some statute law to the particular circumstances of each case.

Under the Occupiers Liability Act (1957), hospital authorities must provide safe premises, so that if patients are admitted to wards or to hospitals where there is a known outbreak of infection, the hospital authorities might be made responsible for the death of a patient or for permanent injury suffered by a patient as a result of such infection. Nursing and medical staff therefore have a duty to report, at the earliest possible opportunity, such infection when it is discovered, and the infection control doctor or team must decide immediately what steps should be taken to prevent a spread of the infection. There is a further duty of the hospital authorities to ensure that no staff are employed at the hospital who may transmit serious infection to others; if it becomes known to the hospital authorities that a particular member of staff is a carrier of organisms that cause typhoid fever or other dangerous infectious diseases, then the hospital authorities must take steps either to terminate that person's employment or to deploy him where there is minimal risk of infection to other members of the staff or patients. These restrictions must not be applied in the case of less dangerous organisms (e.g. *Staph. aureus*) which are often carried by healthy persons; special precautions should, however, be taken when these less dangerous organisms cause an outbreak of clinical infection (see p. 000).

In the case of tuberculosis, tuberculin testing of staff should be carried out routinely and BCG should be given where there is a possibility of nursing and other staff coming into contact with patients suffering from the disease. If this is not done, the hospital may be sued by a nurse who contracts tuberculosis on the grounds that the hospital is not providing a safe system of work. Immunization against other diseases which can be prevented in this way should, in some circumstances, be offered.

A patient in a hospital cannot be held liable either for introducing infection or for spreading it in the hospital, but it is clear that the hospital authorities must take care, by all reasonable precautions, including some kind of isolation, if necessary, to prevent the spread of infection. Similarly, a claim against the hospital authorities in respect of infection caused by a member of the hospital staff, either to another member of the staff or to a patient or visitor, would be rational only if the hospital had known about it and had failed to take any appropriate action. If it is known that a visitor is suffering from an infection which he is likely to communicate to hospital staff or to patients, there might be a responsibility upon the hospital to stop the visiting, but the hospital authorities cannot really be held responsible for every infection which may be either caused or spread by a visitor. A hospital authority can be, and has been, held legally responsible when a patient was discharged from a hospital suffering from a specific infectious disease which he subsequently communicated to another person. In that case it was held that there was negligence on the part of the hospital authorities in discharging somebody into the community who was likely to infect other members of the community; such a patient should have been kept in hospital and isolated until he was judged to be no longer infectious.

When patients become infected through some error in aseptic techniques or hospital hygiene, the hospital authorities may be held responsible. If, for example, it could be demonstrated that it was the accepted practice to sterilize certain containers (e.g. of saline solutions) and the hospital fails to sterilize and maintain sterility of the fluid in the bottle before distribution to patients, then the hospital authorities may be held liable if contamination of the fluid has taken place at any time before it is actually used. On the other hand, if a practice is not universally adopted (e.g. provision of 'ultraclean' air systems for total hip replacement operations) and the hip becomes infected, it could be argued that the hospital authorities were not liable, as their failure to provide such an enclosure (if antibiotic prophylaxis was used) did not constitute failure to provide a reasonable standard of care in the treatment of the patient in accordance with current practice in this country.

2.5.1   HEALTH AND SAFETY AT WORK ACT (1974)

Under this Act responsibilities are placed upon health authorities to provide and maintain plant and systems of work that are, so far as is reasonably practicable, safe and without risks to health of employees; and to arrange for ensuring, as far as is reasonably practicable, safety and absence of risks to health of employees in connection with the use, handling, storage and transport of articles and substances. Safety representatives may be appointed by staff, and, if they require it, health authorities must establish safety committees under the Safety Representatives and Safety Committees Regulations (1977). If this has not been done, it should be done immediately as there are additional responsibilities on health authorities under the Act towards patients so that they are not exposed to risks to their health and safety. The Department of Health and Social Security (1974) circular HC(78)30 states that in view of the liabilities imposed by the Act on health authorities and their employees, each authority should establish a general structure of responsibility which makes it clear who is responsible for the discharge of particular aspects of the general duties imposed by the Act. It also states, however, that the role of the control of infection committee and team recommended in a much earlier circular (RHB (51) 100) need not be affected. It also sets out the responsibilities of management to have advisers and safety officers for specialist departments, safety liaison officers and, where staff require them, safety committees.

The Health and Safety Executive has stated that, while it would be prepared to consider the systems in force in hospitals to provide health and safety at work for employees, it would not necessarily be bound by those systems if it is considered that they were in any way inadequate.

Under the Unfair Contract Terms Act (1977), a supplier of any goods, which will include drugs, dressings, equipment, etc., or a servicing contractor, can no longer disclaim liability for negligence in the supply of the goods, the making of the equipment or the servicing of the equipment if the patient dies or suffers personal injury.

2.5.2   CONTROL OF SUBSTANCES HAZARDOUS TO HEALTH (COSHH) REGULATIONS (1988)

'This Act' has been in force since October 1989 and introduces a framework for controlling exposure of personnel to hazardous substances arising from work activity (DoH 1989; Harrison 1991). It includes micro-organisms as well as toxic substances. The employer is responsible for assessing health risks created by the work and of the measures required to protect the health of the workers. These regulations are particularly relevant to infection control staff and are likely to involve such hazards as glutaraldehyde in endoscopy units, ethylene oxide sterilizers in the SSD, disinfectants and detergents, transport of laboratory specimens, protection of staff against HBV infection, tuberculosis and Legionnaire's disease. It will obviously have a major application in hospital laborator-ies but requirements for clinical units are uncertain. Most hospitals will already have guidelines for the control of infection which should be adequate for the Regulations involving infection in the clinical units.

2.6   Balance of risks of infection and cost-effectiveness of preventive measures

The application of the Health and Safety at Work Act to infection in hospitals may create problems which are not present in factories or in the general community. The interpretation of the Act in terms of infec-tion in patients is uncertain, since it is not intended to interfere with the clinical responsibility of medical or nursing staff. The interpretation 'as far as is reasonably practicable' is difficult to define. Hospitals are establishments for treating sick people, many of whom are admitted with an existing infection or will acquire an infection during their stay. The diagnosis of an infection may take several days and noninfective conditions can closely mimic infection. Susceptibility of the patient and techniques of treatment are important factors in the emergence of infec-tion. Most hospital infections are unlikely to be transferred to staff and the incidence of acquired infection in staff is usually very low, particu-larly if the common upper respiratory infections are excluded. Although every effort is made to minimize risks, staff should accept that a high standard of personal hygiene is necessary, and most accept that there is some risk of acquiring an infection during the course of their normal duties. It is important that infected patients, irrespective of the infection (e.g. AIDS) receive the best possible treatment and that this is not impaired because of their infection. The spread of infection between patients, or between patients and staff, cannot be eliminated but can be reduced by simple methods such as handwashing. Expensive measures, which may involve uneconomic use of staff and resources, may achieve little more than these simple basic measures. All grades of hospital staff are responsible for carrying out measures to reduce the likelihood of spread of infection and this personal responsibility cannot be passed on to the employing authority. Some departments, for example intensive care or isolation units, may be potentially more hazardous than others due to the types of patient treated and methods of treatment required. All patients and equipment should be considered to be possibly infective, and special measures may be recommended by infection control staff for known transmissible infections. The increased risks of infection should also be recognized by visitors, and, where appropriate, visitors should be made aware of these possible hazards.

Decisions on measures required in a particular situation must be made in terms of possible benefit to patients, benefit to the hospital community, and the cost of the measures. Cost benefit is obviously not a term to be used lightly when considering infection in patients or staff, but it is unfortunately a necessity. The occasional failure of soundly based, commonly accepted measures is not necessarily due to negligence. If legal or other authorities criticize staff without well-founded evidence, infection control staff are likely to adopt a defensive approach which is detrimental to patient care and to the NHS as a whole. Some examples of difficult decisions for infection control staff will be described.

A common problem is the management of a chronic salmonella carrier, either a member of staff or a patient. Person-to-person spread of salmonella is rare except in infant nurseries. The staff carrier could still, with reasonable safety, return to work after the cessation of symptoms provided he/she does not handle food, drugs or babies and is conscientious in matters of personal hygiene (Pether and Scott 1982). A patient can, with reasonable safety, be sent home or to convalescence while still excreting salmonella if he/she is otherwise fit to be discharged and provided that suitable instructions as to personal hygiene are given. If spread of infection occurs in either of these situations the hospital could be held legally responsible, but any other course of action would have been unrealistic. Similarly, a member of the medical or nursing staff who is a known HBV carrier or whose blood is positive for HIV antibody should be allowed to continue work, provided he/she takes reasonable hygienic precautions; nevertheless, there is a small risk of transfer of hepatitis B and a lesser risk of HIV (Chapter 10). The risk depends on the nature of the work. Spread to a patient is more likely to occur from a surgeon than from a ward nurse.

The inanimate environment is not a major factor in the spread of infection and structural alterations can be costly. Care is necessary not to embark on expensive structural changes on the basis of infection hazard because of an apparent legal requirement rather than on evidence of efficacy in the prevention of infection. A good selective surveillance system is likely to be more cost-effective in the prevention of infection than routine environmental monitoring, or routine screening of faeces of catering staff or noses of theatre staff; routine monitoring of air or surfaces in operating theatres or pharmacies is an example of a test method which is not related to the risk of infection.

Routine screening of staff means keeping staff unnecessarily off duty without evidence that the organisms they carry are likely to infect others. A large proportion of the staff will, if screened, be found to carry *Staph. aureus* in their noses, and a much smaller proportion may be found to carry Group A β-haemolytic streptococci in the throat or salmonella in the faeces, and most of them are unlikely to cause clinical infection. Screening for nasal staphylococci is reasonable only in an outbreak of staphylococcal infection, when carriers of the epidemic strain will be sought by phage typing, withdrawn from ward duty, given nasal antimicrobial treatment if this is thought desirable, and monitored for removal of the epidemic strain before returning to ward duty.

Routine screening of staff for Hb_sAg or HIV antibody should similarly be avoided. In particular, the consequences of a positive test should be considered prior to testing for HIV antibody. If testing is considered necessary, agreement is required from the member of staff concerned before the sample is taken. Some members of staff will be offered immunisation against hepatitis B. The vaccine is still relatively expensive and the incidence of carriage or infection in the general population is low. Health authorities may offer the vaccine only to certain high-risk groups at the present time and failure to offer cannot be considered negligent unless the incidence of hepatitis B in the group of patients treated is unusually high. Similarly, a member of staff cannot be considered negligent if he does not accept the offer of vaccination. The availability of a cheaper, genetically engineered vaccine has extended the groups recommended for vaccination, although the actual risk still remains generally low.

Assessment of risk of spread should be based as far as possible on scientific evidence. A source, a route of spread, and a portal of entry of sufficient numbers of organisms to a susceptible host are required for an infection to occur. If these conditions are not met, spread is not possible – for example, a surgical dressing from a patient with an HIV infection is not a risk if sealed in a plastic bag or handled with gloves. If the HIV seropositive rate in a hospital is low (e.g. 0.1%), the risk of acquiring infection is extremely low; only 0.4% of personnel receiving a needle-stick injury from a known infected person will acquire infection and even less from a mucous membrane or skin exposure.

Measures to control infection can be expensive and time-wasting for staff and patients and should not be introduced unless evidence of their potential value is available.

2.7   Quality control and audit

The necessity for improved quality control in health services is now generally accepted and is an obvious requirement for controlling infection. Although the preparation of overall infection rates is the obvious approach of the epidemiologist, for reasons explained above, this is not generally practical or cost-effective. Nevertheless, data can be presented to the infection control committee on infections in high risk areas, isolation of 'alert' organisms (see p. 35) and measures taken to control infections. Evidence of implementation of policies can be obtained by surveys of wards, kitchens and other units and by questionnaires to determine improvement in staff knowledge. It is important that these are both useful, do not take up too much staff time and that they are taken into consideration when determining staffing levels. The quality control procedures should be concerned with processes which are likely to influence the acquisition of infection and not on irrelevant testing such as routine air sampling of operating theatres. Clinical audit is an aspect of quality control which is likely to involve infection control staff. Computerization of all patient records should enable more accurate infection rates to be reported. All complications, including infections, should be included in the audit and discussed by the clinicians on a regular basis. Infection control staff should be invited to attend these sessions. However, the problem of accurate recording of data, especially the follow-up in the community, remains.

2.8   Notification of infectious diseases

Some diseases are notifiable by law to the CCDC; the doctor who diagnoses the infection is responsible for the notification. There are some differences in the lists of diseases notifiable in England and Wales, in Scotland and in Northern Ireland (see Appendix 2.1).

Although there is no statutory obligation to notify the detection of symptom-free carriers of bacteria that cause notifiable disease, it is recommended that persistent carriers of typhoid bacilli and other salmonellae should be reported to the CCDC.

Appendix 2.1   Diseases notifiable to the Consultant in Communicable Disease control or other appropriate medical officer

ENGLAND AND WALES

Acute encephalitis
Acute poliomyelitis
Anthrax
Cholera
Diphtheria
Dysentery
Food poisoning (or suspected
   food poisoning)
Lassa fever
Leprosy
Leptospirosis
Malaria
Measles
Meningitis
Meningococca septicaemia
   (without meningitis)
Mumps

Ophthalmia neonatorum
Paratyphoid fever
Plague
Rabies
Relapsing fever
Rubella
Scarlet fever
Smallpox
Tetanus
Tuberculosis (all forms)
Typhoid fever
Typhus
Viral haemorrhagic fever (e.g.
   Ebola fever)
Viral hepatitis
Whooping cough
Yellow fever

SCOTLAND

Anthrax
Chickenpox
Cholera
Diphtheria
Dysentery
Erysipelas
Food poisoning
Legionellosis
Leptospirosis
Leprosy
Malaria
Scarlet fever
Smallpox
Tuberculosis – respiratory and
   non-respiratory
Tetanus
Typhoid fever

Measles
Meningococcal infection
Mumps
Paratyphoid fever A and B
Plague
Poliomyelitis – paralytic and non-
   paralytic
Puerperal fever
Rabies
Relapsing fever
Rubella
Typhus
Viral haemorrhagic fevers (e.g.
   Ebola fever)
Viral hepatitis
Whooping cough

NORTHERN IRELAND

Acute encephalitis
Acute meningitis
Anthrax
Chickenpox
Cholera
Diphtheria
Dysentery
Food poisoning (all sources)
Gastro-enteritis (persons under 2 years of age only)
Hepatitis A, Hepatitis B, Hepatitis unspecified (viral)
Legionnaire's disease
Leptospirosis
Malaria
Measles
Mumps
Paratyphoid fever
Plague
Poliomyelitis – paralytic and non-paralytic
Rabies
Relapsing fever
Rubella
Scarlet fever
Smallpox
Tetanus
Tuberculosis – pulmonary and non-pulmonary
Typhoid fever
Typhus
Viral haemorrhagic fevers
Whooping cough
Yellow fever

References and further reading

Casewell, M.W. (1989) Control of hospital infection: enhancing present arrangements. *British Medical Journal*, **298**, 203.

Control of Substances Hazardous to Health Regulations. (1988) HMSO, London.

Department of Health and Social Security (1974) *Health Services Management, Health and Safety at Work etc. Act.* Health Circular HC(78)30, HMSO, London.

Department of Health and Social Security (1988a) *Public Health in England. The Report of an Enquiry into the Future Development of the Public Health Function.* HMSO, London.

Department of Health and Social Security (1988b) *Hospital Infection Control: General Management Arrangements.* HMSO, London.

Department of Health (1989) *The Control of Substances Hazardous to Health: Guidance for the Initial Assessment in Hospitals.* HMSO, London.

Harrison, D.I. (1991) Control of Substances Hazardous to Health (COSHH). Regulations and hospital infection. *Journal of Hospital Infection*, **17** (Supplement A) 530.

Haley, R.W., Culver, D.H., White, J.W., *et al.* (1985) The efficacy of infection surveillance and control programs in preventing nosocomial infection in US hospitals. *American Journal of Epidemiology*, **121**, 182.

Howard, A.J. (1988) Infection control organization in hospitals in England and Wales, 1986. Report of a survey undertaken by a Hospital Infection Society Working Party. *Journal of Hospital Infection*, **11**, 183.

Pether, J.V.S. and Scott, R.J.D. (1982) Salmonella carriers. Are they dangerous? Study to identify finger contamination with salmonella by convalescent carriers. *Journal of Infection*, **5**, 81.

Wenzel, R.P. (1987) Epidemics – identification and management. In *Prevention and Control of Nosocomial Infections*. Williams and Wilkins, Baltimore.

Williams, R.E.O., Blowers, R., Garrod, L.P. and Shooter, R.A. (1966) *Hospital Infection: Causes and Prevention*, 2nd edn. Lloyd Luke, London.

3 Surveillance, records and reports

In most hospitals the overall incidence of infection is unknown; the methods of surveillance (i.e. discovery and recording of infection) are variable and infection records, when kept by the ward staff, are often inaccurate. Surveillance has been defined as 'the continuing scrutiny of all aspects of occurrence and spread of a disease that are pertinent to effective control' (Benenson 1985). Surveillance of infection in hospital is necessary for the following reasons:

1. to recognize, by any unusual level or change in level of incidence, the existing or impending spread of an outbreak, and to identify the appearance of any particularly dangerous organism;
2. to judge the desirability of introducing special measures to control an outbreak, or threatened outbreak, and to assess the efficacy of such measures;
3. to assess the efficacy of the regular preventative measures in use in the hospital;
4. to reduce the level of avoidable infection and to identify high risk patients so that selective measures can be introduced and to ensure control efforts have their maximum and most cost effective outcome.

Of major importance is early recognition of an impending outbreak, or of possible hazards, such as contaminated incubators, which might be followed by infection.

Surveillance and record keeping must not be regarded as an end in themselves, but as an instrument for measuring the effectiveness of an infection control programme and for giving an early indication of outbreaks or problem areas. The main purpose of recording infections is to provide information for action to be taken. Administrative managers should not expect infection rates to be recorded for the whole hospital, since it is not a cost-effective procedure and does not necessarily improve quality control. Keeping records is time consuming and should be kept to the essential minimum unless more detailed records are required for a research project. However, the 'Study on the Efficacy of Nosocomial Infection Control' (SENIC) carried out in the USA indicated that a highly efficient surveillance and infection control system could reduce the infection rates by one third. Feedback to clinicians was considered to be of particular importance in reducing wound infection (Haley *et al*. 1985). The optimal surveillance system is unknown and several methods will be described below (American Society for Microbiology 1987; Castle and Ajemian 1987; Ayliffe 1988).

In addition to obtaining information on infections in patients, surveillance of staff, the environment and certain equipment may sometimes be required, but routine microbial screening of staff or the environment is not, in general, recommended.

3.1 Methods of surveillance of infection in patients

3.1.1 DAILY SCRUTINY OF LABORATORY RECORDS BY LABORATORY OR INFECTION CONTROL STAFF

This is a minimal requirement in all hospitals. It is simple and requires no extra staff or recording methods. Impending outbreaks can usually be detected at an early stage. The storage of laboratory data, particularly of antibiotic sensitivity patterns, on a computer and the regular examination of printouts will aid the detection of less obvious cross-infection.

The incidence of clinical infection cannot be calculated from laboratory records and the limited usefulness of this method depends on the taking of bacteriological samples from all suspected cases of infection. Infections from which bacteriological samples cannot be obtained will be missed if laboratory records are the only method of surveillance.

3.1.2 LABORATORY RECORDS AND ROUTINE VISITS TO THE WARDS

This is the preferred method in the UK. The infection control nurse examines the laboratory records every morning and discusses results with the laboratory technicians and infection control doctor. The nurse completes the necessary information on the infected patient by visiting the ward. The nurse can then determine whether this is a true clinical infection, whether it is hospital-acquired, and decide on the relevant action. If the ward staff does not send samples to the laboratory: this method may be no more effective than laboratory surveillance alone, but if frequent visits are made to the ward the nurse can encourage the ward staff to send samples from all patients with suspected infections and can also obtain information on possible infections which have not had a bacteriological investigation. The ward staff must also be encouraged to telephone the infection control nurse or doctor when an infection is suspected (e.g. a patient with diarrhoea in a maternity unit) so that early action can be implemented before microbiological results are available. In addition, the ward sister might be encouraged to keep a daily note of any infection or infection-related problem. This can be examined by the infection control nurse if the ward sister is busy at the time of the visit. Similarly, managers of relevant departments (e.g. SSD, catering) should contact the infection control nurse or doctor if a member of the staff develops an infection.

It may not be possible to visit all the wards and units daily, but special risk units, such as intensive care, should be visited regularly, preferably daily, even if none of the patients is known to be infected.

3.1.3   OTHER METHODS

Visiting wards and units daily or several times a week, examining all patient records and recording all clinical infections is a technique used in many hospitals in the USA. This may be complemented by visits to the laboratory. Recording of patients receiving antibiotics has also been used as an aid for detecting infections. Continuous clinical surveillance of all patients is not possible for one nurse in a busy general hospital and is an inefficient use of limited resources which should be concentrated on areas of high risk or on 'high risk' patients.

Techniques for risk assessment are being developed and are discussed elsewhere in the chapter (page 36). Increased length of stay may also be a useful measurement particularly if cost of infection is being considered.

A prevalence survey may be useful for a recently appointed infection control nurse to obtain knowledge of the hospital and its problems (Meers *et al*. 1981). Some hospitals may also carry out an annual survey to provide a prevalence rate to supplement other surveillance techniques, but this is of little use in the routine day to day control of infection. Prevalence surveys could also be made by a regionally-based team in hospitals without their own infection control team. A prevalence survey in a ward or hospital may also be useful to determine the extent and spread of antibiotic-resistant organisms or to ensure that these have been eliminated.

The prevalence rate is higher than the incidence rate because it takes into account length of stay, and infected patients tend to stay in hospital longer than noninfected patients.

3.2   Records of infection

Records of infection in a ward book kept by the nursing or medical staff are not usually an effective method of surveillance. Similarly, the completion by the ward staff of cards containing relevant information which are sent to the laboratory with the specimen is a method some-times used (see previous edition of this book), but this also provides additional work for the ward staff and is not usually an effective method.

Computerization of patients' notes may enable additional data on infection to be recorded. This has the disadvantage of variable accuracy, depending on who is responsible for collecting data, and possible failure to detect problems promptly. However, rapid developments in com-puterization are taking place and advances in this technique are likely. The requirements for clinical audit should improve the accuracy of data since the clinicians will be responsible for recording details of all major complications, including infections.

For day-to-day recording of infection, a board showing all the wards in the hospital can be kept in the office of the infection control doctor or nurse. Coloured flags indicate the location of infections and the colours and shapes of the flags can indicate different organisms, phage-types and sites of infection. Although such a board gives an immediate visual impression of the current state of infection in the hospital, it requires constant attention to keep up-to-date. This method is particu-larly useful during an outbreak of infection.

Various other methods of keeping records are available, but one of the most useful is a 'Kardex' or similar system (see Appendix 3.3). A separate page is kept for each ward or unit and it is easy to detect a problem in a particular area. However, this method is being replaced by computerized records with daily printouts.

Most hospitals have a system for detecting particularly hazardous, transmissible or highly antibiotic-resistant organisms. These 'alert organisms' are initially detected by experienced laboratory staff who pass on the information promptly to the infection control nurse. If the laboratory records are computerized a 'flagging' system ensures that these organisms are not missed. A computer program can also be pro-duced to detect changes in levels of infection. This is particularly useful for recognizing changes over long periods which might otherwise not be recognized. An example of the basic data to be collected is shown in Appendix 3.2. All infections in special units are recorded, but additional information may be collected on wounds or other infections – either routinely or over a specified period. If additional data are recorded routinely, this may be time consuming and it is important to decide whether the additional effort is worthwhile in terms of prevention of infection. However, variations in definition can influence the rate and scoring systems are sometimes used (Wilson *et al.* 1990). Even decisions by different observers on the presence or absence of pus, particularly in mild infections, can be variable.

3.3   Wound infection

The wound infection rate must be defined if comparisons are to be made within a hospital or between hospitals. A list of all operations performed may be obtained from the operating theatre and should at least be classified into clean, clean-contaminated or contaminated (see below), but even in these categories there can be a wide difference in infection rates in different types of operations. A meaningful single overall infection rate for all types of wound is not possible, since the likelihood of infection differs in each of these categories and numbers may be too small for comparison. It is useful also to record the severity of infection in each type of wound, the presence or absence of pus and whether the wound was drained or not drained. Accuracy may be further improved by comparing individual types of operation (e.g. hernia), and introducing 'risk' factors into the calculation (Cruse and Foord 1973). Using a computer model, incidence or prevalence can be corrected for 'risk' factors such as age, sex, type of operation, (clean, clean-contaminated or contaminated), pre-operative stay, wound drainage and special factors such as diabetes (Bibby *et al.* 1986, Garibaldi *et al.* 1991). However, other models are available and differ in some respects (see for example Simchen *et al.* 1984; 1988). Haley *et al.* (1985) have suggested four factors:

1. operation on abdomen;
2. length of operation over 2 hours;
3. contaminated or dirty wound;
4. three or more underlying diagnoses.

Further work is needed to define a model which only requires readily obtainable information. Infections occurring after discharge from hospital must also be included if accurate rates are to be obtained. The infection rate should be based on clinical and not bacteriological findings. Only operations in which there has been a breach in the skin should be included in the assessment; endoscopies, manipulations and examinations under anaesthesia, vaginal operations, and also incisions of abscesses, should not be included in the total operations at risk for acquired infection. Cystoscopies should be considered separately as there are certain special problems concerned with the sterilization or disinfection of the instruments used. Infection following cystoscopy is important but should not be included under wound infection.

In recording the incidence or prevalence of wound infection the following descriptions, definitions and information are useful.

1. The type of operation, and whether the wound is drained or not.
    Operations are further classified as:

(a) clean – an operation not transecting gastrointestinal, genitourinary or tracheobronchial systems and not performed in the vicinity of any apparent inflammatory reaction (e.g. a hernia repair);

(b) clean-contaminated – an operation transecting one of the above systems where bacterial contamination could occur but is usually not abundant and where evidence of definite contamination is not available (e.g. operations on the stomach or gall-bladder);

(c) contaminated – an operation transecting systems where bacteria are known to be present (and usually abundant), or in the vicinity of apparent inflammatory reactions (e.g. operations on the colon, mouth or perforated appendix);

2. Presence or absence of pus.
3. Sepsis and degree of severity:
   (a) mild sepsis – small or superficial area of inflammation with minimal discharge;
   (b) moderate sepsis – superficial inflammation of whole wound (or over one third) with a serous or small amount of purulent discharge, or a deeper infection involving a small area (one third or less) usually with a purulent discharge;
   (c) severe sepsis – a deep purulent infection, with or without sinuses or fistulae, or widespread cellulitis, or wound breakdown with an obvious inflammatory reaction and pus.
4. Organisms and antiobiotic sensitivity.
5. Other information – which can be collected as required by the individual hospital (e.g. operating theatre, surgeon, length of operations, number of primary diagnoses, antibiotic treatment, probable origin of infection, time of dressing of wound, etc.)

3.4   Probable place of infection

It would be advantageous to know where the infection was acquired and the following points may be helpful.

3.4.1   INFECTION ACQUIRED IN OPERATING THEATRE

This may be indicated by the following:

1. deep infection in a clean, undrained wound at any time;
2. infection occurring within three days of the operation, or prior to first dressing in a clean wound;
3. supporting evidence includes:
   (a) pyrexia;
   (b) staphylococcus of same type not isolated from any patient in the ward;

(c) staphylococcus of same type isolated from a member of operating staff and not present in the ward;

(d) staphylococcus of same type in different wards from patients operated on in the same operating theatre.

3.4.2   INFECTION ACQUIRED IN THE WARD

This is indicated by superficial infection in a wound (usually drained), occurring after first dressing. Culture is initially negative. Deep infection may develop later in a drained wound. Supporting evidence is staphylococcus of same type isolated from other patients or members of the staff in the ward.

3.4.3   PLACE OF ACQUISITION OF INFECTION NOT KNOWN

This applies where there is superficial infection in any wound after first dressing and no available evidence from bacteriology in favour of theatre or ward infection.

3.4.4   INFECTION ACQUIRED FROM PATIENT'S OWN BACTERIAL FLORA

These include infections due to *Staph. epidermidis* or *Staph. aureus* that was present in patient's nose prior to, or at time of, surgery. However, resistant strains may have been acquired by the patient in the ward before the operation.

Infections due to antibiotic-sensitive Gram-negative bacilli, usually *Escherichia coli* and *Bacteroides* spp.

3.5   Other acquired infection

Other acquired infections may be included in the routine records, but the relevance of this information to the control of infection, except in the case of urinary tract infection, is rather doubtful because it is often impossible to tell whether the infection is acquired in hospital – for example, laboratory records of sputum examinations are rarely helpful in determining the incidence of acquired chest infection. Hospital-acquired or 'associated' infection is assessed mainly from clinical information and an agreed definition must be used for each site of infection. This is especially important in prevalence surveys. The definitions used in the national survey carried out in 1980 (Meers *et al.* 1981), were modifications of those used by the Centres for Disease Control and are as follows.

3.5.1 DEFINITION OF HOSPITAL ACQUIRED INFECTION

An infection found to be active or under active treatment at the time of the survey, which was not present on admission to hospital. (With patients recently admitted it is necessary to judge whether any infection was being incubated on admission, and to mark such as not hospital-acquired (i.e. 'community-acquired'). Similarly, a patient who is read-mitted with established infection which has resulted from an earlier admission is recorded as suffering from hospital-acquired, not community-acquired, infection.

3.5.2 CRITERIA FOR DIAGNOSING THE PRESENCE OF AN INFECTION (WHETHER HOSPITAL OR COMMUNITY-ACQUIRED)

Urinary tract infection   A patient being treated for a bacteriologically or clinically diagnosed infection, or in whom a bacteriological diagnosis has been made without treatment being given.

Respiratory tract infection
Upper   A patient with acute coryzal symptoms, or a significant sore mouth or throat with inflammation, but excluding sufferers from an allergy.
Lower   New or increased purulent sputum production with chest signs and/or X-ray changes not attributed to embolus, heart failure or aspiration.

Skin infection   Skin conditions showing evidence of inflammation with or without the production of pus in skin or subcutaneous tissue. Include infected (not merely colonized) ulcers or pressure sores.

Bacteraemia   Positive blood cultures (excluding contamination, but accepting as positive multiple isolations, of, for instance, a coagulase-negative staphylococcus when supported by symptoms or signs).

Ear infection   New purulent discharge.

Eye infection   Significant new purulent discharge.

CNS infection   Positive culture, or exudate diagnostic of a virus infection.

Genital tract   New purulent discharge.

Gastrointestinal infection
Generalized   Symptoms, preferably with a report of culture of a recognized pathogen causing gastroenteritis.
Localized   Diverticulitis, appendicitis, cholecystitis, ano-rectal sepsis, dental abscess or other local infection.

Bones or joints   Evidence of osteomyelitis or septic arthritis.

Other   Any other significant infection, including specific ones, such as measles, hepatitis.

It is equally important to take 'risk' factors into consideration when comparing incidence rates of infections other than wounds. Indwelling catheterization, length of time of catheterization and antibiotic therapy should all be recorded when investigating urinary tract infection. Patient factors, such as chronic bronchitis and smoking, will influence hospital-acquired respiratory infection. Computer models for improving comparisons in these groups are being developed. Although the incidence rate is usually based on infections/100 patients discharged over a month or other defined interval, a more realistic result can be obtained by using patient days. This may be calculated by dividing the number of infections by the number of days spent by patients in hospital to arrive at, for example, the rate per 100 patient days.

3.6   Presentation of reports

Information on infections, e.g. wound and neonatal infections, is presented to the infection control committee at monthly or three monthly intervals. Individual results may be presented to surgeons on their own operations. The course of outbreaks should be followed, either by using a board with flags (see p. 35) or by using appropriate charts (Appendix 3.2). The infection rate in clean undrained wounds is useful as a measure of acquired infection in the operating theatre and the total operations in each category, i.e. clean, clean-contaminated and contaminated, can usually be obtained from operating theatre records. However, these are not always accurate and must sometimes be supplemented from the patients' notes. This can be time-consuming and it may be sufficient to report the total infections in each category provided the number of operations is reasonably constant. Early discharge of patients from hospital provides some difficulties in compiling accurate wound infection rates, but the information can be obtained (usually with difficulty) from the community health services and outpatients department.

Reports should be simple and preferably expressed graphically, so that the current situation in wards or theatres can be immediately assessed. This is more readily achieved if the data is computerized. Commercially produced 'software' packages are now available, but comparisons between surgeons or hospitals can be invalid unless 'risk' factors are taken into consideration. Many hospitals will prefer to develop their own systems. The ward staff are always interested to know the results of studies made on their wards and particularly in the results from their own nasal swabs. Reports should always be sent to the ward concerned, following a bacteriological survey. Since antibiotic therapy for individual patients is often required before the results of sensitivity tests are available, the medical staff should be provided with information on prevalent pathogens and their sensitivity patterns in the hospital (see Chapter 13).

3.7 Surveillance of infection in staff

Surveillance of infection amongst members of staff, in close cooperation with the occupational health department, is also important. This includes enteric and other community-acquired infections, septic lesions, carriage of multi-resistant *Staph. aureus*, and hospital-acquired infections (see Chapter 14).

Treatment and management of these infections can usually be decided in discussion between infection control officer and the occupational health (or staff) medical officer.

3.7.1 DETECTION OF STAPHYLOCOCCAL CARRIERS

As approximately 20–30% of healthy staff are nasal carriers of *Staph. aureus*, and as there is no accepted laboratory test for virulence of the organism, routine nasal swabbing of staff in wards and operating theatres is rarely indicated. Routine nasal swabs from staff may be required during outbreaks of infection and as a follow-up after treatment of a carrier on the staff. If an identifiable strain of known virulence or a strain with unusual resistance to antibiotics is responsible for an outbreak of infection, routine nasal swabbing may be required for a limited time as part of a programme to eradicate the organisms from the unit. It is of greater importance to exclude staff with skin lesions or sepsis from wards or theatres than to spend time unnecessarily on the routine examination of nose swabs.

3.7.2 DETECTION OF CARRIERS OF GROUP A β-HAEMOLYTIC STREPTOCOCCI (*STREPTOCOCCUS PYOGENES*)

The incidence of puerperal infection caused by Group A β-haemolytic streptococci (formerly the major hazard) is now so low that routine nose and throat swabbing is no longer obligatory in maternity units. Swabs must be taken from staff and patients when an infection occurs in the unit and is not of endogenous origin (Chapter 9).

3.7.3 DETECTION OF FAECAL CARRIERS OF *SALMONELLA* OR *SHIGELLA* SPP.

Experience has shown that it is impracticable to demand routine bacteriological examination of faeces of food-handling staff; this measure is not recommended, unless specifically indicated by past history or recent visits to areas where enteric infections are endemic (see Chapters 9 and 12).

3.7.4 DETECTION OF HBV CARRIERS AND OF PATIENTS WITH HIV ANTIBODIES

Since carriers are not excluded from working, routine screening is inadvisable. If tests for HIV are required, permission should be obtained from the staff concerned. Arrangements should be made for counselling before tests are carried out, and again if the results are positive.

3.8 Routine monitoring of environment and equipment

3.8.1 ENVIRONMENT

Unless there is an outbreak of infection, routine bacteriological sampling of floors, walls, surfaces and air is rarely indicated. If sampling is done, quantitative or semi-quantitative techniques should be used. Results should be reported as numbers of organisms per unit area or volume. Random swabbing of areas of unspecified size will give results which are not comparable with each other or with previous results and are difficult to interpret. The non-quantitative isolation even of known pathogens may also be misleading. Selective and/or indicator media should be used for counting pathogens such as *Staph. aureus* or *Clostridium perfringens*. Standards for counts on surfaces are rarely valid; numbers of organisms on a surface vary according to the amount of recontamination from the air, and on floors also from shoes and trolleys. However, counting organisms on a surface may be useful for teaching and research purposes. The number of organisms in the air of wards or theatres depends mainly on the number of people in the room and their activity, and on the airflow (air changes per hour), which is rarely standardized except in operating theatres. Routine checking of airflow in a ventilated area is a more reliable guide to the efficiency of a ventilation system than bacteriological tests. Nevertheless, if air to the theatre is recirculated, as in laminar flow systems, filters must be regularly checked and occasionally bacteriological tests may be required. Although of doubtful value, air sampling is often suggested before opening a new operating suite or after major repairs or maintenance. A total count of not more than 35 cfu/m^3 in the supply air is suggested as acceptable (Arrowsmith 1985). Inspection of ducts, testing of air flows and patency of filters are more accurate criteria. Air sampling (settle-plates, or other quantitative methods, e.g. slit-sampling) may be useful in recognizing the presence of staphylococcal dispersers in a ward or theatre and in testing individuals suspected of being dispersers. Contact plates from floors, other surfaces or bedding, may similarly be used to detect dispersers. Contact plates from floors are also useful to determine whether a ward is free from dispersers at the end of an outbreak.

3.8.2   EQUIPMENT

Routine monitoring of sterilization and some disinfection processes is necessary. Physical or chemical measurement of the efficiency of the process is generally preferable to bacteriological assessment. The results of bacteriological tests are available only after 1–5 days, depending on the organisms and the method of treatment. Sampling of treated equipment or fluids is of less value than process control, since initial contamination may be low and a large proportion of samples may be sterile. If sampling of the treated product is required, tests should be made in laboratories skilled in this type of work and statistically valid results produced.

Sterilization or disinfection by heat is preferable to chemical methods and monitoring should, when possible, be carried out with correctly placed thermometers or thermocouples. Records of temperature and time should be obtained for every cycle (see Chapter 4). Initial bacteriological tests of the process may sometimes be useful and routine bacteriological monitoring may be necessary for some equipment when varying loads or materials are treated. Good and regular maintenance of equipment is as important as routine tests for efficiency.

Monitoring of sterilization processes is described in Chapter 4. Disinfection processes are often less well controlled. Heat disinfection of infant feeds, crockery, cutlery, laundry and bedpans, as well as pasteurization processes should, if possible, be controlled by regular temperature-time measurements. Initial bacteriological testing of the process is advisable, and in some instances (e.g. expressed breast milk used in a bank) routine bacteriological tests are also advisable.

Disinfection by chemical methods also requires regular monitoring. Chemical tests of the process may sometimes be made, for example to assess presence and amount of hydrogen peroxide, formaldehyde and ethylene oxide. For most disinfectants, occasional bacteriological in-use testing may be necessary, since disinfectants vary in stability and may be inactivated to a varying extent by materials; dilutions and time of application are less readily controlled than are heating methods. After chemical disinfection of certain special equipment (e.g. respiratory ventilators) it may be advisable to confirm by bacteriological sampling that no pathogens can be found, but this is not necessary if the process is well controlled.

Appendix 3.1   Example of an outbreak: number of infections occurring over a two-week period

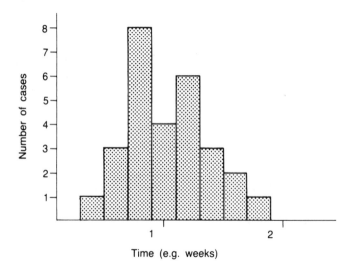

Time (e.g. weeks)

Appendix 3.2   Example of infections routinely recorded

'ALERT' ORGANISMS

1. *Strep. pyogenes, Salmonella* and *Shigella* spp., enteropathogenic *E. coli, M. tuberculosis,* rotavirus, *Ps. aeruginosa, N. meningitidis, Legionella* spp.
2. Highly-resistant strains of *Staph. aureus* (e.g. resistant to methicillin, gentamicin, fusidic acid, mupirocin).
   Highly-resistant strains of Gram-negative bacilli (e.g. resistant to gentamicin, third generation cephalosporins, ciprofloxacin).

(contd. on page 46).

Appendix 3.3   Example of 'Kardex' record

Ward Date specimen	Patient	Month and year Date of birth	Date of admission	Consultant	Operation/ diagnosis	Date of operation	Type	Organism	Antibiotic resistance	Comments
1/1 W/S	John Smith	1.1.01	1.1	RS	Varicose ulcers	–	–	*Strep.* Gp A	Sens	Present on admission
10/1 W/S	John Jones	10.10.10	1.1	RS	Append-ectomy	6.1	C/C	*Bacteroides*	Sens	
25/1 W/S	John Doe	2.2.22	20.1	RS	Lumbar sympathectomy	23.1	Clean	*Staph. aureus*	PT	Phage type 80/81 drained

Abbreviations
W/S: Wound swab
Sens: Sensitive to all antibiotics tested
C/C: Clean/Contaminated
P: Penicillin-resistant
T: Tetracycline-resistant

(contd. from page 44).
3. Strains showing unusual resistance (e.g. penicillin-resistant *Str. pneumoniae*).
4. Blood culture isolates.

CLINICAL INFECTIONS

1. All infections from the special care baby unit, intensive care unit, paediatric wards and other high risk areas.
2. Communicable diseases.
3. Wound or other selected infections, e.g. urinary tract infections.

References

American Society for Microbiology (1987) Proceedings of the Annual Meeting of the American Society for Microbiology Seminar on Surveillance Methodology. *Infection Control*, **8**, 448.

Arrowsmith, L.W.M. (1985) Air sampling in operating theatres. *Journal of Hospital Infection*, **6**, 352.

Ayliffe, G.A.J. (1988) Hospital infection surveillance in the United Kingdom. *Infection Control and Hospital Epidemiology*, **9**, 320.

Benenson, A.S. (1985) *Control of Communicable Diseases in Man*, 14th edn. *American Public Health Association, Washington.*

Bibby, B.A., Collins, B.J. and Ayliffe, G.A.J. (1986) A mathematical model for assessing postoperative wound infection. *Journal of Hospital Infection*, **8**, 31.

Castle, M. and Ajemian, E. (1987) *Infection Control – Principles and Practice*, 2nd edn. John Wiley, New York, Chichester, Brisbane.

Cruse, P.J.E., and Foord, R. (1973) A five year prospective study of 23 649 surgical wounds. *Archives of Surgery*, **107**, 206.

Garibaldi, R.A., Cushing, D. and Lerer, T. (1991) Predictors of intraoperative acquired surgical wound injections. *Journal of Hospital Infection*, **18** (Supplement A), 289.

Haley, R.W., Culver, D.H., Morgan, W.M., *et al*. (1985) Identifying patients at high risk of surgical wound infection: a simple multivariate index of patient susceptibility and wound contamination. *American Journal of Epidemiology*, **121**, 206.

Meers, P.D., Ayliffe, G.A.J., Emmerson, A.M. *et al*. (1981) Report on the National Survey of Infection in Hospitals 1980. *Journal of Hospital Infection*, Supplement 2.

Simchen, E., Stein, H., Sacks, T.G. *et al*. (1984) Multivariate analysis of determinants of postoperative wound infection in orthopaedic patients. *Journal of Hospital Infection*, **5**, 137.

Simchen, E., Wax, Y., Pevsner, B. (1988) The Israeli study of surgical infections, (ISSI) ii Initial comparisons among hospitals with special focus in hernia operations. *Infection Control and Hospital Epidemiology*, **9**, 241.

Wilson, A.P.R., Weavill, C., Burridge, J. and Kelsey, M.C. (1990) The use of the wound scoring method 'ASEPSIS' in postoperative wound infection surveillance. *Journal of Hospital Infection*, **16**, 297.

4 *Sterilization and physical disinfection*

Microbial contaminants can be removed by cleaning with a detergent and water, or destroyed by sterilization or disinfection. Cleaning followed by drying of surfaces other than those of the body can be almost as effective as the use of a disinfectant.

Sterilization means treatment which achieves the complete killing or removal of all types of microorganisms, including the spores of tetanus and gas gangrene bacilli which are resistant to most disinfectants and more resistant to heat than non-sporing micro-organisms. **Disinfection** means treatment which reduces the numbers of vegetative micro-organisms (e.g. staphylococci, salmonella), and viruses – but not necessarily bacterial spores or 'slow' viruses – to safe or relatively safe levels. A **disinfectant** is a chemical compound which can destroy vegetative micro-organisms and viruses; the word **antiseptic** is often used for disinfectants which are applied to the skin or to living tissues, but since the purpose of antiseptics is to disinfect (one speaks of 'skin disinfection'), the word antiseptic might seem superfluous; it is, however, useful as an indication that the compound can be safely applied to tissues. The word **sterilant** has sometimes been used for the small range of chemical compounds (ethylene oxide, formaldehyde and glutaraldehyde) which, under controlled conditions, can kill sporing bacteria. All items to be sterilized should be physically cleaned before they are subjected to a standard sterilizing process. Methods of sterilization are summarized in Appendix 4.2. (See also Appendix 6.2, Chapter 6).

All surgical instruments, dressings and other objects or solutions which are introduced into traumatic or operation wounds or by injection must be provided sterile (i.e. sterilized and adequately protected against subsequent contamination). The same applies, in general, to materials introduced into other areas normally sterile, though disinfection by 'pasteurizing' or boiling, which destroys vegetative bacteria and most viruses, is accepted as adequate for cystoscopes and some other endoscopes that cannot tolerate heat sterilization. However, there is a slight possibility of clostridial infection arising after operations on the genito-urinary tract, and manufacturers should be encouraged to develop equipment able to withstand autoclaving.

Laboratory discard materials should be transported in robust containers without spillage and stored in a safe manner while awaiting sterilization. The Advisory Committee on Dangerous Pathogens (1990) recommends four levels of containment for discard material, the method of disinfection and sterilization being dependent upon the level of microbiological risk associated with the discard materials. An autoclave with an effective containment system for high risk items has been described (Oates *et al.* 1983).

4.1   Methods of sterilization (see also Appendix 4.2)

Sterilization can be achieved by moist heat at raised atmospheric pressure, by dry heat at normal pressure, by ionizing radiation (gamma radiation or electron beams), by 'sterilants' such as ethylene oxide and glutaraldehyde, or by filtration. It can also be obtained by steam and formaldehyde at sub-atmospheric pressure. If the article to be sterilized is not damaged by heat, heat sterilizing methods should always be used in preference to other methods because they are more reliable and can be more effectively monitored.

4.1.1   HEAT STERILIZATION AND DISINFECTION

Heat sterilization depends on the temperature to which articles are exposed and on the time of exposure; the higher the temperature, the shorter the time required for sterilization. Two factors must be taken into account in deciding the time of exposure:

1. **the penetration time**, i.e. the time required for the least accessible part of the load to reach the selected sterilizing ('holding') temperature;
2. **the holding time**, i.e. the period of exposure to the selected sterilizing temperature. These times will vary with different types of load.

Dry heat is less effective than moist heat and therefore requires a higher temperature and longer time at that temperature.

Dry heat   Red heat from a Bunsen burner is of value in the laboratory, but is not suitable for sterilizing surgical instruments: the 'flaming' of a scalpel, dipped in spirit, is not satisfactory. For sterilization of certain hospital supplies the hot air oven is appropriate.
There are two main types of hot air sterilizers.

1. The fan oven – heat is produced by electric elements in the walls of the oven and a fan circulates the hot air evenly. The oven works at 160–180° with a holding time of 30–120 min, and with a total cycle

time of 2.5–5 hours depending upon the degree of cooling. It can be used for mixed loads of glass and metal instruments and also some sharp instruments used in ophthalmic surgery. Fats, oils and powders which are impervious to steam are also sterilized by this method. The main disadvantage is the long cycle time. All hot air ovens should be fitted with a door lock and a temperature chart recorder, which are mandatory requirements in the UK (DHSS 1980). Ovens without a fan are unsatisfactory.

2. The conveyor oven – formerly popular for sterile syringe services but, since the general introduction of disposable syringes, this method has been little used. The articles to be sterilized pass slowly along a conveyor system under an infra-red heat source. The oven works at 180°C with a holding time of 7.5 min.

Moist heat   Steam or water boiling at atmospheric pressure, and at a temperature of 100°C will not sterilize, but exposure at this temperature for 5–10 minutes may be sufficient treatment of specula for which disinfection is generally considered adequate (Central Sterilizing Club Working Party No. 1 1986). Washing machines are available which clean and disinfect equipment. Recommended temperatures for disinfection are 71°C for three minutes or 80°C for one minute. To ensure the destruction of bacterial spores by moist heat, a temperature above 100°C is required. In the autoclave (or pressure steam sterilizer), the boiling point of water and the temperature of the steam produced are raised in proportion to the increase in pressure. At a pressure of 1.03 bar (15 lb/in^2) above atmospheric pressure the boiling point of water is 121°C and at a pressure of 2.2 bar (32 lb/in^2) the boiling point is 134°C. Steam at these temperatures will sterilize objects in fifteen minutes and three minutes respectively.

To sterilize effectively, steam must come into direct contact with the surfaces to be sterilized. The latent heat which is given out when steam condenses to water increases the sterilizing efficiency of steam, but this effect occurs only if the steam is not superheated – i.e. raised to a temperature higher than that at which water boils under the pressure present in the autoclave. It is essential to remove all air from the autoclave; this can be done by admitting steam into the upper part of the chamber, from which it will descend, pushing the air through an outlet in the floor of the chamber. This 'downward displacement' method is suitable for unwrapped instruments, bowls and bottled fluids. Air can also be removed effectively by the use of a high vacuum pump before the admission of steam; the high vacuum autoclave should be used for sterilization of porous loads (packs). Improved removal of air can be obtained by the use of pulsed steam (i.e. alternating vacuum with steam injection for 5–8 pulses); this method is especially useful when a small load is being sterilized in a large autoclave. Removal of steam and drying of the load in an autoclave with a vacuum pump is achieved by drawing a vacuum after the sterilization stage. The complete cycle for a high vacuum autoclave is approximately 20 minutes.

4.1.2   IONIZING RADIATION

These methods are not suitable for use in hospitals, but are used commercially. The process may damage some plastic materials and advice should always be sought before reprocessing any item. Equipment made of or containing metal, polythene, paper, wool, cotton, polyvinyl chloride, nylon, terylene and polystyrene are usually unaffected. Rubber varies in its response, but butyl and chlorinated rubber are not suitable for sterilization by these methods. Electron beams (β-particles from a linear accelerator) or gamma radiation (from cobalt–60, at a dosage of 2.5 Mrad (25 000 Gy) is used. This dosage gives good penetration and leaves no residual radioactivity. Units used for radiotherapy in hospital are not suitable for sterilization purposes.

4.1.3   CHEMICAL METHODS

Ethylene oxide   Heat-sensitive articles may be sterilized by ethylene oxide gas. Ethylene oxide (EO) is extremely penetrative, non-corrosive and an effective sterilizing agent. Unfortunately, it is toxic, irritant, and explosive when mixed with air at concentrations greater than 3%. It is also odourless and leaks may therefore go unnoticed. Despite these disadvantages, EO is widely used commercially for sterilizing heat-sensitive items. It is also used in some hospitals, especially by those offering a specialist or regional facility for processing heat-sensitive items (Central Sterilizing Club Working Party Report No. 2 1986).

During a typical cycle, air is removed from the load by drawing a vacuum and the chamber and its contents are heated to the desired temperature (37°C or 55°C). As air removal reduces the humidity, which is an essential prerequisite for sterilization, sub-atmospheric steam is introduced to rehumidify the load. Gas is then introduced from a cylinder or single-use canister and the temperature and pressure maintained for the sterilization period. Finally, gas is removed and the chamber and its contents are flushed with filtered air. The holding time is dependent on temperature, pressure, humidity and gas concentration. The design of sterilizers is therefore related to these parameters and the requirements of the user, i.e. temperature/pressure tolerance of the items processed, size of load, time available for processing, etc.

The most commonly used hospital EO sterilizers in the UK are those of the sub-atmospheric type but high pressure types are also available.

By adopting a higher pressure (80 psi, 5.5 bar), it is possible to maintain lethal concentrations of EO using mixtures of EO with inert substances, such as carbon dioxide and freon. This reduces the risk of flammability or explosion but increases the risk of leaks. Sub-atmospheric sterilizers utilize pure EO, but the risk of leaks is minimized as the entire cycle is below atmospheric pressure (Babb *et al.* 1982). Sub-atmospheric EO sterilizers are usually much smaller than high pressure models, but they may be used to sterilize items which are sensitive to high pressures, e.g. flexible fibreoptic endoscopes.

The effectiveness of EO as a sterilizing agent may be influenced by other factors, such as the presence of salt crystals and packaging. All items must therefore be scrupulously clean. For packaging, paper, polypropylene or polyethylene bags are suitable, but nylon must not be used. Packages should be heat-sealed or sealed with tape. Indicator tape or packaging should be used to indicate those items processed. The sterilizing process must be controlled by spore tests supplemented by indicator tests (p. 54).

Ethylene oxide and its residues are toxic and irritant, and materials exposed to it should be thoroughly aerated before use. Aeration time is dependent on the absorbency of the items processed, the temperature, and the air exchange rates in the storage facility. Those with large capacity sterilizers or a greater throughput should use a separate aeration room with exhaust ventilation and open shelving to allow good air circulation. Very absorbent items, or those required soon after sterilization, may be aerated in a heated exhaust, ventilated cabinet. Aeration at 55°C greatly enhances the elution of EO, and consequently much shorter aeration periods may be used. Preliminary aeration is usually carried out in the chamber itself in order to protect staff from exposure during removal. Aeration at 55°C for 24 hours, or 3–7 days at room temperature, is normally considered adequate.

As much concern has recently been expressed over the toxicity of EO, the Health and Safety Executive (HSE) has adopted a control limit of exposure of persons at work to 5 ppm EO over an eight hour time-weighted averaged period, but further reductions in accepted levels are possible in the future. There is at present no maximum short-term limit, but many users have adopted a standard of their own (e.g. 5–75 ppm) as an interim measure. Exposure can be minimized by installing the sterilizer in a separate exhaust ventilated suite of rooms, by carrying out preliminary aeration in the chamber, and by installing an exhaust hood above the sterilizer door. It is recommended that access to the sterilizer, plant room and aeration facility be restricted to trained personnel who are fully conversant with the hazards associated with the process and that emergency procedures are clearly displayed in the work area.

Irradiated articles should not be subsequently treated with ethylene oxide unless known to be safe after such treatment.

Glutaraldehyde (p. 71)   Immersion of equipment in a fluid is generally a less reliable method of sterilization (or disinfection) than exposure to heat or to EO, and it has the disadvantage that thorough rinsing is necessary after processing. All materials must be clean and only surfaces wetted by glutaraldehyde will be satisfactorily treated. Glutaraldehyde, when used in a 2% solution, can be relied upon to sterilize in ten hours, but for practical purposes three hours should provide an adequate sporicidal effect (Babb *et al.* 1980). Treatment for shorter periods, (e.g. 20 min) only disinfects, but some spores (e.g. *Cl. difficile*) are rapidly killed (Dyas and Das 1985). Glutaraldehyde is potentially toxic and appropriate precautions are required when used (p. 96).

Low temperature steam and formaldehyde (LTSF)   This method is an alternative to EO and may be preferable, as it is a much safer process and prolonged aeration is not required. Formaldehyde alone is unacceptable for sterilizing heat-labile items because of its poor penetration and its slow sporicidal activity. If, however, it is used in conjunction with sub-atmospheric steam (Hurrell 1980; Alder 1987) it becomes a far more reliable process and sterilization is more rapidly achieved. Most LTSF sterilizers operate at a temperature of 73°C and 3–5 hours are required for the sterilizing process. A vacuum of 40 m bar is generally required during the air removal and pulsing stages to ensure adequate penetration, removal of formaldehyde, and a dry load. Steam is usually pulsed, but the best conditions for admitting formaldehyde at its optimal concentration have not been clearly established. Commissioning and routine testing methods are now available (DHSS 1980; Central Sterilizing Club Working Party No. 2 1986) which, if satisfactory, should ensure a high probability of sterilization. Many machines at present manufactured do not reach the required standard without some modification and need considerable attention from skilled engineers and microbiologists. The problems include excessive condensation, poor temperature control, variable formaldehyde concentrations in the chambers, and inadequate removal of residual formaldehyde or paraformaldehyde at the end of the cycle. Temperature variability tends to be less in smaller machines, and improved design, such as the inclusion of a complete heated jacket, may be necessary. As some of the equipment processed is expensive and heat-sensitive, it is particularly important that a high temperature cut-out mechanism is fitted. This is usually set at a maximum of 80°C.

Formaldehyde is an irritant substance and care should be taken to avoid undue exposure, especially during filling of the reservoir, on removing the load and during maintenance, particularly if a failure occurs during the cycle. Gloves should be worn to protect against skin contact, and as the eyes are particularly vulnerable protection is advised when filling reservoirs from stock solutions. Fortunately, formaldehyde is detected by smell at relatively low concentrations and well below the 2 ppm maximum exposure limit recommended by the HSE (1991). Formaldehyde is rarely absorbed into processed items, providing they are suitably packed and condensate is not allowed to accumulate. This can be done by placing packages vertically and processing tubing with open ends downwards. Processing should be carried out by trained personnel who are fully conversant with the hazards and emergency procedures.

Most of the difficulties with LTSF sterilizers are associated with the use of formaldehyde. However, LTS without formaldehyde is a very reliable disinfection process and 10 minutes at 71–75°C will meet most requirements in the hospital service. An advantage over the use of disinfectants is that equipment is dry at the end of processing and may be wrapped. There is also no problem with residual disinfectant. Routine microbiological tests are required for the use of LTSF, but not for LTS alone. A daily chamber leak test is required for both processes.

Low temperature steam, with or without formaldehyde, is a suitable process for heat-sensitive items which will tolerate moisture, a vacuum of at least 40 m bar, and temperatures of 80°C.

4.2 Tests for effectiveness of sterilization

4.2.1 AUTOCLAVES; STEAM AT HIGH TEMPERATURE (POROUS LOADS)

On commissioning a new sterilizer and at regular three monthly intervals the chamber temperature and steam penetration should be checked with standard thermocouples (DHSS 1980). A load dryness test should be undertaken when new sterilizers are commissioned (British Standards Institution 1990; and see Appendix 4.1). The temperature and pressure records for each cycle should be examined; a Bowie-Dick test and a chamber leak test should be carried out daily on all porous load autoclaves (see Appendix 4.1). Although a weekly leak test is sometimes suggested, a daily test is preferable. The satisfactory functioning of the automatic device detecting the presence of air or gas should be checked weekly and its performance verified annually (see Appendix 4.1). These tests may be supplemented with indicator systems, e.g. Browne's tubes and indicator tape, which should be stored under manufacturer's recommended condition and not used if out of date. It must be recognized that these indicator tests provide evidence of physical conditions required for sterilization, not of sterilization. Spore tests are not recommended for routine use in the UK, but are routinely used (e.g. weekly) in the US and some European countries. However, spore tests may be of use in checking packaging where penetration may be in doubt, and if there is any suspicion of infection occurring due to failure of an autoclave. Although they are often variable, spores strips containing approximately 10^6 *Bacillus stearothermophilus* produced by a recognized method and well controlled should be reasonably reliable.

4.2.2   BOTTLED FLUID AUTOCLAVES

Detailed commissioning and regular testing of loads with multiple thermocouples are required. Charts or hard copy printout for each cycle should record temperature from a thermocouple in the load, as well as from the chamber drain. These records must be compared with master charts of that particular load made during commissioning (DHSS 1980).

4.2.3   HOT AIR STERILIZERS

These are tested by thermocouples; Browne's tubes or other indicators may also be used. A chart recorder or printer is required.

4.2.4   GAS STERILIZERS

The physical and chemical parameters of gas sterilization are difficult to control and vary with the type of sterilizer and nature of the load. Until such time as these can be fully established, biological validation is necessary using bacterial spores.

4.2.5   ETHYLENE OXIDE

One or more spore-strips containing 10^6 *B. subtilis* var. *niger* and conforming to DHSS specification TSS/S/330.012, should be used. In the absence of a mandatory test procedure, it is recommended that each cycle should be monitored using at least one spore strip contained in a protective envelope and placed either in a centrally placed package or in the free chamber space. It is also recommended that those using large capacity machines include additional spores strips, up to ten for a chamber size of 5 000 litres. Tests should also be made on new items which may present problems of cleaning or gas penetration. Spore tests can be reduced if cycles are shown to be consistently reliable. Ethylene oxide indicators are useful for identifying processed items but should not be used as an indication of sterility.

4.2.6 LOW TEMPERATURE STEAM AND FORMALDEHYDE

On commissioning, tests should be made for steam penetration and air tightness of the chamber (DHSS 1980; British Standards Institution 1990, Part 1). If formaldehyde is used, tests should be made with *B. stearother-mophilus* spore strips (NCTC 10003), and produced to DHSS specification TSS/S.330.016. For routine testing and spore disc and formaldehyde indicator paper are inserted in the capsule of a test helix (Line and Pickerill 1973) which is placed in the top of the load and centre of the chamber. Following sterilization, this is removed for culture, the temperature record compared with the master temperature record and the paper examined for formaldehyde penetration. Providing these tests are satisfactory, the cycle is accepted as one of sterilization. Spores should be incubated in at least 15 ml of tryptone soya broth (bottle caps loose) in an incubator at 56°C for at least five days but for commissioning and routine maintenance tests incubation for 14 days is recommended.

As with other sterilizers, commissioning and maintenance tests should include electrical and other checks, for example high temperature cutout.

Additional tests are necessary periodically, and on commissioning. These include tests of distribution and penetration, hospital load, environmental and residual formaldehyde vapour tests (DHSS 1980; Central Sterilizing Club Working Party No. 2 1986).

Distribution and penetration tests   Spore strips are removed from their envelopes, mounted on cotton threads and placed at 27 locations within the chambers, at the top, centre, bottom, front, middle and back. Also included are two helices, each containing a spore strip. These are placed halfway up the chamber at one-third and two-third intervals from the door. Formaldehyde-sensitive indicator papers may be included at each spore site, and may help to identify the reason for spore failures. The test is considered satisfactory if no growth is observed from the test spores after 14 days incubation. Positive and negative controls should be included with each batch.

Hospital load tests   Eight 10 ml glass syringes, each loaded with a spore strip and indicator paper and adjusted to 0.5 ml volume and with a 24 swg needle and cover attached, are used as test pieces. Syringes should be packed in Post Office approved cardboard boxes (111 mm × 48 mm × 35 mm), lined and double-wrapped in crepe sterilization paper. These are mounted near each corner of the chamber. In addition, two cardboard instrument trays (300 mm × 50 mm cross section) are lined with crepe sterilization paper and loaded with mixed instruments. The loaded boxes are then double-wrapped with crepe sterilization paper and loaded into the sterilizer. Following sterilization, the spores and indicator strips are recovered and examined in the manner previously described.

Environmental and residual formaldehyde vapour tests At the end of the cycle, the door should be opened to a gap of 25 mm and a gas sample taken 100 mm in front of the gap at the operator's breathing zone. This test should be carried out without the exhaust ventilation hood operating. Hospital load test packs should be removed from the sterilizer and left unopened for ten minutes. Packs are then opened and left for a further five minutes before measuring the gas concentrations. The load with the highest potential for retaining gas is checked for residual formaldehyde.

The levels of gas measured in the above tests should not exceed those limits laid down by the HSE in guidance note EH40, i.e. 2 ppm (1991).

Advice should be sought from sterilizer engineers and microbiologists when contemplating the purchase of new equipment to ensure that it will do the job required of it and that it is known to operate competently elsewhere.

Appendix 4.1 Autoclave tests

BOWIE-DICK AUTOCLAVE TAPE TEST FOR POROUS LOAD
AUTOCLAVES (DHSS 1980; AND BRITISH STANDARDS
INSTITUTION 1990: PART 3)

The principle is very simple. A standard test pack is made up from huckaback towels. In the centre is placed a piece of paper to which has been fixed a cross of approved autoclave tape which has been stored according to the manufacturer's recommendations. This tape shows a colour change when exposed to steam. The test pack is now autoclaved in the usual way. **If all the air has been removed** the steam will penetrate rapidly and completely and the tape will show a uniform colour change. **If all the air has not been removed**, when steam is admitted for the sterilizing stage the air will be forced into the centre of the pack, where it will collect as a 'bubble'. The tape will not change colour in the region of the bubble because it has not been exposed to steam and this will show up when the paper with the tape cross is removed at the end of the run (see Fig. 4.1).

If the test is to be a reliable guide to the safe working of the sterilizer it must be carried out exactly as described.

Performance of the test Up to 36 huckaback towels, 36 x 24 in, comply-

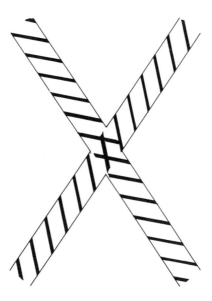

Figure 4.1 A satisfactory Bowie-Dick test, with an even colour change along the strips of tape.

ing with BS 1781 TL.5 are required (British Standards Institution 1967). The towels should be washed before being used for the first time, and whenever they are soiled or discoloured.

Between tests they should be unfolded and hung out to air for at least an hour.

Each towel should be folded into eight thicknesses and placed one above the other to form a stack 10–11 inches (250 mm) high. The exact number of towels needed will depend on how often they have been used, but 25–36 may be needed to attain the recommended weight of 4.7 to 5 kg. A piece of paper, approximately 12 in × 12 in, to which approved autoclave tape has been applied in the form of a St Andrew's cross, is placed in the middle of the stack; greaseproof or waxed paper should not be used. The stack may be placed in a dressing casket – such as that described in BS 3281 (British Standards Institution 1960) – or in a box made of cardboard or metal, so long as it is not airtight. If preferred, the stack can be wrapped, in fabric or paper, or it can be secured with tape. All that matters is that the towels should stay in position when the test pack is handled.

The test pack must be placed in the sterilizer by itself with appropriate Chamber furniture to support it above the base and subjected to a standard sterilizing cycle. The 'holding' or 'sterilizing' time must not be more than 3.5 min at 134°C. If the automatic cycle is set for a longer holding time this must be cut short, for purposes of the test, to 3.5 min at 134°C by using the manual control. Should there be any doubt about how to do this the engineer should be asked for advice.

Reading the test   When the cycle is finished the pack should be taken out and the paper with the tape cross should be examined.

After a satisfactory run the tape will show a colour change **which is the same at the centre as at the edges** (Fig. 4.1).

If the tape at the centre is paler than it is at the edges it means that there was a bubble of air there and that the sterilizer was not working properly. If this happens the matter should be reported at once (Fig. 4.2).

The paper with its tape cross from each test can be marked with the date and other particulars and kept for reference.

The towels should be aired and folded ready for the next test.

Comments   Unless the test is carried out exactly as described it may not be truly reliable. In particular the following points should be noted.

1. The more air there is to remove, the more exacting will be the test – that is why the test pack is used by itself in an otherwise empty chamber.

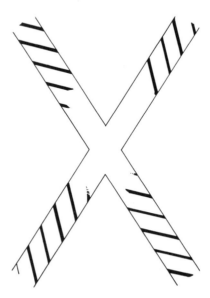

Figure 4.2   A failed Bowie-Dick test. The tapes have failed to change colour in the central area.

2. The exact colour change shown by the processed tape may depend on the storage conditions. The requirement is to determine whether the colour change occurs at the centre and differs from the edges.
3. The contrast in colour change from centre to edge will be reduced to an unreadable level if long 'holding' periods are used. That is why the holding period must not exceed 3.5 min and the temperature must be 134°C. Even an extra minute or two may seriously affect a comparison of results.
4. Because of this it is important to realize that if a sterilizer fails to pass the Bowie-Dick test as described, it cannot be made safe merely by increasing the holding time until a uniform colour change is produced. Such a sterilizer is in urgent need of skilled attention.
5. The test should be viewed in parallel with results of the chamber leak rate test (daily).

Alternative test packs   Alternatives to the huckaback towel test packs are available – for example, the Lantor cube (Deverill *et al.* 1987). Only test packs complying with Department of Health specification TSS/S/330.017 should be used.

CHAMBER LEAK RATE TEST

This test is only applicable to autoclaves which are capable of creating a vacuum, and it should be performed daily. There are two reasons why air leaking into the autoclave is unacceptable; these are, firstly, that the presence of air prevents penetration of the load by steam and, secondly, that the air will not have passed through the bacteria-retentive filter and therefore there is a potential risk of recontaminating the load.

The test involves the drawing of a vacuum in the autoclave chambers, followed by the closure of all valves leading to the chamber, stopping the vacuum drawing system and observation of the chamber pressure for a timed period. The manufacturer's instructions should be followed and, in case of doubt, the advice of the sterilizer engineer should be sought.

At the start of the leak test the chamber pressure (P1) should be less than 40 m bar. Five minutes after the start of the test the chamber pressure (P2) should be noted, and the chamber pressure (P3) noted again after a further ten minute period. During this 10 minute period the chamber pressure (P3-P2) should not be greater than 13m bar for porous load sterilizers or 5m bar for low temperature steam disinfectors, low temperature steam and formaldehyde and ethylene oxide sterilizers.

Considerable care and knowledge must be applied in the interpretation of the results (British Standards Institution 1990: Parts 3 and 5).

Both the maximum leak rate and maximum vacuum level which gives an indication of the performance capability of the air removal system should be recorded in the sterilizer log book.

The leak rate test and the Bowie-Dick tape test for porous load sterilizers are complementary tests. A sterilizer which fails to meet the requirements of either of these tests must not be used until the fault(s) has been rectified and the sterilizer satisfies both of these tests.

AIR DETECTOR TEST FOR POROUS LOAD STERILIZER

The air detector is tested after the satisfactory completion of the leak rate test. For this series of tests a variable air flow device should be connected to a valved port at high level adjacent to the chamber door.

When the sterilizer is commissioned, and annually thereafter, an air detector **performance** test should be undertaken with a small and full load.

Firstly a Bowie-Dick pack is located in the chamber and thermocouples inserted into:

1. the geometric centre of the pack;
2. the active chamber discharge;
3. the chamber free space.

During an operating cycle the air detector should indicate a fault if (a) the chamber pressure rise exceeds 10 m bar per minute on (b) at the commencement of the sterilization hold period the temperature at the geometric centre of the Bowie-Dick pack is more than 2°C below the temperature of the active chamber discharge.

Secondly, in addition to the Bowie-Dick pack the chamber is fully loaded with fabric materials (cotton or linen containing not more than 20% of synthetic fibre) aired with a mean density 150 kg/m^3 to 170 kg/m^3. The fabric should be freshly laundered without the addition of starch or fabric conditioner.

During an operating cycle the sensitivity of the air detector is demonstrated to be similar to that found during the small load test. To undertake this test it may be necessary to increase the chamber pressure rise to a value greater than 100 m bar in 10 minutes.

At weekly intervals the operation of the air detector should be checked by undertaking a **function** test. For this test a Bowie-Dick pack is introduced into the chamber and the same air flow leaked into the chamber that was used during the small load function test described above. The result is satisfactory if during an operating cycle the sterilizer indicates a fault. If a fault is not indicated the sterilizer should be withdrawn from service and the air detector performance test should be undertaken.

LOAD DRYNESS TEST

The load dryness test is performed using a Bowie-Dick test pack without test papers or temperature sensors. The test pack should be aired for at least one hour as described above. Three towels are selected, marked, each placed in a polyethylene bag constructed in sheets of thickness not less than 250 μm. The minimum bag size should be 350 x 250 mm. Each bag/towel assembled is weighed on scales with an accuracy of + or − 0.1 g and the mass recorded. The towels are removed from the bags and replaced in the Bowie-Dick test pack, one in the centre, the others as the fourth towel from either end of the test pack. With the test pack inserted into the chamber an operating cycle is initiated within 60 seconds. The operating cycle should not include extended drying.

Within 60 seconds after the completion of the operating cycle the test pack is removed from the chamber. Remove the three marked towels and immediately place in the three corresponding marked bags. Each bag is sealed by turning its open end over several times. The total time from the completion of the operating cycle to sealing the bags should not exceed three minutes.

The towels in the polyethylene bags are allowed to cool and weighed. The means of the mass gain should not be greater than 1% (m/m).

Appendix 4.2 Methods of sterilization and physical disinfection

Category	Operating conditions (temperature and/or time for sterilizing)	Process time (approx.)	Application
1. Steam – DD			
(a) Laboratory autoclave	121°C/15 min	2–12 h	Cultures, media glassware
(b) Instrument sterilizer	126°C/10 min 134°C/3.5 min	20–60 min 5–15 min	unwrapped instruments and bowls
(c) Bottle sterilizer	121°C/15 min 126°C/10 min 115°C/30 min	2–12 h	bottled fluids
2. Steam – HVHT			
Porous loads	134°C/3–3.5 min	20–25 min	dressings, wrapped instruments

(continued)

Appendix 4.2 *Continued*

Category	Operating conditions (temperature and/or time for sterilizing)	Process time (approx.)	Application
Laboratory discard	134°C/3–3.5 min	2–12 h	glass and bottled fluids
Laboratory discard	134°C/3–3.5 min	50–60 min	small plastic items
3. Steam – HVLT * (a) Without formalin	73°C/10 min	15–30 min	heat sensitive equipment
(b) With formalin	73°C/1–3 h	1–3 h	heat sensitive equipment
4.* Hot water	70–100°C/5–10 min	5–10 min	heat sensitive equipment
5. Hot air (a) Fan oven	160°C/60 min 180°C/30 min	2–4 h	glass, metal instruments
6. 2% glutaraldehyde	3 h (for disinfection see Appendix 16.2)		heat sensitive equipment
7. Ethylene oxide	20–60°C 1–6 atm P 200–1000 mg 10–100% Eo	2–24 h	heat sensitive material or equipment

HVHT– high vacuum high temperature
HVLT– high vacuum low temperature
  DD– downward displacement
    *– disinfects only

References and further reading

Advisory Committee on Dangerous Pathogens (1990) *Categorisation of Pathogens According to Hazard and Categories of Containment*. 2nd edn, HMSO, London.
Alder, V.G. (1987) The formaldehyde/low temperature steam sterilizing procedure. *Journal of Hospital Infection*, **9**, 194.

Babb, J.R., Phelps, M., Downes, J. *et al.* (1982) Evaluation of an ethylene oxide sterilizer. *Journal of Hospital Infection*, **2**, 385.

Babb, J.R., Bradley, C.R., and Ayliffe, G.A.J. (1980) Sporicidal activity of glutaraldehydes and hypochlorites and other factors influencing their selection for the treatment of medical equipment. *Journal of Hospital Infection*, **1**, 63.

Bowie, J.H., Kelsey, J.C. and Thompson, D.R. (1963) Bowie and Dick autoclave tape test. *Lancet*, **1**, 586.

British Standards Institution (1960) *BS 3281: Specification for rectangular metal boxes for use in high vacuum steam sterilizers.*

British Standards Institution. (1966) *BS 3421: Performance of Electrically Heated Sterilizing Ovens.* BSI, London.

British Standards Institution. (1967) *BS 1781: Linen Textiles for use by Government Departments, Hospitals and Local Authorities.*

British Standards Institution. (1988) *BS 2646: Autoclaves for Sterilization in Laboratories.*

British Standards Institution. *BS 3970: Sterilizing and Disinfecting Equipment for Medical Products.* BSI, London.

British Standards Institution. (1990) *BS 3970: Sterilizing and Disinfecting Equipment for Medical Products.*

Part 1.   Specification for general requirements.

Part 2.   British Standards Institution (1966) BS 3970: Sterilizers for bottled fluids.

Part 3.   Specification for steam sterilizers for wrapped goods and porous loads.

Part 4.   Specification for transportable steam sterilizers for unwrapped instruments and utensils.

Part 5.   Specification for low-temperature steam disinfectors.

* Part A.   Specification for steam sterilizers for fluids in sealed rigid containers.

* Part B.   Specification for steam sterilizers for fluids in unsealed vented containers.

* Part C.   Specification for steam sterilizers for fluids in sealed non-rigid containers.

* Part D.   Specification for sterilizers using low-temperature steam with formaldehyde.

* Part E.   Specification for steam sterilizers using ethylene oxide or ethylene oxide mixtures.

* Part F.   Specification for steam sterilizers for unwrapped utensils, instruments and holloware.

(* Being drafted)

British Standards Institution. *BS 2745: Washer Disinfectors for Medical Purposes.* (Being drafted)

Russell, A.D., Ayliffe, G.A.J. and Hugo, W.B. (1991) *Principles and Practice of Disinfection, Preservation and Sterilization.* 2nd edn. Oxford, Blackwell Scientific Publications.

Campbell, M. and Cripps, N.F. (1991) Environmental control of glutaraldehyde. *Hospital Estates Journal*, **45**, 2.

Central Sterilizing Club Working Party No. 1 (1986) *Washer/Disinfector Machines.* Central Sterilizing Club UK. Obtainable from Hospital Infection Research Laboratory.

Central Sterilizing Club Working Party No. 2. (1986) *Sterilization and Disinfection of Heat-Labile Equipment. Central Sterilizing Club UK.* Obtainable from Hospital Infection Research Laboratory.

Department of Health and Social Security. (1980) *Hospital Technical Memorandum (HTM) No. 10: Steam sterilizers.* HMSO, London. (Being updated)

Department of Health, specification for Biological Monitors for Control of Ethylene Oxide sterilization, TSS/S/330/012.

Department of Health and Social Security. *Specification for indication test tape for use in the Bowie Dick test (for porous load steam sterilizers)* TSS/S/330/013; TSS/S330/014.

Department of Health specification for Biological Monitors for the control of low temperature steam and formaldehyde sterilization TSS/S/330/016.

Department of Health. *Specification for Total Pack Systems for Use as a Replacement for the Bowie and Dick Test (for Porous Load Sterilizers)*, TSS/S/330.017.

Deverill, C.E.A., Cripps, N.F., Roberts, M. *et al.* (1987) The Bowie/Dick test: An alternative way. *Journal of Sterile Services Management*, **5**, 21.

Dyas, A. and Das, B.C. (1985) The activity of glutaraldehyde against *Clostridium difficile. Journal of Hospital Infection*, **6**, 41.

Health and Safety Executive Guidance Note (1991) EH 40/91 Occupational Limits, HMSO.

Hurrell, D.J. (1980) Low temperature steam disinfection and low temperature steam/formaldehyde sterilization. *Sterile World*, **2**, 13.

Gardner, J.F. and Peel, M.M. (1991) *Introduction to Sterilization, Disinfection and infection control.* 2nd edn. Churchill Livingstone, Edinburgh.

Line, S.J. and Pickerill, J.K. (1973) Testing a steam-formaldehyde sterilizer for gas penetration efficiency. *Journal of Clinical Pathology*, **26**, 716.

Oates, K., Deverill, C.E.A., Phelps, M. and Collins, B.J. (1983) Development of a laboratory autoclave system. *Journal of Hospital Infection*, **4**, 181.

5 *Disinfection: Types of chemical disinfection and formulation of policy for disinfection*

Most hospitals have produced a policy for the use of disinfectants, but it is still possible to find inappropriate disinfectants being used at inadequate concentrations. Expensive and ineffective disinfectants are still in use when cheaper or more effective agents are available, or when a disinfectant is not required at all. There remains a need for some degree of regional, if not national, standardization; a sound disinfectant policy should considerably increase the cost-effectiveness of disinfection in hospitals.

5.1 Types of chemical disinfectants

5.1.1 PHENOLICS (see Table 5.1)

Phenols and cresols are usually derived from the distillation of coal tar, but mixtures of synthetic phenols may be used. Chlorinated fractions and petroleum residues may also be added.

1. Black and white fluids These are crude coal tar derivatives. Black

Table 5.1 Phenolic disinfectants for environmental use

Disinfectant	Type*	Routine use dilution %	Strong concentration %	Manufacturer
'Stericol'	CSPD	1.0	2	Sterling Industries Ltd.
'Hycolin'	CSP	1.0	2	Wm. Pearson Ltd.
'Clearsol'	CSPD	0.625	1	Coventry Chemicals Ltd.
'Izal'	W	1.0	2	Sterling Industries Ltd.

* CSP= Clear soluble phenolic
D= Contains added detergent
W= White fluid

fluids (e.g. 'Jeyes fluid') are solubilized in soap and are toxic and irritant to the skin. White fluids (e.g. 'Izal') are emulsified suspensions and tend to precipitate on surfaces, making subsequent cleaning more difficult. These disinfectants, especially white fluids, are sometimes used for environmental disinfection in hospitals, but have largely been replaced by clear soluble phenolics.

2. Clear soluble phenolics (e.g. 'Stericol', 'Hycolin', 'Clearsol') Like other phenolics, these compounds are active against a wide range of bacteria, including *Pseudomonas aeruginosa* and tubercle bacilli. They are fungicidal, kill some viruses, but show no useful activity against bacterial spores. They are relatively cheap, stable, and not readily inactivated by organic matter. They often contain a compatible detergent.

Uses are mainly confined to environmental disinfection, since they are too corrosive for instruments and too toxic to be applied to the skin. They are, however, occasionally used to disinfect postmortem instruments and equipment contaminated with tubercle bacilli if heat treatment is not available. These and other phenolics should not be used in food preparation areas or on equipment likely to contact mucous membranes.

5.1.2 CHLOROXYLENOLS (e.g. 'DETTOL', 'IBCOL')

These are non-irritant but are readily inactivated by organic matter and hard water, and high concentrations are required (2.5–5%). Chloroxylenols are effective against Gram-positive bacteria but poorly active against Gram-negative bacteria. The addition of a chelating agent (EDTA) increases the activity of chloroxylenols against Gram-negative bacilli.

5.1.3 PINE OIL DISINFECTANTS

These compounds are non-toxic and non-irritant, but are relatively ineffective against many organisms, in particular *Ps. aeruginosa*. They should not be used as disinfectants in hospitals.

5.1.4 HALOGENS (COMPOUNDS OR SOLUTIONS RELEASING CHLORINE, BROMINE, OR IODINE)

Chlorine-releasing agents These are cheap and effective disinfectants which act by release of available chlorine. They are rapidly effective against viruses, fungi, bacteria and spores. They are particularly recommended for use where special hazards of viral infection exist. Solutions are unstable at use-dilutions and should be prepared daily. They are readily inactivated by organic matter (e.g. pus, dirt, blood, etc.) and may damage certain materials (e.g. plastics, rubber, some metals and fabrics). Chlorine-releasing agents are not compatible with some detergents, and should not be mixed with acids – including acidic body fluids such as urine – since the free chlorine produced may be harmful, particularly in a confined space. Solutions may be stabilized with alkalis or sodium chloride. Chlorine-releasing agents disinfectants at low concentrations are non-toxic and are particularly useful for water treatment, babies' feed bottles and food preparation areas, but may also have other uses in the hospital environment. Uses and recommended concentrations are shown in Table 5.2.

Table 5.2   In-use concentrations of chlorine-releasing agents

Uses	AVAILABLE CHLORINE	
	%	mg/1 (ppm)*
Blood spillage from patient with HIV or HBV infection	1.0	10 000
Laboratory discard jars	0.25	2 500
General environmental disinfection	0.10	1 000
Infant feeding bottles and teats Food preparation areas	0.0125	125
Eradication of legionella from water supply system depending on exposure time		50) 5)
Hydrotherapy pools – routine		1.5–3.00
– if contaminated		6–10
Routine water treatment		0.5–1

* Undiluted commercial hypochlorite solutions contain approx 10% 100,000 ppm av Cl$_2$

Preparations of chlorine or bromine releasing agents include the following.

1. Strong alkaline hypochlorite solutions (e.g. 'Chloros', 'Domestos', 'Sterite') containing approximately 10% (100 000 ppm av Cl$_2$). Similar solutions in the US are supplied at 5% (50 000 ppm av Cl$_2$). The concentrated solutions are corrosive. Dilute solutions may be used with a compatible detergent and will only reliably disinfect clean surfaces.
2. Hypochlorite solutions containing 1% (10 000 ppm av Cl$_2$) and stabilized with sodium chloride (e.g. 'Milton' or a preparation of comparable properties). These solutions are usually diluted 1:80 (125 ppm av Cl$_2$) for the disinfection of infant feeding bottles and catering

equipment. The low chlorine content is inactivated by very small amounts of organic matter and in-use solutions have a narrow margin of safety.

3. Hypochlorite/hypobromite powders (e.g. 'Septonite', 'Diversol BX'). Solutions of these powders (0.5–1.0%) are used in the same way as other hypochlorite preparations, and are rather less corrosive. The powder may be used for cleaning baths and sinks where an abrasive preparation is not desirable.

4. Abrasive powders containing hypochlorites (e.g. hospital scouring powder, 'Vim', 'Ajax' etc.)

5. Non-abrasive powders (e.g. 'Titan') containing hypochlorites are now usually preferred to abrasive powders for cleaning and disinfecting hospital baths and sinks.

6. Other chlorine releasing compounds include sodium dichloroisocyanurate (NaDCC) tablets (e.g. 'Sanichlor', 'Haztab' 'Multichlor', 'Presept') tablets. These compounds are stable during storage and more convenient for dispensing, but the prepared solutions deteriorate quickly. They tend to be slightly more effective and less corrosive than hypochlorite solutions but care is still necessary with metals. The cost of preparing solutions with a low concentration (e.g. 100–200 ppm av Cl_2) is comparable to that of liquid hypochlorite preparations, but the use of tablets for preparing high concentrations (e.g. 10 000 ppm av Cl_2), is expensive.

NaDCC powders or granules may be applied directly to spillage of blood from suspected HBV or HIV patients and are convenient and effective alternatives to solutions (Coates 1988; Bloomfield and Miller 1989). However, their use should be avoided with large spillage (> 30 ml), as excessive chlorine may be produced.

Other preparations include compounds releasing chlorine dioxide, and chloramine T. These compounds are infrequently used at present as hospital disinfectants.

Iodine and iodophors A 1% solution of iodine in 70% alcohol is an effective pre-operative skin antiseptic. Skin reactions may occur in some individuals; for this reason 0.5% alcoholic chlorhexidine or an alcoholic iodophor solution is usually preferred.

Iodophors are complexes of iodine and 'solubilizers' which possess the same activity as iodine, but are non-irritant and do not stain the skin. Iodophors are mainly used for hand disinfection, for example povidone-iodine (PVP–I) ('Betadine', 'Disadine', 'Videne' 'Phoraid') detergent preparations or 'surgical scrubs'. These contain 7.5% PVP–I (equivalent to 0.7% available iodine) and are effective for this purpose. Alcoholic preparations containing 10% PVP–I (1% available iodine) are suitable for pre-operative preparation of the skin at the operation site. Some iodophors may also be used for disinfection of the environment, but they are expensive and cannot be recommended for general disinfection in hospital.

Iodine is the only antiseptic which has been shown to have a useful sporicidal action on the skin; when applied as an iodophor it can be left on the skin long enough to remove a large proportion of *Cl. perfringens* spores when these are present, but this is of uncertain clinical value (see Chapter 7).

5.1.5 QUATERNARY AMMONIUM COMPOUNDS, SUCH AS BENZALKONIUM CHLORIDE (e.g. 'ROCCAL', 'ZEPHIRAN', 'MARINOL' AND CETRIMIDE ('CETAVLON')

These are relatively non-toxic antibacterial compounds with detergent properties; they are active against Gram-positive organisms but much less active against Gram-negative bacilli and are readily inactivated by soap, anionic detergents and organic matter. Quaternary ammonium compounds (QACs) at higher dilutions inhibit the growth of organisms (i.e. they are 'bacteriostatic') but do not necessarily kill them (i.e. they do not show a 'bactericidal' effect). For this reason, their effectiveness has often been exaggerated. Their use in hospital is limited because of their narrow spectrum of activity, but they may be useful for cleansing dirty wounds (e.g. cetrimide). Apart from possible uses in food preparation areas, QACs should not be used for environmental disinfection. Contamination of a weak solution of a QAC with Gram-negative bacilli is a possible hazard which can be prevented by avoidance of cork closures or of 'topping-up' stock bottles. Incorporating a chelating agent enhances the activity of QACs against Gram-negative bacilli. However, QACs are ineffective against the HBV, tubercle bacilli and spores and show variable activity against HIV. They should only be used for between-patient cleaning of endoscopes prior to disinfection with 70% ethanol in cases of glutaraldehyde sensitivity and low infection risk (Chapter 6).

5.1.6 CHLORHEXIDINE ('HIBITANE')

This useful skin antiseptic is highly active against vegetative Gram-positive organisms, but less active against Gram-negative bacilli. It also has good fungicidal activity but has little or no activity against tubercle bacilli, viruses and bacterial spores. It is relatively non-toxic but is inactivated by soaps. Its use in hospital should be restricted as much as possible to procedures involving contact with skin or mucous membranes; it is too expensive for environmental use.

Detergent solutions containing 4% chlorhexidine gluconate are available (e.g. 'Hibiscrub'; 'Hibiclens'). These have been found highly effective in disinfection of surgeons' hands prior to operating and have a good persistent effect due to residue on the skin after rinsing and drying. Some alternative preparations show inadequate bactericidal effects and are irritant to the skin. Trials are necessary before introducing new products even if they contain similar concentrations of chlorhexidine gluconate.

'Savlon' is a mixture of chlorhexidine and cetrimide. The hospital concentrate contains 15% cetrimide and 1.5% chlorhexidine. It is usually used at a concentration of 1%. At this concentration the antimicrobial activity of the chlorhexidine is poor. However, cetrimide is a good cleansing agent and enhances the activity of chlorhexidine. 'Savlon' is expensive; if used, it should be reserved for clinical procedures, such as cleansing dirty wounds, and not used for instruments or environmental disinfection.

Low concentrations of antiseptics are likely to become contaminated during use. The provision of pre-sterilized single-use sachets ('Hibidil', 'Savlodil' – Chapter 7) reduces this risk.

'Hibisol' is a 0.5% solution of chlorhexidine in 70% isopropanol, for disinfection of clean, intact skin (e.g. hands); 0.5% chlorhexidine gluconate in 70% ethanol (or isopropanol) is used for disinfection of the operation site.

5.1.7 HEXACHLOROPHANE

This compound is highly active against Gram-positive organisms but less active against Gram-negative. It is relatively insoluble in water, but can be incorporated in soap or detergent solutions without loss of activity. It has a good residual effect on the skin. These solutions are prone to contamination with Gram-negative bacteria unless a preservative is included in the formulation. Potentially neurotoxic levels may occur in the blood if emulsions or other preparations of hexachlorophane are repeatedly and extensively applied to the body surface of babies. This product, though very effective, is now infrequently used for skin disinfection in hospitals, and can be obtained for use only on medical advice. It may be used for washing of hands of staff during staphylococcal outbreaks or for surgical hand disinfection. Toxic levels are not approached when a hexachlorophane dusting powder (Sterzac) is used on the umbilical stump of neonates, and this method, which has been found highly effective in the control of staphylococcal infection, may still be considered to have a role in hospital practice.

5.1.8 TRICLOSAN (IRGASAN DP300 – e.g. 'STERZAC' BATH CONCENTRATE, 'MANUSEPT', 'pHisoMed', 'ZALCLENSE', 'CIDAL', 'AQUASEPT', 'GAMOPHEN')

Triclosan-containing products have properties and a spectrum of activity similar to that of hexachlorophane, but exhibit no toxicity to neonates. They are now widely used as an alternative to hexachloro-phane in hand rubs, soaps and bath concentrates. In-use concentrations vary from 0.3–2.0%. Antimicrobial tests and trials for tolerance are required before use of individual products, as these are variable and generally less effective than chlorhexidine preparations.

5.1.9 ALCOHOLS

Ethyl alcohol 70% (ethanol) and 60–70% isopropyl alcohol (isopropanol) are effective and rapidly acting disinfectants and antiseptics with the additional advantage that they evaporate leaving the surfaces dry, but they have poor penetrative powers and should only be used on clean surfaces. They are active against mycobacteria but not against spores. Activity against viruses is variable, and non-enveloped viruses (e.g. poliovirus) tend to be more resistant, particularly to isopropanol. The recommended concentration of ethanol (70%) is optimal *in vitro* for killing organisms, and is more effective than absolute alcohol. Alcohol, or alcohol impregnated wipes, may be used for the rapid disinfection of smooth clean surfaces, e.g. trolley tops, thermometers, probes and electrical/electronic equipment which cannot be safely immersed in aqueous disinfectants. If the item is contaminated with blood or secretions, prior cleaning is advised. It is commonly used for skin disinfection (e.g. without additives for treating skin prior to injection). With the addition of 1% glycerine or other suitable emollients, 70% alcohol rubbed on until the skin is dry is an effective agent for the rapid disinfection of physically clean hands, especially where handwashing facilities are unsuitable or not immediately available. The addition of other bactericides to alcohol does not appreciably increase its immediate effect as a skin antiseptic, but the repeated use of alcohol solutions may lead to lower equilibrium levels of bacteria on the skin. The addition of non-volatile antiseptics (e.g. chlorhexidine, PVP–I and tri-closan) may provide a residual antiseptic action on the skin.

5.1.10 ALDEHYDES: FORMALDEHYDE, GLUTARALDEHYDE ('CIDEX', 'ASEP', 'TOTACIDE' 28, 'SPORICIDIN') AND SUCCINE DIALDEHYDE ('GIGASEPT')

Though formaldehyde is required in some instances for fumigation and may sterilize if used with sub-atmospheric steam, solutions of formaldehyde are too irritant for use as general disinfectants. Glutaraldehyde is preferred to other disinfectants for heat-sensitive items; it is non-damaging to metals, plastics and rubber and is effective against vegetative organisms, viruses (including HBV and HIV) and fungi. Activity against tubercle bacilli is relatively slow (e.g. 20–60 minutes exposure time may be required). Aldehydes are more active against spores than other commonly used chemical agents with the exception of ethylene oxide and buffered hypochlorites (Babb *et al.* 1980). Glutaraldehyde may be irritant to the eyes, skin and respiratory mucosa and can cause sensitization. Alkaline solutions such as 'Cidex' require activation; once activated they remain stable for only 2–4 weeks depending on the preparation. To ensure sporicidal activity, an exposure period of at least three hours is required, although shorter times may be sufficient to kill some pathogenic spores, such as *Cl. difficile* (Dyas and Das 1985). Acid solutions of glutaraldehyde are more stable and do not require activation, but usually have a slower sporicidal effect. They may be more suitable for the occasional or small user. Their activity is improved by use at a temperature of 50–60°C, although this can be associated with an increase in vapour levels. Glutaraldehyde is particularly useful for the disinfection or sterilization of heat-sensitive items, such as endoscopes, but it is expensive. Other aldehydes, e.g. succine dialdehyde ('Gigasept') have similar properties to glutaraldehyde. The addition of a phenolic compound to 2% glutaraldehyde ('Sporicidin') improves the sporicidal action, but the advantages are marginal for routine disinfection. Most of the tests have been made on 2% aldehyde solutions and higher dilutions are less effective over the same time period.

5.1.11   HYDROGEN PEROXIDE AND RELATED COMPOUNDS

Hydrogen peroxide (3% or 6%) is infrequently used as a hospital disinfectant in the UK. It is used for disinfection of tonometers and soft contact lenses, and the disinfection of ventilators. It has been added to urinary drainage bags. Frequent use has been associated with corrosion of certain metals. Peroxygen compounds (e.g. Virkon) are virucidal and less corrosive than hypochlorites and are likely to play an increasing role in the disinfection of equipment and environmental surfaces. Virkon powder can be used as a less corrosive alternative for decontamination of spillage. Peracetic acid is used for disinfection of certain types of equipment, e.g. patient isolators, and for the disinfection of endoscopes. It is sporicidal and claimed to be relatively non-toxic or corrosive in the concentrations used but requires further evaluation.

5.1.12 AMPHOLYTIC COMPOUNDS (e.g. 'TEGO')

These compounds combine detergent and antibacterial properties. They are similar to the QACs and may be of value in the food industry, but are expensive; there are few indications for their use in hospitals.

5.1.13 OTHER ANTIMICROBIAL COMPOUNDS

Many other antimicrobial compounds have been used. Among these are the acridine and triphenyl methane (crystal violet and brilliant green) dyes, which were at one time widely used as antiseptics for skin and for wounds. Silver nitrate and other silver compounds (e.g. silver sulphadiazine) have a valuable place as topical antiseptics in prophylaxis against infection of burns. 8-Hydroxy-quinoline has been found effective as a fungicide. Mercurial compounds have poor bactericidal powers, but they are strongly bacteriostatic; phenyl mercuric nitrate has been used as an effective preservative for ophthalmic solutions. Other compounds are described by Block (1983) and Russell *et al.* (1991).

5.2 The formulation of a disinfection policy

The general principles for formulation of a policy are summarized below (see Ayliffe *et al.* 1984). The hospital infection control committee should prepare the disinfectant policy and decide on the types of disinfectants used; this requires consultation between the microbiologist, infection control doctor, infection control nurse, pharmacist, supplies officer and representatives of medical, nursing and domestic staff. Demands for disinfectants come from many departments of the hospital and there are many sources of supply. All requests for disinfectants should be approved by the hospital pharmacist who can check whether they are in agreement with the hospital policy.

5.2.1 PRINCIPLES

1. List all the purposes for which disinfectants are used, then check requisitions and orders to ensure the list is complete.
2. Eliminate the use of chemical disinfectants when heat can reasonably be used as an alternative, when sterilization is required, where thorough cleaning alone is adequate, or where disposable equipment can be used economically. There should be few remaining uses for disinfectant fluids.
3. Select the smallest practicable number of disinfectants for the remaining uses, i.e. one routine disinfectant for each field of use (the

environment, skin and equipment), plus an alternative for use where patients or staff are sensitive to the routine disinfectants, for instruments which may be damaged by the disinfectant, and for use when the routine disinfectant happens to be unavailable, or is inappropriate for a particular purpose.

4. Arrange for the distribution of disinfectants chosen at the correct use-dilution or supply equipment for preparing and measuring disinfectants at the site of use.

5. All potential users of disinfectant should receive adequate instruction in their preparation and use. This should include information on:
   (a) the correct disinfectant and concentration to be used for each task;
   (b) the shelf-life of the disinfectant at the concentration supplied, the type of container to be used and the frequency with which the solution should be changed in use;
   (c) substances or materials which will react with or neutralise the disinfectant;
   (d) an assessment of toxic or other risks to employees using the disinfectant or detergent is required; also the measures required for protection of employees (COSHH Regulations 1988). Personal safety measures, e.g. should rubber gloves be worn, how can the product be safely opened and mixed, what action is required if the product comes in contact with the skin or eye?

6. The policy should be monitored to ensure that it is and continues to be effective. Occasional in-use tests and chemical estimations of concentration may be required.

5.2.2 \SELECTION OF DISINFECTANTS (see also Rutala *et al.* 1990)

Antimicrobial properties Where compatible with other requirements, disinfectants used should be bactericidal rather than bacteriostatic, active against a wide range of microbes and not readily inactivated. The manufacturer can supply information on the properties of the disinfectant, but independent antimicrobial tests are also required. The Kelsey-Sykes test (Kelsey and Maurer 1974) is commonly used in the UK, but it seems likely that in the future it will be replaced by European tests such as a standardized suspension test (Council of Europe 1987) and possibly others. The AOAC surface test in the US has been criticized for lack of reproducibility and it is hoped that some international standardization of tests will be possible in the future.

Other properties The properties of the disinfectants chosen should be considered in terms of acceptability as well as antibacterial activity. Stability, toxicity and corrosiveness should be assessed by the pharmacist with the aid of relevant information obtained from manufacturers. Acceptability and cleaning properties should be assessed by the domestic superintendent or other user. Cost is clearly important and a regional contract for one or two generally acceptable disinfectants should considerably reduce costs. A trial period of possibly three months might be introduced and an assessment of all relevant factors should be made before the policy is permanently introduced.

5.3 Recommended disinfectants and use-dilutions

5.3.1 ENVIRONMENT

A chlorine-releasing agent and a phenolic disinfectant should be sufficient for most environmental hospital requirements.

Hypochlorites and other chlorine releasing agents (see Table 5.2, p. 67) have the disadvantages and advantages already mentioned. They may be incorporated in a powder (abrasive or non-abrasive) for cleaning baths, toilets, washbasins. Solutions (1000 ppm av Cl_2) may be used for disinfecting clean surfaces and, when necessary, for food preparation areas. Chlorine-releasing agents should be used if disinfection of virus-contaminated material is required. However, routine or too frequent use can cause expensive corrosion and damage to equipment and some surfaces. Other less corrosive antiviral agents are required. (see Chapters 18 and 19).

A clear soluble phenolic disinfectant (e.g. 'Stericol', 'Hycolin', 'Clearsol') is often chosen as one of the disinfectants for routine use (see Appendix 7.2). There is little to choose between these compounds in terms of effectiveness at the recommended use-dilutions. For most purposes the concentration required for light contamination will be adequate (i.e. 'Clearsol' 0.625%; 'Stericol', 'Hycolin', 'Izal' 1%). This provides a reasonable margin of safety and should be used unless otherwise indicated. The strong concentrations, i.e. x 2, should be used for heavily contaminated areas or if contamination with tubercle bacilli is likely (disinfection by heat or use of disposables is particularly important for dealing with contamination by tubercle bacilli). Phenolics are not usually suitable for use against viruses and the increasing anxiety about HIV is responsible for a reduction in their routine use.

Narrow spectrum or expensive disinfectants are mainly used for clinical purposes and are not recommended for general environmental use, but may sometimes be required for special equipment. Glutaraldehyde should be available for disinfection of immersible metal objects contaminated with HBV or HIV, but chlorine-releasing agents may be occasionally used if the equipment is thoroughly rinsed after disinfection. Alternatively this may be immersed in alcohol or cleaned and disinfected using a disposable alcoholic wipe. NaDCC compounds tend to be less corrosive than hypochlorites.

5.3.2   DILUTION AND DISTRIBUTION OF DISINFECTANTS

Ineffective cleaning and inadequate concentration is the commonest cause of failure of a disinfectant to kill organisms, and survival of contaminants in the disinfectant is unlikely if it is at the recommended use-dilution. It is therefore preferable for the pharmacist to supply departments with containers of disinfectant already prepared at the correct use-dilution. Containers should have the date of issue and the date after which the disinfectant should not be used (e.g. one week after issue); they should be clearly labelled 'do not dilute', 'use undiluted' or with a similar instruction. Containers should be thoroughly washed and preferably disinfected by heat before refilling. If heating is not possible, thorough drying after washing should be adequate as this will kill most of the bacteria likely to be present. Corks must not be used; containers should have plastic closures which can be easily cleaned.

The main disadvantage of this method of dispensing is the transport of large quantities of fluid (mainly water), particularly if large amounts of disinfectants are used and as some disinfectants (e.g. chlorine-releasing agents) are unstable when diluted. The alternative method is to supply undiluted disinfectant to the department where dilutions are prepared when required. A suitable and relatively fool-proof measuring system is required for both disinfectant and water. A measuring device attached to the container is commonly used, but unless staff are well trained, dilutions will be inaccurate. A measured amount of undiluted disinfectant in a bottle, tablet or sachet is an alternative, but the water must also be measured. The strong disinfectant solution requires careful handling to avoid damage to the skin or the eyes of the operator. Gloves and a plastic apron should be worn and eye protection is necessary if splashing is likely.

5.3.3   TRAINING AND STAFF INSTRUCTION

Whichever system of supplying disinfectants is used, all personnel handling or using them must be adequately trained and supervised.

5.3.4   IN-USE TESTS

Since disinfectants are used under a variety of conditions, it is essential to test their effectiveness under actual conditions of use. Contamination of a disinfectant solution is a particular hazard, and 'in-use' tests (Ayliffe *et al*. 1984) should be carried out when a new disinfectant or different concentration of an existing disinfectant is introduced. Repeat tests should be carried out occasionally to ensure that no changes in the recommended policy have occurred or that resistant bacterial strains are not selected. If the cleanliness of the equipment immersed in the disinfectant is uncertain (e.g. mops and brushes), the surface of the equipment should also be examined by a microbiological surface sampling technique (e.g. cotton wool swabs, contact plates). Routine testing is probably unnecessary if staff are well trained in disinfection procedures.

5.4 Review of policy

This should be considered annually. Defects of the current system should be noted and changes introduced where necessary.

References

Ayliffe, G.A.J., Coates, D. and Hoffman, P.N. (1984) *Chemical Disinfection in Hospitals*. Public Health Laboratory Service, London.

Babb, J.R., Bradley, C.R., and Ayliffe, G.A.J. (1980) Sporicidal activity of glutaraldehyde and hypochlorite and other factors influencing their selection for the treatment of medical equipment. *Journal of Hospital Infection*, **1**, 63.

Block, S.S. (1983) *Disinfection, Sterilization and Preservation*, 3rd edn. Lea & Febiger, Philadelphia.

Bloomfield, S.F. and Miller, E.A. (1989) A comparison of hypochlorite and phenolic disinfectants for disinfection of clean and soiled surfaces and blood spillages. *Journal of Hospital Infection*, **13**, 231.

Coates, D. (1988) Comparison of sodium hypochlorite and sodium dichloroisocyanurate disinfectants. Neutralization by serum. *Journal of Hospital Infection*, **11**, 60.

Control of Substances Hazardous to Health Regulations (1988). HMSO, London.

Council of Europe (1987) *Test Methods for the Antibacterial Activity of Disinfectants*. Council of Europe, Strasburg.

Dyas, A. and Das, B.C. (1985) The activity of glutaraldehyde against *Clostridium difficile*. *Journal of Hospital Infection*, **6**, 41.

Kelsey, J.C. and Maurer, I.M. (1974) An improved Kelsey-Sykes test for disinfectants. *Pharmaceutical Journal*, **213**, 528.

Russell, A.D., Hugo, W.B., and Ayliffe, G.A.J. (1991) *Principles and Practice of Disinfection, Preservation and Sterilization*, 2nd edn. Blackwell Scientific Publications, Oxford.

Rutala, W.A. (1990) APIC guidelines for selection and use of disinfectants. *American Journal of Infection Control*, **18**, 99.

6 *Decontamination of the environment, equipment and the skin*

The choice of method of decontamination – i.e. cleaning, disinfection, sterilization – depends on many factors, but the initial choice can be based on infection risks to patients. These can be classified as high, intermediate, low and minimal risks (Ayliffe *et al*. 1984). However, there is an overlap between these categories and requirements for decontamination may vary within a category.

6.1 Infection risks to patients from equipment, materials and the environment

6.1.1 HIGH RISK

Items in close contact with a break in the skin or mucous membrane or introduced into a sterile body area (see p. 93) (e.g. surgical instruments, dressings, catheters and prosthetic devices) – sterilization is required. (If sterilization is not practically achievable, high level disinfection, although not optimal, may be adequate.)

6.1.2 INTERMEDIATE RISK

Items in contact with intact mucous membranes, body fluids or contaminated with particularly virulent or readily transmissible organisms, or if the item is to be used on highly susceptible patients or sites – disinfection is required, (e.g. gastroscopes, respiratory equipment).

6.1.3 LOW RISK

Items in contact with normal and intact skin – Cleaning and drying usually adequate, (e.g. washing bowls, toilets and bedding).

6.1.4 MINIMAL RISK

Items not in close contact with the patient or his/her immediate surroundings. Unlikely to be contaminated with a significant number of pathogens or to a susceptible site – cleaning to transfer organisms and drying usually adequate, (e.g. floors, walls, sinks).

6.2 Hospital environment

The inanimate environment of the hospital (i.e. minimal risk) is of little importance in the spread of endemic hospital infection (Ayliffe *et al.* 1967; Maki *et al.* 1982) but may occasionally have a role in outbreaks. Recommendations for decontamination are shown in Appendices 6.1 and 6.2.

6.2.1 WARD

A ward surface (floor, furniture, equipment or wall) that is physically clean and dry is unlikely to represent an appreciable infection risk. A clean environment is necessary to provide the required background to good standards of hygiene and asepsis and to maintain the confidence of patients and the morale of staff (Maurer 1985). Wet surfaces and equipment are more likely to encourage the growth of microorganisms and to spread potential pathogens. Cleaning equipment and used cleaning solutions may be heavily contaminated with microbes and should be removed from patient treatment or food preparation areas as soon as cleaning is completed. Thorough cleaning will remove microorganisms and the material on which they thrive. This will render most items relatively free of infection risk and safe to handle. Disinfectants are not usually required and should only be used as part of a properly controlled policy. Disinfectants should be accurately diluted, freshly prepared for each task and disposed of promptly after use. Antimicrobial agents are sometimes included in cleaning solutions not described as disinfectants. These may be highly selective and adversely affect the microbial ecology and should therefore be avoided wherever possible. Where cleaning services are contracted to an industrial organization, the cleaning solutions and equipment should conform to hospital policy.

6.2.2 DUTIES AND RESPONSIBILITIES OF DOMESTIC SERVICES STAFF

The Domestic Services Manager is usually responsible for hospital domestic staff and should ensure they are properly trained and supervised. Routine cleaning of the environment, including floors, toilets, baths, wash basins, beds, locker tops and other furniture, should be the responsibility of the domestic service in all wards and departments. Domestic staff specially trained and aware of possible infection hazards should be available to clean and, if necessary, disinfect the rooms occupied by infected patients. The cleaning procedures in use should be agreed with the infection control staff and should include a list of the contents of the room to be cleaned or disinfected, methods for disposal of waste material, and methods of disinfection of cleaning equipment. Nursing and other patient care staff should, wherever possible, be relieved of cleaning tasks. Surfaces or equipment contaminated with potentially infectious material require immediate attention. Nurses should continue to clean and disinfect these items unless specifically trained domestic staff are available. If there is an unusual infection risk associated with the presence of a particular patient (e.g. in cleaning blood spillage from an HBV or HIV infected patient, or in a high risk department), the ward sister should ensure that the domestic staff are aware of that risk. It may be considered that the task could be performed more safely by a trained nurse. Cleaning should be carried out in a planned manner and cleaning schedules should be drawn up for each area to include all equipment, fixtures and fittings. New items should be added to schedules as commissioned. Cleaning schedules should be sufficiently detailed to specify the method, frequency, timing where relevant, the equipment to be used, where equipment is to be stored and how it is to be cleaned. The responsibility for each task should be indicated and should include the maintenance of paper towel cabinets and soap or dispensers, and replacement of cleaning materials and linen. The schedules should be agreed with the persons in charge of the area to be cleaned and, in high risk areas, the infection control staff.

6.2.3 FLOORS

The bacteriological advantages of using a disinfectant rather than a detergent solution, or a wet rather than a dry method, are marginal in routine hospital cleaning. In a busy ward, recontamination from airborne settlement or transfer from shoes and trolley wheels is rapid. Levels of bacterial contamination on floors may be restored to their original level within two hours of cleaning, whether disinfectants are used or not (Ayliffe *et al.* 1966). Infection rates are not influenced by the use of a disinfectant and a detergent alone will normally suffice (Danforth *et al.* 1987). Disinfectants should only be used where there is a known or predictable risk of contamination with specific human pathogens (e.g. *Salmonella* spp., tubercle bacilli, HBV or HIV). Disinfection of floors and other surfaces may also be included in cleaning policies for specific areas (e.g. clean rooms, isolation units, etc.) and where recommended by the microbiologist to deal with a particular risk. However, the risks of acquiring infection from floors and other environmental sites in these areas, including operating theatres, is low and cleaning alone is usually adequate.

6.3 Dry cleaning

Brooms re-disperse dust and bacteria into the air and should not be used in patient treatment or food preparation and service areas; suitable methods are a vacuum cleaner or dust-attracting mop. Vacuum cleaners should meet the requirements of BS 5415. The inner paper bag should be checked before use and discarded if more than half full. Bag exchange should be made away from patient treatment areas with the minimum dispersal of dust. Filters should be inspected at regular scheduled intervals (e.g. monthly) and changed if dirty or blocked.

The dust-attracting mop, although less efficient, may be used either as a supplement or as an alternative to a vacuum cleaner. Dust-attracting mops may be either impregnated with or manufactured from a dust-attracting material, and may be disposable or re-processable. If used for an excessive period without replacement, they will fail to retain the dust and may disperse it into the air. An acceptable period of use should be decided for each area. To avoid dispersal during use the head should remain in contact with the floor during sweeping and should not be lifted at the end of each stroke. Dry-cleaning removes only soil and will not remove stains or scuff marks.

6.4 Wet cleaning

Wet cleaning is required at intervals to remove stains and scuff marks. Sluice rooms, toilets and other moist areas require wet cleaning at least once daily. A neutral detergent is usually adequate and should be freshly prepared and accurately diluted for each task. Mops and other equipment should be cleaned, drained where appropriate, and stored dry. Buckets should be rinsed and stored inverted to assist drying. Mops are difficult to dry completely and are frequently contaminated with Gram-negative bacilli. Although these may be transferred to the surface during cleaning, they will disappear rapidly as the surface dries. Floors transiently contaminated in this way do not appear to cause infections in general surgical and medical wards. Mops require disinfection after use in rooms of infected patients and possibly before use in rooms occupied by immunosuppressed patients. Laundering in a machine with a heat disinfection cycle is the preferred method, but rinsing followed by a soak in 1% bleach or an alternative chlorine-releasing agent (1000 ppm available chlorine) for not more than 30 minutes, re-rinsing and allowing to dry, is an acceptable alternative. Where disinfection is not required mops should be kept clean, and laundering is the preferred method.

All cleaning equipment should be examined at regular scheduled intervals and cleaned if soiled. Worn or damaged equipment should be repaired or replaced. Cleaning solutions should be changed frequently to prevent the accumulation or multiplication of bacteria and discarded or removed from the patient treatment area as soon as cleaning is completed. A two-compartment bucket or a wheeled stand containing two buckets (which allows the used water from the mop to be discarded into a separate bucket or compartment) is an advantage. Surfaces should be left as dry as possible after cleaning. Poorly designed or inadequately maintained mechanical cleaning equipment may increase the bacterial count of the cleaned surface or the surrounding air and should not be introduced into high-risk areas without consultation with the microbiologist or infection control staff. The cleaning and maintenance of all new equipment should be agreed before putting it into use. Protocols should indicate the acceptable area of use for the equipment, and any attachments. It may be permissible to use a scrubbing machine in more than one area, but separate pads should be used. Preferably, scrubbing machines with integral tanks which cannot be totally drained should not be used in patient treatment areas. Where a machine has a solution storage tank it should be drained as completely as possible at the end of the day's session and kept dry until required.

6.5   Spray cleaning

It is important to ensure that solutions sprayed in patient treatment areas are not heavily contaminated with Gram-negative bacilli. Solutions should be freshly prepared and spray bottles not in use should be stored dry.

6.6   Carpets (or other soft flooring materials) in hospital wards

Although bacteria are usually present in larger numbers and survive longer than on hard floors, there is no evidence that carpets are associated with infection (Ayliffe *et al*. 1974). Nevertheless, it is still reasonable to minimize potential infection hazards by selecting carpets with specifically desirable properties. If installed in surgical wards or other clinical areas, the carpets should have a waterproof backing and joints should be sealed. Pile fibres should be water-repellent and non-absorbent. Ease of cleaning and rate of drying are improved by having a pile of short upright fibres. The carpet should be washable, and if possible, not damaged by application of commonly used disinfectants. Spillage of blood, particularly from patients at high risk of blood borne infection, may require disinfection with chlorine-releasing agents which damage most carpets. Alternatives to chlorine-releasing compounds (e.g. per-oxygen powders) which are less damaging to carpets are available. However, spillage can usually be safely removed by thorough washing with a detergent solution, provided gloves are worn by the operator. It is important, before buying a carpet, to ensure that it is resistant to the agents likely to be applied in the ward and that stains can be easily removed. Carpets should be vacuum cleaned daily and periodically wet cleaned with specially designated equipment (e.g. steam cleaners with a vacuum extraction).

The decision as to whether or not to fit carpets in clinical areas is difficult and is not based only on infection risk. Carpets in wards with frequent or large volume spillage (e.g. units for the mentally handicapped) are usually inadequately maintained, and are therefore not recommended in these areas (Collins 1979). Other clinical areas, such as surgical and obstetric wards may also frequently be contami-nated with blood and other body fluids, and routine cleaning again may be inadequate. Problems of smell and staining have been responsible for the removal of carpets in many clinical areas. In general, it would seem preferable to avoid carpets in these areas, since attractive, alternative flooring is now available. Washable floors are advisable in isolation wards, since carpets may prolong the survival of certain organisms such as multi-resistant strains of *Staph. aureus* (e.g. MRSA). If it is still decided to fit carpets in clinical areas, it is of major importance to ensure that, in addition to buying suitable carpets and cleaning equipment, the cleaning schedules are agreed before the carpet is bought, and that they are achievable. Cleaning guidelines provided by manufacturers are often not possible to carry out, as ward areas need to be evacuated during the procedure. Facilities should also be available for the prompt removal of spillage. Absorbent powders are particularly useful for this purpose followed by either vacuum cleaning or the spot application of a suitable carpet compatible detergent. As it is usually not possible to use a disinfectant because of possible damage to the carpet, protective clothing (i.e. gloves and a plastic apron) should be worn when removing spillage.

6.7 Spillage

Cleaning with a detergent and water may be adequate for most spillage (e.g. food, urine etc.). A disinfectant should be used for spillage containing potentially hazardous organisms. Disposable gloves should always be worn for cleaning known contaminated spillage. If there is danger of contaminating clothing, a disposable plastic apron should also be worn. A sprinkler may be used to cover small amounts of the spillage with sufficient chlorine-releasing granules or powder to absorb any moisture. When the fluid is completely absorbed, a disposable paper wipe should then be used immediately to remove residue and discarded into a plastic bag. Finally the surface is washed using a disposable paper wipe and dried. Discard all waste, wipes, disposable gloves, and apron if worn, seal and dispose of as clinical waste. Powders or granules should be used on wet spillage only. Liquid disinfectants (phenolics or chlorine-releasing agents) can also be used and may be necessary for a large spillage (i.e. >30 ml). Chlorine-releasing powder, granules or fluids containing 10 000 ppm av Cl_2, should be used for blood or body fluid spillage known or suspected to be contaminated with HIV or HBV. If chlorine-releasing agents are added to acidic body fluids (e.g. urine), this may result in a rapid release of toxic levels of chlorine. At these concentrations chlorine-releasing agents are toxic and corrosive and likely to damage or decolourize many surfaces; 1000 ppm can be used for other spillage or precleaned surfaces. If the surface is likely to be damaged by chlorine-releasing agents, other agents with antiviral activity (e.g. peroxygen compounds) may be more appropriate. Universal precautions indicate that all blood and certain body fluids are potentially infectious and routine disinfection before cleaning is often recommended. This would seem to be excessive (particularly in hospitals where the infection rate with HBV or HIV is low) and unnecessary provided gloves and a plastic apron are worn and hands are washed. Thorough cleaning alone is usually sufficient. A clear soluble phenolic is less likely to damage surfaces and is suitable for bacterial contamination (e.g. with enteric organisms or mycobacteria).

6.8 Walls and ceilings

Only very small numbers of bacteria adhere to clean, smooth, dry, intact walls (Ayliffe *et al.* 1967). These surfaces are unlikely to be a significant infection hazard. Ceilings show an even smaller number of bacteria. The cleaning of walls and ceilings should be carried out sufficiently often to prevent the accumulation of visible dirt, but intervals between cleaning should not usually exceed 12–24 months in patient treatment areas or six months in operating theatres.

Disinfection is not required unless known contamination has occurred. Splashes of blood, urine or known contaminated material should be cleaned promptly. When cleaning walls, the surface should be left as dry as possible. Damaged paint work exposes plaster which cannot be effectively cleaned or disinfected, and may become heavily colonized with bacteria if it becomes moist (e.g. through condensation). Damaged wall surfaces should be promptly repaired and redecorated, particularly in operating theatres. A moist surface may encourage growth of fungi, especially aspergillus.

6.9 Other surfaces

Locker tops should be wiped daily with a freshly-prepared detergent solution using disposable wipes. Other furniture should be similarly cleaned as required. Shelves and ledges should be damp-dusted weekly or more often if dust accumulates. Disinfection is not required, unless the surface is contaminated with infected body fluids and other potentially infectious material.

6.9.1 BATHS, SINKS AND WASH BASINS

Baths and wash basins should be cleaned at least daily by the domestic staff, and patients should be encouraged to clean the bath after each use. Detergent is adequate for routine cleaning. A cream cleaner may occasionally be required to remove scum, but should not be used on fibreglass baths unless approved by the manufacturer. It is necessary to disinfect baths after use by infected patients, or before use by patients with open wounds. A non-abrasive chlorine-releasing powder can be used for this purpose. Abrasive powders are effective, but they damage porcelain surfaces and must never be used on fibreglass.

Alternatively, solutions of chlorine-releasing agents may be used with a detergent, but only if the detergent is known to be compatible. No attempt should be made to disinfect sink traps or outlets, since disinfection of these sites is usually ineffective. Plugs should not be used in wash-hand basins.

6.9.2 TOILETS AND DRAINS

Toilet seats and handles should be cleaned at least once daily, and when visibly soiled. A detergent solution should be used for routine cleaning. Disinfection with a clear soluble phenolic or a chlorine-releasing agent may be required if the seat is obviously contaminated, or after use by patients with gastrointestinal infection. If a disinfectant is used, the seat should be rinsed with water and dried before use. Pouring disinfectant into lavatory pans or drains is unlikely to reduce infection risks.

6.9.3 CROCKERY AND CUTLERY

Centralized arrangements for machine washing and drying of all crockery and cutlery is preferred to washing on individual wards (see also: Dishwashing in Hospital Wards 2: Domestic Service Management Advice Note 1976). A washing machine with a final rinse temperature of 80°C for one minute or other appropriate time/temperature combination (e.g. 70°C for three minutes) is a satisfactory alternative in ward kitchens (see the section on kitchen hygiene, Chapter 12, p. 235) and is desirable in isolation wards.

6.10 Cleaning materials

Single-use wipes should, wherever possible, be used for cleaning surfaces (e.g. baths, sinks, bowls, mattresses, beds, furniture, etc.). They should also be used for mopping up spillages from a known source of infection and for cleaning cubicles occupied by infected patients. If disposables are not available in other areas because of cost, the following alternatives can be used.

1. A nylon brush, which can be dried quickly, may be used for cleaning baths. Absorbent cotton mops or bristle brushes become heavily contaminated and are difficult to disinfect and should not be used.
2. If non-disposable cloths are used for cleaning, these should be washed after use, preferably in a washing machine with a disinfection cycle, and dried. Separate cloths should be used in the kitchen, sluice and other ward areas. A colour code may be used to distinguish areas of usage.
3. Toilet brushes should be rinsed well in the flushing water of the lavatory pan; after shaking off excess water, they should be stored dry.

Sponges dry slowly, are difficult to disinfect and should not be used.

6.11 Disinfection of rooms with formaldehyde gas

Formaldehyde disinfection may be required for rooms that have been occupied by patients with viral haemorrhagic fevers, although the necessity is doubtful. The method is not required or recommended for terminal disinfection of rooms occupied by patients with the common range of infectious diseases or hospital-acquired infections. If required expert supervision should be available, since formaldehyde is a toxic gas.

The windows should be sealed and formaldehyde generated by addition of 150 g of potassium permanganate to 280 ml of formalin for every 1000 ft³ (28.3 m³) of the room volume. The ratio of formalin to potassium permanganate should be strictly adhered to.

This reaction may produce a considerable amount of heat: a heat-resistant container must be used and the container should stand on a heat-resistant surface. Temperature and humidity should be controlled and should not fall below 18°C and 60%, respectively. To ensure adequate humidity, it may be necessary to nebulize water into the air. After starting the generation of formaldehyde vapour, the door should be sealed and the room left unopened for 48 hours.

6.12 Decontamination of non-clinical equipment (see also Appendix 6.1)

6.12.1 WASHING AND SHAVING EQUIPMENT

Plastic wash-bowls The bowls should be thoroughly washed with a detergent and hot water after each use and dried. It is important to remove residual fluid remaining in the bowl after cleaning, and the bowls should, if possible, be stored separately and inverted. Each patient should preferably have his own washing bowl, particularly in intensive care or other high risk units. The bowl should be terminally disinfected, by heat or with a chlorine-releasing agent or clear soluble phenolic before it is issued to the next patient. Thorough cleaning and drying is probably sufficient in general wards. A hanging basket is convenient for storage of washing bowls under the bed.

Nailbrushes Nailbrushes frequently become contaminated with Gram-negative bacilli even when stored in a disinfectant solution, and their use should be avoided except for special procedures (e.g. first scrub of the day in an operating theatre). Nylon brushes kept in a dry state are less often contaminated than bristle brushes, but brushes should be avoided if possible. If nailbrushes are required in patient treatment or food production areas they should preferably be supplied sterilized or heat disinfected by the SSD.

Soap dishes and dispensers Soap dishes are rarely necessary, and may encourage bacterial growth. If used, they should be washed and dried daily. The nozzle of liquid soap dispensers should be cleaned daily to remove residues, and the outside cleaned and dried. Disposable cartridge-type refills with an integral nozzle are preferred, but tend to be expensive. If non-disposable reservoirs are used topping-up should be avoided and the inside of containers should be cleaned and dried before re-filling. In cartridge-type dispensers the channel and reservoir between the refill and nozzle, if not disposable, require periodic cleaning. Liquid soaps used in hospitals should contain a preservative (e.g. 0.3% chlorocresol) which should prevent bacterial growth during periods of use.

Razors For pre-operative shaving, a disposable or autoclavable razor is preferred. Communal razors used by the hospital barber should be wiped clean and disinfected after each shave using 70% alcohol. Electric razor heads should also be immersed in 70% alcohol for five minutes.

6.12.2 BEDS AND BEDDING

Bed frames Bed frames are rarely an infection risk and, unless visibly soiled, routine cleaning is unnecessary after discharge of a patient. However, bed frames should be included in cleaning schedules and should be wiped with detergent solution and dried. If disinfection is considered necessary, a clear soluble phenolic is usually suitable. Expensive antiseptics should not be used.

Mattresses and pillows Mattresses and pillows cannot readily be disinfected if they become contaminated. They should be enclosed in a waterproof cover and additional waterproof draw sheets used if body fluid contamination is likely. Wiping the cover with a detergent solution and thorough drying, usually provides adequate decontamination. Avoid excessive wetting during cleaning. Disinfectants, particularly clear soluble phenolics, can make covers permeable and should be avoided if possible. If disinfection is required, use a chlorine-releasing (1 000 ppm av. Cl_2) solution and then rinse well (DOH, 1991).

It may be possible to disinfect some pillows and patients' supports by low temperature steam. Silver nitrate used for topical treatment of burns will also damage mattress covers. Stained mattress covers are often permeable to fluids and should be changed. All mattresses should be routinely inspected for damage.

Duvets Duvets with a waterproof outer surface and covered with a launderable outer fabric cover are now used in some hospitals, but some patients find them uncomfortable, particularly in hot weather. Provided the duvet does not become soiled or wet, replacement of the outer fabric cover of the duvet between patients is usually adequate. Cleaning of the plastic surface will be required if it becomes soiled or contaminated. Thoroughly wiping the outer surface of the duvet with a detergent solution and allowing it to dry completely will usually be sufficient. If disinfection is required after spillage or use by an infected patient, proceed as described for mattresses and pillows. Launderable duvets without a waterproof outer surface are available, but routine disinfection of the whole duvet in the laundry could be a problem and the possible implication should be carefully considered after discussion with the laundry manager before they are introduced (e.g. an outbreak of MRSA may require laundering of all duvets in a ward at the same time). Duvets are not recommended for incontinent patients nor if gross contamination with body fluids is likely.

Bedding Bedding can become heavily contaminated with colonized skin scales in a few hours. Frequent changing is therefore of limited value in controlling the spread of infection. Procedures for laundering are described in Chapter 12.

Cotton blankets should be used and should be changed on discharge of the patient or if they become soiled or contaminated with potentially infectious spillage.

Sheets should be changed on discharge of the patient and at least twice weekly intervals, also if soiled, wrinkled, stained or contaminated with potentially infectious material.

Curtains The level of microbial contamination on curtains is related to the level of dispersal by patients in the immediate vicinity and if changed will rapidly regain that level. Curtains should therefore be washed when obviously soiled or every six months. The curtains in the vicinity of a disperser of an epidemic strain of *Staphylococcus aureus* may remain heavily contaminated for some hours and should be changed if the area is to be re-occupied by a susceptible patient within 24 hours. The degree of microbial contamination is not usually related to the type of material used or the time the curtains were last changed.

Bed-cradles These should be kept clean and maintained in good condition. Disinfect only after use by an infected patient; then the cradle may be wiped over with a clear, soluble phenolic, or chlorine-releasing solution and rinsed. They should not be stored in patient treatment areas.

6.12.3 TOYS

Disinfection is rarely necessary. Contaminated, solid toys may be wiped over with a clear soluble phenolic or a chlorine-releasing agent and rinsed, or with 70% alcohol. Soft toys may be disinfected using low temperature steam or hot water. If grossly contaminated, they should be destroyed.

6.12.4 DRESSING-TROLLEY TOPS

To clean, use a detergent solution and a disposable paper wipe, then dry. To disinfect, wipe with 70% alcohol or a clear soluble phenolic.

6.12.5 INSTRUMENTS, BOWLS, ETC. FOR CLINICAL PROCEDURES

These should be supplied packed and sterilized by the SSD. Sterilization or disinfection of instruments at ward level should rarely be required. If it is necessary to sterilize instruments at ward or clinic level, a small autoclave should preferably be used. Boiling water baths do not sterilize, but if used correctly are a more reliable method of disinfection than most chemical agents. In an emergency, instruments can be disinfected, but not sterilized, in boiling water for 5–10 min. Immersion of clean instruments in 70% alcohol, or 2% glutaraldehyde for ten minutes will disinfect, but is not as reliably effective as hot water or steam. Instruments immersed in glutaraldehyde should be thoroughly rinsed in water to remove irritant residues before use. Sterile water should be used for invasive items. The use of glutaraldehyde in wards or clinics should be avoided if possible. Wiping with 70% alcohol is a rapid, but less certain method of disinfection of instruments such as scissors, and is particularly useful for surfaces. Cheatle forceps should preferably not be used for aseptic techniques. If there are circumstances requiring their use (e.g. in hospitals without an SSD) forceps, complete with container, should be cleaned and autoclaved or boiled daily; during periods of use, the forceps should stand in a freshly prepared solution of clear soluble phenolic.

Used instruments should be transferred to a paper or plastic bag which is placed in a rigid container and returned without further treatment to the SSD.

6.12.6 THERMOMETERS

Oral thermometers Oral thermometers should be stored dry, since growth of Gram-negative bacilli is possible if they are kept in a disinfectant. If a separate thermometer is used for each patient, it may be disinfected by wiping with an alcoholic wipe before returning to its holder. It should be disinfected by immersion in 70% alcohol or 2% clear phenolic solution (Stericol) for ten minutes when the patient is discharged. If not kept for individual patients, thermometers may be immersed in alcohol at the end of the round, and stored dry.

Rectal thermometers Disposable sleeves will reduce the risk of contamination and, if used, the sleeve should be removed and the thermometer treated as for oral thermometers. If a sleeve is not used, remove all traces of lubricant by wiping with an alcohol wipe, then disinfect as above.

6.12.7   BEDPANS

To prevent transfer of faecal contamination, the hands should always be washed after handling a used or re-usable bedpan, even if it is apparently clean.

Re-usable bedpans   Bedpans should, where possible, be washed and disinfected in a bedpan washing machine with a heat disinfection cycle. A heat disinfection cycle should ensure that all surfaces reach 90°C or are raised to 80°C and held at that temperature for at least one minute. The cycle should be checked at least every six months to ensure that the required temperature is reached. Washing machines without a heat disinfection cycle are acceptable in most situations, but not on urological wards, infectious diseases wards or where enteric infections are likely to occur. They should be replaced by machines with a heat disinfection cycle when a new machine is required. If washers are not available, emptying the bedpan into the sluice, washing and allowing to thoroughly dry before re-use is also acceptable for non-infected patients.

Alternative methods of disinfection   Bedpans may be placed in boiling water for 5–10 minutes but this should rarely be necessary. Chemical disinfection is not usually practical. Immersion tanks should preferably be avoided as they may be ineffective if not well-maintained and can encourage the growth of resistant strains of Gram-negative bacilli. Wiping the entire surface of a cleaned bedpan with a clear soluble phenolic (or a chlorine-releasing solution, though this may damage stainless steel bedpans), rinsing and allowing to dry is an alternative, but is not as effective as heat disinfection, and should only be used in an emergency or in countries with limited facilities.

Disposable bedpans   Single use paper-pulp bedpans disposed of in a purpose-built macerator are an alternative to washer disinfectors. To minimize the risk of blockages, the horizontal course of the soil pipe above ground should not be greater than 20 ft (7 m) and should have an overall fall of 1 in 40. (Leakage and possible aerosol production round the lid was a fault in some early models but this problem has now been overcome). Paper-pulp bedpans require a non-disposable support. These supports become contaminated in use and require washing after use. If heavily contaminated with faeces, they should be washed and wiped with a clear soluble phenolic. An individual support is recommended for each patient. This may be disinfected if soiled and on discharge of the patient.

6.12.8 COMMODES

The container used in the commode should be treated as a bedpan. Containers which fit bedpan washers are preferred. If the seat becomes soiled or is used by a patient with an enteric infection, it should be disinfected with a clear soluble phenolic, or chlorine-releasing agent, rinsed and dried before re-use. Disposable wipes should be used for cleaning and disposable gloves and a plastic apron should be worn. Hands must be washed at the end of the task even if gloves are worn.

6.12.9 URINE BOTTLES

Bedpan washers will also accommodate urine bottles and recommendations are as for bedpans. Washers with a heat disinfection cycle are strongly recommended for urology and infectious diseases wards. Urine bottles not disinfected by heat should always be regarded as contaminated and hands should be washed after contact. If heat disinfection is not available, a separate labelled urine bottle should be supplied to patients with urinary tract infections and should be rinsed after each use and disinfected on discharge of the patient as described for bedpans.

Disposable paper-pulp urine bottles for disposal in bedpan macerators are available but may not be suitable for urology wards if direct visual examination of the urine is required.

6.13 Decontamination of medical equipment (Central Sterilizing Club – Working Party Reports 1 and 2 1986)

See also Appendices 6.1 and 6.2.

6.13.1 HIGH RISK ITEMS

Most of the items in this category (e.g. surgical instruments, prosthetic devices, dressings, surgical drapes and gowns, parenteral fluids etc.) can be sterilized by steam at high temperature. Dry heat can be used for sterilizing some of the instruments used in ophthalmic and dental surgery, glass syringes, oils and powders. Single use items, such as catheters, plastic syringes, needles, grafts and internal pacemakers are usually sterilized by the manufacturer by ethylene oxide or irradiation. Inexpensive items, especially those which are difficult to clean, should not be re-used. All reprocessed equipment should be cleaned thoroughly before sterilization prior to re-use. The manufacturers should state which methods of decontamination can be used for any reusable item of equipment. Non-disposable items should preferably be able to withstand moist heat at 134°C (or at least 80°C). If items are damaged at these temperatures or if they cannot be cleaned easily their use should be discouraged. Some expensive items, such as flexible endoscopes, are heat sensitive and must be decontaminated by less effective methods, such as immersion in disinfectants.

Operative endoscopes (e.g. arthroscopes, laparoscopes, ventriculo-scopes) Since an increasing amount of operative surgery will be carried out in the future with an endoscope, autoclavable instruments are preferred. However, many of the new instruments are flexible and damaged by heat. Clean thoroughly and if possible sterilize with ethylene oxide or low temperature steam and formaldehyde (LTS/F). Since these methods may not be available or practicable, immersion in 2% glutaraldehyde for three hours is an acceptable alternative, but this method is less reliable due to the possible presence of air bubbles and recontamination on subsequent rinsing. Shorter immersion times (10–20 minutes) are usually used because of limited availability of instruments. This process is referred to in the USA as high level disinfection (it is effective against vegetative bacteria, viruses, fungi and *Mycobacterium tuberculosis*, but not usually bacterial spores, or some atypical mycobacteria (Rutala, 1990)). Provided the endoscope is well cleaned before disinfection the risk of infection is small, although the remote risk of an infection due to spore forming organisms cannot be excluded.

Cystoscopes High level disinfection is usually used, i.e. 2% glutaraldehyde for 10–20 minutes. The longer exposure time of 20 minutes is required if an effect against *M. tuberculosis* is required (Best *et al.* 1990). The concentration of glutaraldehyde in the solution should not be allowed to fall below 1.5% and solutions should be changed after processing about 100 cystoscopes. Solutions should not be used beyond the manufacturers recommended post – activation use life (e.g. 14–28 days). If sufficient instruments are available, autoclaving or low temperature steam may be used. Pasteurization in a water bath at 70–80°C for 10 minutes is an alternative to chemical disinfection but the manufacturer should be consulted on heat tolerance if hot water or steam is used. Another alternative is 70% ethanol for five minutes, but this may damage the instrument if immersion is prolonged beyond that agreed by the manufacturer.

6.13.2   MISCELLANEOUS HIGH RISK ITEMS

Catheters   Single use is preferred. Some cardiac catheters are too expensive for single use and reprocessing may be necessary although it is not usually recommended by regulating authorities in the wealthier countries. They may be re-sterilized with ethylene oxide provided the cleaning process is efficient and the structure and function remain unimpaired. The clinician involved in the procedure should take the responsibility for re-using catheters since damage to materials is a greater risk to the patient than infection.

Grafts (heart valves, arterial grafts, joints and other implants)   Autoclave if possible; if heat labile use ethylene oxide. Sterilization of these items in the hospital should not usually be necessary unless the package containing the device has been opened and it has not been immediately used.

Cryoprobes   Autoclave if possible; if heat labile use LTSF or ethylene oxide. Immersion in 2% glutaraldehyde or 70% alcohol may be necessary if cryoprobes are heat labile and gaseous sterilization is not available.

Transducers and blood monitoring equipment   These may be a source of infection. Disposable or ethylene oxide or LTSF. High level disinfection (e.g. 2% glutaraldehyde or 70% ethanol) may sometimes be necessary.

Haemodialysis equipment   See Chapter 18.

6.13.3   INTERMEDIATE RISK ITEMS

Non-invasive endoscopes   *Ps. aeruginosa* and other Gram-negative bacilli, including salmonella, have been transferred from one patient to another on inadequately decontaminated flexible fibreoptic endoscopes (Ayliffe 1988). Reports on the transfer of mycobacteria and HBV are rare and there has been no evidence of transfer of HIV. Nevertheless, care is necessary to avoid the possibility of spread of any infection by ineffective decontamination. Endoscopic retrograde cholangiopancreatography (ERCP) is a particularly vulnerable procedure and severe Gram-negative infections have been reported. Thorough cleaning and disinfection is important with this procedure. Potential pathogens such as the Gram-negative bacilli can grow overnight in the channels of the endoscope and the water bottle, and disinfection is required at the beginning of the list as well as after each patient. The time available for processing between patients is often short (15–20 minutes). However, vegetative bacteria and most viruses are killed or inactivated by 1–2 minutes' exposure to 2% glutaraldehyde (Sattar *et al.* 1989; Hanson *et al.* 1989, 1990; Tyler *et al.* 1990). Preliminary studies with duck hepatitis B viruses suggest that they are inactivated in 2½ minutes by glutaraldehyde preparations (Murray *et al.* 1991). A variety of automatic cleaning and disinfection machines are available (Babb *et al.* 1984). Most of these are effective, but preliminary brushing of the suction/biopsy channel and wiping the insertion tube is still required. All channels should be cleaned and disinfected. The glutaraldehyde concentration is reduced during repeated use particularly in automated systems and the solution should be changed regularly (e.g. after 20 procedures). The rinse water should also be changed regularly to avoid any build-up of glutaraldehyde. Infection has been reported from Gram-negative bacilli growing in the rinse water tank. This should be routinely disinfected.

Before changing the method of decontamination, it is advisable to consult the manufacturer and give him details of the method to be used. Many disinfectants are corrosive and may damage the endoscope. It should also be noted that low temperature steam may reach 80°C and ethylene oxide 55°C with pressures up to 80 lb/in^2 (5.5 bar).

Flexible gastrointestinal endoscopes (Babb and Bradley 1989, 1991)   Two per cent alkaline activated glutaraldehyde ('Asep', 'Cidex', 'Sporicidin', 'Totacide 28'), succine dialdehyde (Gigasept) are the disinfectants of choice (Ayliffe *et al.* 1986). The British Society of Gastroenterology (1988) recommend thorough cleaning of all channels and external surfaces followed by four minutes' immersion in 2% glutaraldehyde for between patient decontamination. Endoscopes used on patients known or suspected of having pulmonary tuberculosis should be immersed for one hour. Known AIDS patients are managed as immunocompromised patients and the endoscope should be disinfected for one hour before and after the procedure. This is to protect patients from opportunistic pathogens, some of which (e.g. *M. avium-intracellulare*) are relatively resistant to glutaraldehyde.

Cryptosporidia are resistant to glutaraldehyde, but thorough cleaning should be adequate.

Although glutaraldehyde is recommended, an alternative, less irritant agent may be required. Cleansing with a detergent followed by 70% ethanol is recognized as an alternative, but less effective, between patient method. Immersion of the endoscope for longer than five minutes in ethanol may damage epoxy lens cements. Other agents are being investigated including peroxygen compounds (e.g. Virkon) and peracetic acid.

Flexible bronchoscopes   The British Thoracic Society (1989) recommend that bronchoscopes are immersed in 2% glutaraldehyde for 20 minutes between patients and for one hour after a known or suspected case of pulmonary tuberculosis (Best *et al*. 1990). The risk of recontamination of the instrument with environmental mycobacteria derived from the rinse water is high in some areas. It is therefore recommended that the instrument is rinsed in sterile water, or tap water followed by 70% alcohol, particularly before use on an immunocompromised patient.

Endoscope accessories   Many of the accessories (e.g. biopsy forceps, brushes, snares, water bottles etc.) are now autoclavable. These should be dismantled, cleaned thoroughly (preferably using ultrasonics) dried, reassembled and processed, either in the Sterile Services Department (SSD) or using a bench top sterilizer. Non-autoclavable accessories should be dismantled, cleaned and immersed in 2% glutaraldehyde.

Use of 2% glutaraldehyde   Although microbiologically effective, glutaraldehyde is irritant and sensitizing. Gloves impermeable to glutaraldehyde (e.g. nitrile) should always be worn. Solutions should be stored and used in covered containers. The glutaraldehyde levels in the air should not exceed 0.7 mg/m^3 (0.2 ppm) either for long term (eight hours) or for short term (ten minutes) exposure. It is likely that this standard will be reduced to below 0.1 ppm in the foreseeable future. Glutaraldehyde users are strongly advised to provide an extraction system which is available as a mobile trolley if a permanent system is impracticable. The use of less concentrated solutions may reduce the irritant effect but longer immersion times will be required to maintain the antimicrobial effect. Similar irritancy and sensitization problems are likely also with other aldehydes. It is important to rinse thoroughly all items immersed in glutaraldehyde.

6.13.4   RESPIRATORY EQUIPMENT

Ventilators   Many types of ventilator are available, most of which can be adequately protected by filters so minimizing the necessity to decontaminate the ventilator itself. Some ventilators have a removable internal circuit which can be autoclaved or disinfected using low temperature steam. Chemical disinfection may sometimes be required. Most methods of chemical disinfection suitable for ventilators will not work efficiently in the presence of organic matter, and none of the methods is entirely reliable. Of the methods available, nebulization with hydrogen peroxide (a modification of the method described by Judd *et al*. 1968) for 'Cape ventilators' is chosen but the method will require further modification depending on the type of ventilator. The method is quick; the peroxide readily breaks down and is not toxic to patients or staff. If the ventilator is visibly contaminated, it must be stripped down and cleaned prior to disinfection. The method is described in Appendix 6.3 and should be followed particularly for machines with inspiratory and expiratory circuits. An alternative method of disinfection is by the use of formaldehyde (Benn *et al*. 1973). This method can be used only on machines with closed circuits and great care is necessary to remove residual formaldehyde and protect SSD staff. Formaldehyde cabinets are also effective provided the ventilator is kept running during the cycle. If the patient is known or suspected to be suffering from pulmonary tuberculosis the use of the formaldehyde method is advisable. Nebulized hydrogen peroxide may be used on machines with single circuits, though these may often be dismantled more easily, washed and disinfected by heat or by 2% glutaraldehyde. Small machines, for example infant ventilators, may sometimes be treated with ethylene oxide. If gaseous methods are used care should be taken to ensure that all toxic residues are removed by flushing with air or oxygen before the ventilator is reused.

The preferred method of patient humidification is either with a water bath or a heat-moisture exchanger. Less condensation is produced in the tubing with the latter method, therefore reducing the risk of contamination with Gram-negative bacilli. The ventilator external circuitry and humidifier (if used) can be decontaminated using a washing machine or low temperature steam. Some circuits are autoclavable although this may reduce the life of the equipment. If water humidification is used it is recommended that the circuits are changed every 48 hours in adult patients (Craven *et al*. 1982) and between patients, or weekly, in neonatal units. Although filters are hydrophobic, moisture traps may be incorporated to protect the filter. If heat-moisture exchangers are used circuits may be changed between patients or weekly (Cadwallader *et al*. 1990).

Humidifiers Humidifiers in which water vapour (not an aerosol) is blown towards the patient, are not a serious infection hazard. They should be changed, together with the ventilator circuit, every 48 hours. The condensate may contaminate the hands of staff and humidifiers should be cleaned and disinfected, preferably by heat, before refilling with sterile water. Chlorhexidine in a final concentration of 0.1% may be used to prevent bacterial growth in the evaporator type of humidifier in infant incubators but not the nebulizer type. However, this should not be necessary if the humidifier is properly maintained. The use of chlorohexidine may select resistant organisms.

Contaminated nebulizers, which produce an aerosol, may be responsible for lung infections caused by Gram-negative bacilli, especially *Ps*.

aeruginosa. Their use should be avoided unless they can be decontaminated by heat daily. Water should be replaced and not topped up. If the nebulizing part of the machine is liable to damage by heat, it should be flushed through with water and dried. If drying is not possible, it should be rinsed in 70% alcohol and allowed to dry; occasional bacteriological tests should be made to ensure the nebulizer is not contaminated.

Oxygen tents   These should be washed and dried after each patient. Oxygen masks and tubing should be disposable. There is no evidence that piped medical gases become contaminated with bacteria providing the lines remain dry.

6.13.5   ANAESTHETIC EQUIPMENT

The anaesthetic machines themselves are unlikely to become significantly contaminated during an operation and routine decontamination is rarely possible or necessary. However, if filters are not used, decontamination may be required after use on a patient with a known or suspected communicable disease (e.g. pulmonary tuberculosis) when formaldehyde gas may be required. In this case the equipment should be returned to the SSD. The external surfaces of the machine should be kept clean and dry. Contamination is most likely to occur in the face mask and tubing nearest to the patient. This equipment (i.e. tubing, reservoir, ambu-bags, face masks, endotracheal tubes and airways), if not single use, should be cleaned and disinfected. The Medical Equipment Cleaning Unit of a SSD is most suitable. Items should preferably be disinfected using hot water (>80°C in a washing machine) or low temperature steam (73°C) as frequent autoclaving at 121°C or 134°C may damage the equipment. It is rational to provide every patient with a decontaminated set of equipment but this is not usually possible. Sessional or daily treatment of tubing and the reservoir bag is reasonable unless the patient has a respiratory infection or pulmonary tuberculosis is known or suspected (Deverill and Dutt 1980). However, all patients should have a decontaminated face mask, airway and endotracheal tube. Disposable face masks, tubing and reservoir bags may be preferred on patients with known or suspected infections such as TB. If not disposable, all items used on such patients should immediately be autoclaved or disinfected using hot water or sub-atmospheric steam.

Laryngoscope blades   Cleaning and drying may be sufficient. An alcohol wipe (70%) may be used for disinfection.

Scavenging equipment   The tubing close to the patient should be autoclaved or, if heat labile, disinfected using LTS or a washer/disinfector. It should be changed regularly (e.g. weekly) and after use on an infected patient.

Suction equipment   In the absence of piped suction, a separate machine should be available for each patient requiring suction. After use the contents should be discarded, the bottle washed and dried and fresh connection tubing attached. Bacterial multiplication may occur in the aspirate if it is allowed to stand for long periods. This can be emptied in the sluice and the bottle washed in detergent solution and dried. Alternatively a washer disinfector may be used. The bottle should be emptied at least daily irrespective of the amount of fluid aspirated. Non-sterile gloves should be worn and hands must be washed after handling bottle contents. A fresh catheter should be used each time a patient undergoes bronchial aspiration. An anti-foaming agent such as Foamtrol may be used to prevent excessive foaming of the bottle contents which may wet the filter and enter the pump mechanism. The filter should be changed if it becomes moist or discoloured. The use of a detergent or disinfectant in the bottle may be responsible for excessive foaming. Some disinfectants are ineffective and may be toxic to the patient. Disinfectants are therefore avoided during suction but if the contents are considered hazardous to the staff, or the suction equipment is used to irrigate instruments, sufficient disinfectant i.e. clear soluble phenolic or a chlorine-releasing agent, to give a final concentration suitable for a 'dirty' situation, may be drawn through the tubing and be added to the bottle and left for at least 10 mins. The tubing should then be flushed and the bottle washed and dried before re-use. Periodically the machine should be returned to the SSD where the pump can be checked, the filter changed and the tubing, lid, non-return valve and bottle autoclaved or processed in a washer/disinfector. If a patient requires suction for more than 24 hours the bottle and tubing should be changed. When the machine is not in use, the bottle should be kept dry and the catheter should not be connected until it is required. Disposable suction bottles are now available, but are expensive. The container itself is disposable or a disposable liner is fitted within a container. If these are in use the waste disposal policy should take into account the difficulties of transport and incineration (i.e. bursting of the canisters or bags).

Infant incubators   Preferably, these are cleaned in the SSD. After discharge of a patient, the inner surface of the incubator should be thoroughly cleaned with a moist paper wipe and detergent and dried. Special attention should be paid to the humidifier, rubber seals and the mattress. Since adequate cleaning and drying is effective, disinfection is rarely necessary and may fail without preliminary cleaning. However, if disinfection is required, the cleaned surface can be wiped with a freshly prepared hypochlorite solution (125 ppm av Cl_2), rinsed and dried. Alternatively surfaces can be wiped with 70% alcohol; care should be taken as alcohol is flammable and the incubator must be aired thoroughly before re-use. Formaldehyde cabinets are used occasionally, but these are expensive and involve the use of a hazardous chemical. Since prior cleaning of the incubator is still necessary the routine use of a cabinet is of rather doubtful value (Babb *et al.* 1982).

Vaginal, and other specula and sigmoidoscopes   Single use instruments may be preferred. If not the instrument should be thoroughly cleaned and autoclaved. Small autoclaves are now available and are appropriate for use in clinics (HEI 196). Boiling water (for 5–10 minutes) is effective but care is necessary to ensure that items are completely immersed and that the instrument is exposed to boiling water for the required time (i.e. at least five minutes). The boiling water bath should preferably have a timing mechanism. The use of chemical disinfectants should be avoided if possible, but immersion in 70% alcohol for 10 minutes should disinfect adequately. Immersion in 2% glutaraldehyde for 10 minutes is also effective, including activity against *Cl. difficile* (Dyas and Das 1985), but it is irritant and its use should be avoided in clinics.

Tonometers   These should initially be rinsed and immersed in a disinfectant solution for at least five minutes. Chlorine-releasing solution for ten minutes (500–1000 ppm av Cl_2) or 3–6% stabilized hydrogen peroxide is recommended by the Centres for Disease Control. Tonometers should be rinsed thoroughly and dried before re-use. Hydrogen peroxide, in particular, is irritant to the conjunctiva and thorough rinsing or neutralization is important. Wiping with 70% ethanol is probably effective, although the exposure time is short and alcohol can damage the conjunctiva if it is still present on the instrument when used. Immersion in 70% alcohol for 5–10 minutes should be effective, but care is necessary to ensure that this does not damage the instrument and that the alcohol has completely evaporated before use.

6.13.6   DECONTAMINATION OF EQUIPMENT USED ON PATIENTS WITH CREUTZFELDT-JACOB DISEASE

The agent causing this disease is commonly referred to as a 'slow virus' or prion. It has not been characterized and has never been grown in the laboratory. It has been transmitted very rarely by corneal transplantation, human growth hormone and brain electrodes. Care is necessary when handling items contaminated with brain tissue, cerebrospinal fluid, and blood from these patients or if the disease is suspected. Spread to health care workers could occur following a 'sharps' injury. The agent is resistant to most disinfectants, including aldehydes and conventional methods of heat sterilization. It can be inactivated by extended autoclaving at 134° for 18 minutes, 121° for at least one hour (US recommendations) or immersion in a chlorine releasing compound (5000 ppm av Cl_2) or in 1N sodium hydroxide solution for one hour.

Surfaces can be disinfected with a chlorine-releasing solution containing 2 500 ppm av Cl_2 or 1N sodium hydroxide. Sodium hydroxide solution (1N) may be applied to the skin for 10 minutes (US recommendations) after washing, or for decontaminating heat labile equipment such as endoscopes (one hour) if the manufacturers of the endoscope endorse disinfectant compatibility.

6.14   Cleaning and disinfection of skin and mucous membranes

6.14.1   PRINCIPLES

There are three principal reasons for removing or reducing the number of microorganisms present on the skin or mucous membranes:

1. to reduce the number of microorganisms present prior to an invasive procedure;
2. to remove or destroy potentially pathogenic microorganisms present on the hands of staff;
3. occasionally to treat a carrier or disperser of resistant, virulent or highly communicable strains of bacteria.

The bacteria present in healthy skin have been classified for practical purposes as follows:

1. resident organisms that colonize the skin;
2. transient organisms that are deposited on the skin, but do not usually multiply there.

The resident organisms consist mainly of coagulase-negative staphylococci, diphtheroids and occasionally *Staphylococcus aureus*. Gram-negative bacilli, e.g. *Klebsiella*, are usually transients but may be temporary residents for periods varying from several days to many weeks. *Acinetobacter calcoaceticus var anitratum* has many of the survival properties of staphylococci and may be considered a true resident.

Most of the transient bacteria can be removed by a wash with soap and water, which may be almost as effective as disinfection. The resident bacteria, on the other hand, are mostly left on the skin after washing with soap and water, but these can be substantially reduced by disinfection. Some naturally acquired bacteria that do not multiply on the skin (e.g. *Clostridium perfringens* present through faecal contamination) may be difficult to remove by washing with soap and water.

Large numbers of bacteria are found as residents of the mucous membrane in the mouth, nose and vagina, but different organisms predominate in different sites. Antiseptics, which are non-irritant or damaging to the tissues, have a limited, though potentially useful effect in reducing these microorganisms. The urethra normally has few commensal bacteria, but is liable to become contaminated on passage of catheters or other instruments; disinfection of the urethra before instrumentation is one of the important features of prophylaxis against infection of the urinary tract (Chapter 7). The conjunctiva also has few bacteria, but these may include *Staph. aureus*.

6.14.2 CLEANING AND DISINFECTION OF HANDS (Lowbury 1991)

Social handwashing is the washing of hands with non-medicated soap or detergent and water. Hygienic hand disinfection means the killing of transient organisms and may be associated with removal of organisms if an antiseptic detergent is used. Surgical hand disinfection means the killing of transient organisms and a substantial number of resident organisms, and may also be associated with removal of organisms if an antiseptic-detergent is used.

There is some confusion with these definitions and many European workers do not accept removal as part of the disinfection process. This means that only alcoholic preparations can be accepted as hand disinfectants (Rotter 1984). It would seem reasonable to include the process of both removal and killing in the definitions, as antiseptic-detergents are commonly used for disinfection of hands in many countries, including the UK and US.

Washing with soap (or detergent) and water helps to remove dead skin squames and the bacteria present on them. Non-medicated bar soap is usually adequate, provided it is not kept in a dish of fluid. Liquid soap or detergent may be preferred provided dispensers are regularly cleaned and maintained. Washing without a disinfectant is sufficient for most ward procedures (Chapter 7). Washing with an antiseptic-detergent preparation is usually more effective in removing transients than non-medicated soap but the differences are often marginal. The agents commonly used are 4% chlorhexidine-detergent (e.g. 'Hibiscrub', 'Hibiclens') or 7.5% povidone-iodine (e.g. Betadine surgical scrub). Triclosan preparations (e.g. 'Aquasept') are also used and are increasingly popular with staff, but they tend to be less effective.

Repeated applications of these agents, particularly chlorhexidine, show a residual effect against transient organisms, but it remains uncertain whether this effect alone would influence the transmission of infection.

A single application of 70% ethanol or 60% isopropanol, with an emollient (e.g. 1% glycerol) and with or without an antiseptic (e.g. chlorhexidine, povidone-iodine, triclosan) is significantly more effective against transients than a soap and water wash (Rotter 1984; Ayliffe *et al.* 1988). Three ml are poured onto cupped hands and rubbed to dryness. It is important that the formulation used is popular with staff and that all areas of the hands are covered with the agent, since certain areas are easily missed (Taylor 1978).

A standard procedure is recommended (Ayliffe *et al.* 1978), as follows: hands are rubbed, five strokes for each movement, backwards and forwards, palm to palm, right palm over left dorsum, left palm over right dorsum, palm to palm fingers interlocked, backs of fingers to opposing palm with fingers interlaced, rotational rubbing of right thumb clasped in left palm and left thumb in right palm, rotational rubbing with clasped fingers of right hand in palm of left hand, and left hand in palm of right hand, complete hands and wrists (see Fig. 6.1).

If the hands are visibly soiled, a preliminary wash with soap or detergent and water is required before application of an alcoholic solution.

Alcoholic solutions may not be effective against some viruses (e.g. enteroviruses) due to the relatively short exposure time of the agent on the hands, and washing with soap and water prior to the use of 70–90% alcohol is therefore preferred if contamination with these agents is likely. However, 70% alcohol is effective against rotaviruses on the hands.

The same antiseptic-detergent or soap preparations (e.g. chlorhexidine and povidone-iodine) are commonly used for surgical hand disinfection as for hygienic hand disinfection (Lowbury and Lilly 1973). The main difference in the procedure is the longer application time (two minutes instead of 10–20 seconds for hygienic disinfection). Triclosan or hexachlorophane preparations are less frequently used, but are still useful if hypersensitivity to other agents develops. Repeated applications of all these agents reduce the residents to low levels.

The antiseptic-detergent should be thoroughly applied to the hands and wrists for two minutes and then rinsed off. A brush may be used for the first application of the day, but continual use is inadvisable as damage to the skin increases the risk of colonization with *Staph. aureus* or with an increase in numbers of residents.

An alternative and more effective method is the application of an alcoholic solution, with or without an antiseptic (Lowbury *et al.* 1974).

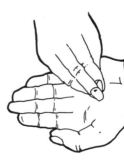

3. Palm to palm fingers interlaced

6. Rotational rubbing, backwards and forwards with clasped fingers of right hand in left palm and vice versa

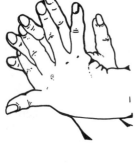

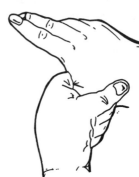

2. Right palm over left dorsum and left palm over right dorsum

5. Rotational rubbing of right thumb clasped in left palm and vice versa

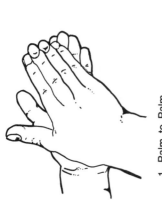

1. Palm to Palm

4. Backs of fingers to opposing palms with fingers interlocked

Figure 6.1 Handwashing technique.
(Ayliffe *et al.* 1978; Lawrence 1985).

Two 5 ml amounts are applied, allowing the first to dry before applying the second, to the hands and wrists using the standardized technique already described and rubbed to dryness. A single application as indicated for hygienic hand disinfection (3 ml applied for 30 seconds) may be adequate for general surgery where the resident flora of the hands is a less frequent cause of infection. Alcohol is also useful for the rapid disinfection of the hands of surgeons following glove puncture during an operation. Alcohol without an added antiseptic surprisingly shows a persistent effect for several hours if gloves are worn. This is probably due to the delayed death of skin bacteria damaged but not immediately killed by alcohol (Lilly *et al.*, 1979).

Since a wide range of preparations are now available, tests for staff acceptability are required before the introduction of a new preparation.

6.14.3 CLEANING AND DISINFECTION OF OPERATION SITE

A rapid reduction of skin flora is required in pre-operative preparation of operation sites. For this purpose a quick-acting antiseptic is desirable. Alcoholic solutions containing chlorhexidine, povidone-iodine or triclosan, are preferred to aqueous solutions for intact skin. The antiseptic should be applied with friction, on a sterile gauze swab over and well beyond the operation site for 3–4 minutes. Application with a gloved hand is more effective. If a gloved hand is used to apply the antiseptic, a second glove should be worn by the surgeon over his operating glove and removed when the preparation of the operation site is complete (Lowbury and Lilly 1975). Alcoholic solutions must be allowed to dry. This is especially important if diathermy is to be used.

The effect of repeated washing or bathing with an antiseptic on infection rates remains controversial (Chapter 11). A single antiseptic bath pre-operatively is unlikely to reduce the risk of infection. Repeated washing and bathing with chlorhexidine-detergent does reduce the level of the resident flora on the skin and could be of value in cardiovascular or prosthetic surgery. However, a single application of alcoholic chlorhexidine rubbed on until the skin is dry, as already described, will reduce the numbers of resident bacteria to levels approaching the low equilibrium obtainable on repeated applications of chlorhexidine-detergent.

Before operations on hands with ingrained dirt (e.g. in gardeners), or operations on the leg of patients with poor arterial supply (e.g. amputations for diabetic gangrene of the foot), a compress soaked in povidone-iodine (e.g. 'Betadine or 'Disadine') solution applied to the operation site for 30 minutes will greatly reduce the numbers of spores of gas gangrene bacilli that present a special hazard in such patients; ordinary methods of disinfection are ineffective against bacterial spores.

However, some spores may remain and antibiotic prophylaxis is still required. Washing with detergents and grease-solvent jellies (e.g. 'Swarfega', 'Dirty Paws') helps to remove ingrained dirt and the dead skin scales on which organisms are carried.

6.14.4 CLEANING AND DISINFECTION OF MUCOUS MEMBRANES

Repeated applications (three or four times a day) of a cream containing 0.5% neomycin and 0.1% chlorhexidine ('Naseptin') to the inside of the nostrils has been shown to remove *Staph. aureus* from a fairly large proportion of nasal carriers; possible alternatives include neomycin-bacitracin ointment or 1% chlorhexidine cream (Williams *et al.* 1967). Mupirocin cream ('Bactroban') is more rapidly effective and more likely to eliminate the staphylococci than other preparations and is particularly useful for treating carriers of methicillin-resistant *Staph. aureus* (MRSA) (see Chapter 9).

Resistance to mupirocin has been described and its widespread use should be avoided since it is the only useful agent for treating carriers of MRSA. *Streptococcus pyogenes* can usually be cleared from the throat by a course of penicillin (injected or given by mouth but not by local application). Erythromycin is effective and should be used in patients who are sensitive to penicillin.

Applications of aqueous solutions of chlorhexidine or povidone-iodine are effective for disinfection of oral mucous membranes, but some dental surgeons consider disinfection to be of doubtful value. Treatment of the vaginal mucosa with obstetric creams containing chlorhexidine or chloroxylenol is considered to have little disinfectant action. An application of a povidone-iodine solution reduces the number of organisms, but the effect on clinical infection is uncertain.

Appendix 6.1 Summary of methods for cleaning and decontamination of equipment or environment

Heat	Autoclave if materials are not likely to be damaged by high temperatures, otherwise use low temperature steam, washer disinfectors or pasteurization
Chemical disinfection	(a) Clear soluble phenolics at concentrations recommended for light contamination, unless otherwise specified
	(b) Chlorine-releasing agents (see p. 67 for concentration)
	(c) 2% glutaraldehyde
	(d) alcohol (use either 60–80% ethyl, or 60–70% isopropyl)

Equipment or site	Routine or preferred method	Acceptable alternative or additional recommendations
Airways and endotracheal tubes	1. Heat sterilize 2. Heat disinfect	3. Chemical disinfection (b) or (d) depending on material. For patients with tuberculosis use disposables or heat
Ampoules	Wipe neck with (d)	Do not immerse
Baths	**Non-infected patients** Wipe with detergent solution or cream cleaner and rinse	**Infected patients and patients with open wounds** Chemical disinfection (b) – Chlorine-releasing detergent solution – Non-abrasive chlorine-releasing powder or granules
Bedding	See section on laundering Heat disinfection: – 65°C for 10 min – 71°C for 3 min	Heat sensitive fabrics, low temperature wash and chemical disinfection (b)
Bedframes	Wash with detergent and dry	After infected patient, disinfectant (a) or (b)
Bedpans	1. Washer disinfector or use disposables. Wash carriers for disposable pans after use	Patients with enteric infections: if (1.) is not possible, heat disinfection after emptying and washing, or chemical disinfection (a). Individual pan for infected patient
Bowls (surgical)	Autoclave	
Bowls (washing)	Wash and dry	For infected patients use individual bowls and disinfect on discharge – Heat disinfection – Chemical disinfection (a) or (b)
Carpets	Vacuum daily; clean periodically by hot water extraction	For known contaminated spillage; chemical disinfection with suitable agent then rinse and dry
Cheatle forceps	Do not use	If used, autoclave daily and store in fresh solution of disinfectant (a)

(continued)

Appendix 6.1   *Continued*

Equipment or site	Routine or preferred method	Acceptable alternative or additional recommendations
Crockery and cutlery	1. Machine wash with rinse temperature above 80°C and dry 2. Hand wash by approved method	For patients with enteric infections or open pulmonary tuberculosis, heat disinfect if possible, or use disposables.
Drains	Clean regularly	Chemical disinfection is not advised
Duvets	Water impermeable cover: wash with detergent solution and dry	Disinfect (b) if contaminated, do not soak or disinfect unnecessarily as this damages the fabric
Endoscopes (gastroscopes), bronchoscopes, laparoscopes, arthroscopes, cytoscopes	1. Clean and heat disinfect or sterilize 2. If heat sensitive, clean and disinfect with (c)	Thoroughly rinse after chemical disinfection (c). A possible alternative is (d) (do not exceed 5 minutes exposure)
Feeding bottles and teats	1. Presterilized or terminally heat-treated feeds	2. Use teats and bottles sterilized and packed by SSD 3. Disinfectants (b) should only be used in small units where other methods are not available
Floors (dry cleaning)	1. Vacuum clean 2. Dust-attracting dry mop	Do not use broom in patient areas
Floors (wet cleaning)	Wash with detergent solution Disinfection not usually required	Known contaminated spillage and special areas, chemical disinfection (a) or (b)
Furniture and fittings	Damp dust with detergent solution	Known contaminated and special areas, damp dust with disinfectant (a) or (b)
Haemodialysis equipment	See p. 366	
Infant incubators	Wash with detergent and dry with disposable wipe	Infected patients – after cleaning wipe with (d) or 125 parts/10^6 (b)
Instruments	Heat	Contaminated instruments should be cleaned before sterilization, preferably in a washer disinfector

Locker tops	See furniture and fittings	
Mattresses	Water impermeable cover, wash with detergent solution and dry	Disinfect (a) or (b), if contaminated; do not disinfect unnecessarily as this damages the mattress (especially a)
Mops (dish)	Do not use	See p. 239
Mops (dry – dust-attracting)	Do not use if overloaded or for more than two days without reprocessing or washing	Vacuuming after each use may prolong effective life between processing
Mops (wet)	Rinse after each use, wring and store dry; heat disinfect periodically	If chemical disinfection is required, rinse in water, soak in 1% (b) (1000 ppm av Cl_2) for 30 min, rinse and store dry
Nail brushes	Use only if essential	A sterile or heat decontaminated brush should be used for all clinical procedures
Pillows	Treat as mattresses	
Razors (safety and open)	Disposable or autoclaved	Chemical disinfection (d)
Razors (electric)	Chemical disinfection (d) Immerse head only	
Rooms (terminal cleaning or disinfection)	Non-infected patients: – wash surfaces in detergent solution and allow to dry	Infected patients: – wash with detergent solution and allow to dry. Use (a) and (b) if disinfection required. Fogging not recommended
Shaving brushes	Do not use for clinical shaving	Autoclave. Use brushless cream or shaving foam
Sputum container	Use disposable only	Non-disposable – should be emptied with care and heat disinfected or sterilized
Suction equipment	1. Clean and dry 2. Heat disinfection or sterilization	If chemical disinfection is required clean and soak in (a) or (b)
Thermometers	1. Individual thermometers: wipe with (d), store dry, terminally disinfect as 2, or use disposable electronic probe	2. Collect after round, wipe clean and disinfect with (a) or (d) for 10 min, rinse (if phenolic), wipe, and store dry

(continued)

Appendix 6.1   *Continued*

Equipment or site	Routine or preferred method	Acceptable alternative or additional recommendations
Thermometers (electronic clinical)	1. Use disposable sleeve 2. Wipe probe with (d) 3. Disposable	Do not use without sleeve for oral or rectal temperatures
Toilet seats	Wash with detergent and dry	After use by infected patient or if grossly contaminated, chemical disinfection (a) or (b), rinse and dry
Tooth mugs	1. Disposable	2. If non-disposable, heat disinfection
Toys	Clean first but do not soak soft toys. If contaminated disinfect: – heat – chemical; wipe surface with (d), (a) or (b)	Expensive or treasured toys may withstand low temperature steam or ethylene oxide; the latter needs long aeration. Heavily contaminated soft toys may have to be destroyed
Trolley tops	1. Clean with detergent and wipe dry	2. Clean first then chemical disinfection (d) or (a) and wipe dry
Tubing (anaesthetic or ventilator)	Heat disinfection: – washer disinfector or – low temperature steam	For patients with tuberculosis or AIDS 1. Use disposable tubing 2. Heat sterilization or disinfection
Urinals	1. Use washer disinfector or use disposables	2. Chemical disinfection (a) or (b). If a tank is used it must be emptied, dried and refilled at least weekly. Avoid if possible
Ventilator (mechanical)	Heat disinfection or disposable circuit Protect machine with filters	If machine is unprotected by filters disinfect with hydrogen peroxide or formaldehyde (for TB) see p. 98
Wash basins	Clean with detergent. Use cream cleaner for stains, scum etc. Disinfection not normally required	Disinfection may be required if contaminated. Use non-abrasive agents (b)
X-ray equipment	Damp dust with detergent solution; switch off, do not over wet, allow to dry before use	Wipe with (d) to disinfect before washing

Appendix 6.2   Decontamination of Equipment

Heat

Method	Temperature (°C)	Holding time (minutes)	Level of decontamination
Autoclave	134	3–3.5	Sterilization
	121	15	Sterilization
Sub-atmospheric steam (LTS)	73	10	Disinfection
Boilers and pasteurizers	70–100	5–10	Disinfection
Washing machines			
Bedpans	80	1	Cleaning/disinfection
Linen	65	10	Cleaning/disinfection
	71	3	Cleaning/disinfection
Others	65–100	Variable	Cleaning/disinfection

Chemical

Method and equipment 2% Glutaraldehyde	Holding time at room temperature	Level of decontamination
Gastroscopes	4 min	Disinfection
Bronchoscopes	20 min	Disinfection*
	60 min	Disinfection (known or suspected mycobacterial infection)
Cystoscopes	10 min	Disinfection
Arthroscopes	20 min	Disinfection*
Laparoscopes	180 min	Sterilization
70% Ethanol		
Gastroscopes	4 min	Disinfection
Other instruments (not endoscopes)	5–10 min	Disinfection

* High level to include M. tuberculosis

Appendix 6.3   Disinfection of cape ventilator with hydrogen peroxide

Method

1. Freshly prepared 20 volume hydrogen peroxide should be used each time. This should be made by diluting a 100 volume hydrogen perox-

ide solution 1:5 with sterile distilled water. Freshly drawn tap water may be used in areas supplied by a high quality soft mains water.

2. A flow rate of 15 l/min is required to drive a suitable nebulizer (e.g. Ohio). The direct oxygen supply can be used if the pressure is sufficient; the valve on the top of the nebulizer is set at 60% to prevent build up of pressure and release of peroxide through safety valve.

3. The ventilator should be switched on and adjusted so that respiratory volume is set at 1000 ml/respiration; the respiration rate is 25 rev/min and expiratory assistance control is set with the black spot exactly in the midway position between minimum and maximum. This is very important; failure to do this will cause a section of the expiratory circuit to remain unexposed to the aerosol. The oxygen inlet should be closed with a cap during decontamination.

   The three drainage taps should be opened and left open with the machine working for 2–3 min, then closed and the drain tap cover door closed. This should remove moisture accumulated in use which may neutralize nebulized hydrogen peroxide.

4. Hydrogen peroxide should be nebulized for 60 min with the nebulizer placed at point A (air intake) and the aerosol allowed to escape directly into the air at point B (inspiratory port). Potassium iodide indicator paper placed at point B should turn deep brown within five minutes of the process commencing.

References

Ayliffe, G.A.J. (1988) Equipment related infection risks. *Journal of Hospital Infection*, **11** (Supplement A), 279.

Ayliffe, G.A.J., Babb, J.R. and Bradley, C.R. (1986) Disinfection of endoscopes. *Journal of Hospital Infection*, **7**, 296.

Ayliffe, G.A.J., Babb, J.R., and Collins, B.J. (1974) Carpets in hospital wards. *Health and Social Services Journal*, **84**, 12.

Ayliffe, G.A.J., Babb, J.R., Davies, J.G. and Lilly, H.A. (1988) Hand disinfections: a comparison of various agents in laboratory and ward studies. *Journal of Hospital Infection*, **11**, 226.

Ayliffe, G.A.J., Babb, J.R. and Quoraishi, A.H. (1978) A test for hygienic hand disinfection. *Journal of Clinical Pathology*, **31**, 923.

Ayliffe, G.A.J., Coates, D. and Hoffman, P.N. (1984) *Chemical Disinfection in Hospitals*. PHLS, London.

Ayliffe, G.A.J., Collins, B.J. and Lowbury, E.J.L. (1966) Cleaning and disinfection of hospital floors. *British Medical Journal*, ii, 442.

Ayliffe, G.A.J., Collins, B.J., and Lowbury, E.J.L. (1967) Ward floors and other surfaces as reservoirs of hospital infection. *Journal of Hygiene (London)*, **2**, 181.

Babb, J.R. and Bradley, C.R. (1989) Decontamination of endoscopes: an update. *Journal of Sterile Services Management*, **7**, 9.

Babb, J.R. and Bradley, C.R. (1991) The mechanics of endoscope disinfection. *Journal of Hospital Infection*, **17** (Supplement A) 130.

Babb, J.R., Bradley, C.R. and Ayliffe, G.A.J. (1982) A formaldehyde disinfection unit. *Journal of Hospital Infection*, **3**, 193.

Babb, J.R., Bradley, C.R., and Ayliffe, G.A.J. (1984) Comparison of automated systems for the cleaning and disinfection of flexible fibreoptic endoscopes. *Journal of Hospital Infection*, **5**, 213.

Benn, R.A.V., Dutton, A.A.C., and Tully, M. (1973) Disinfection of mechanical ventilators: an investigation using formaldehyde in a Cape Ventilator. *Anaesthesiology*, **27**, 265.

Best, M., Sattar, S.A., Springthorpe, V.S. *et al.* (1990) Efficacies of selected disinfectants against *Mycobacterium tuberculosis*. *Journal of Clinical Microbiology*, **28**, 10.

British Society of Gastroenterology. (1988) Cleaning and disinfection of equipment for gastrointestinal flexible endoscopes: interim recommendations of a working party. *Gut*, **29**, 1134.

British Thoracic Society. (1989) Bronchoscopy and infection control. *Lancet*, **ii**, 270.

Cadwallader, H.L., Bradley, C.R. and Ayliffe, G.A.J. (1990) Bacterial contamination and frequency of changing ventilator circuitry. *Journal of Hospital Infection*, **15**, 65.

Central Sterilizing Club. (1986a) *Working Party Report No. 1. Washer/disinfector Infection Machines*. Obtainable from the Hospital Infection Research Laboratory.

Central Sterilizing Club. (1986b) *Working Party Report No. 2. Sterilization and Disinfection of Heat Labile Equipment*. Obtainable from the Hospital Infection Research Laboratory.

Collins, B.J. (1979) How to have carpeted luxury. *Health and Social Services Journal*, September 28th.

Craven, D.I., Connolly, M.G., Lichtenberg, D.A. *et al.* (1982) Contamination of mechanical ventilators with tubing change every 24 or 48 hours. *New England Journal of Medicine*, **306**, 1505.

Danforth, D., Nicolle, L.E., Hume, K. *et al.* (1987) Nosocomial infections on nursing units with floors cleaned with a disinfectant compared with detergent. *Journal of Hospital Infection*, **10**, 229.

Deverill, C.E.A., Dutt, K.K. (1980) Methods of decontamination of anaesthetic equipment: daily sessional exchange of circuits. *Journal of Hospital Infection*, **1**, 165.

Dyas, A. and Das, B.C. (1985) The activity of glutaraldehyde against *Clostridium difficile*. *Journal of Hospital Infection*, **6**, 41.

Hanson, P.J.V., Gor, D., Jeffries, D.J. *et al.* (1989) Chemical inactivation of HIV on surfaces. *British Medical Journal*, **298**, 862.

Hanson, P.J.V., Gor, D., Jeffries, D.J. and Collins, J.V. (1990) Elimination of high titre HIV from fibreoptic endoscopes. *Gut*, **31**, 657.

Judd, P.A., Tomlin, P.J., Whitby, J.L. *et al.* (1968) Disinfection of ventilators by ultrasonic nebulisation. *Lancet*, **2**, 1019.

Lawrence, J.C. (1985) The bacteriology of burns. *Journal of Hospital Infection*, **6** (supplement 13), 3.

Lilly, H.A. Lowbury, E.J.L., Wilkins, M.D. and Zaggy, A. (1979) Delayed antimicrobial effects of skin disinfection by alcohol. *Journal of Hygiene* **82**, 497.

Lowbury, E.J.L. (1991) Special problems in hospital antisepsis in *Principles and*

Practice of Disinfection, Sterilization and Preservation (eds. Russell, A.D., Hugo, W.B., Ayliffe, G.A.J.) Blackwell Scientific Publications. Oxford.

Lowbury, E.J.L. and Lilly, H.A. (1973) Use of 4% chlorhexidine detergent solution (Hibiscrub) and other methods of skin disinfection. *British Medical Journal*, **1**, 510.

Lowbury, E.J.L. and Lilly, H.A. (1975) Gloved hands as applicator of antiseptic to operation sites. *Lancet*, **ii**, 153.

Lowbury, E.J.L., Lilly, H.A. and Ayliffe, G.A.J. (1974) Preoperative disinfection of surgeons hands: Use of alcoholic solutions and effects of gloves on skin flora. *British Medical Journal*, **IV**, 369.

Maki, D.G., Alvarado, C.J. Hassemer, C.A. *et al.* (1982) Relation of the inanimate environment to endemic nosocomial infections. *New England Journal of Medicine*, **307**, 1562.

Maurer, I.M. (1985) *Hospital Hygiene*, 3rd edn. Wright PSG, Bristol.

Murray, S.M., Freiman, J.S., Vickery, K. *et al.* (1991) Duck hepatitis B virus: a model to assess efficacy of disinfectants against hepadnavirus infectivity. *Epidemiology and Infection*, **106**, 435.

Rotter, M. (1984) Hygienic hand disinfection. *Infection Control*, **5**, 18.

Rutala, W.A. (1990) APIC guidelines for selection and use of disinfectants. *American Journal of Infection Control*, **18**, 99.

Sattar, S.A., Springthorpe, V.S., Karim, Y. *et al.* (1989) Chemical disinfection of non-porous inanimate surfaces experimentally contaminated with four human pathogenic viruses. *Epidemiology and Infection*, **102**, 493.

Taylor, L.J. (1978) An evaluation of handwashing techniques. *Nursing Times*, **74** (54), 108.

Tyler, R., Ayliffe, G.A.J., and Bradley, C.R. (1990) Virucidal activity of disinfectants: studies with the poliovirus. *Journal of Hospital Infection*, **15**, 339.

Williams, J. D., Waltho, C. A., Ayliffe, G.A.J. and Lowbury E.J.L. (1967) Trials of five antibacterial creams in the control of nasal carriage of *Staphylococcus aureus*. *Lancet*, **2**, 390.

7 Prevention of infection in wards I: Ward procedures and dressing techniques

7.1 Introduction

This chapter and the next deal with the methods by which patients in hospital wards can be protected against microorganisms from various sources, in particular from other patients, and transmitted by staff, by contaminated objects (fomites) and by air. Surgical patients are exposed to special hazards of infection during the relatively short period of the operation, and the prevention of these hazards is the subject of Chapter 11. Infection may occur also in the ward, where the period of exposure of some unhealed wounds may be prolonged. A clean, closed wound is unlikely to become infected after 24 hours following the operation, and exposure for change of dressing is usually short; but the risk may be greater and more prolonged in some patients, especially those with drained or open wounds and with burns. Patients with septic lesions and other infective conditions will often be nursed in the same ward as patients who are at special risk of infection because of inadequate natural defences. The largest reservoir of infective microorganisms is among patients, and the most important mode of transfer is by the staff who have contact with them. It is therefore important to ensure that adequate measures of protection are used.

Control of infection in wards, as in operating theatres, involves the application of the principles of aseptic and hygienic techniques in the numerous details of patient care. It involves also the design, equipment and ventilation of the ward in such a way that patients may, when necessary, be placed in isolation, to prevent infection passing from them or to them. Research and experience have shown that good buildings, though important, are less vital to the prevention of infection than good aseptic and hygienic procedures; but patient isolation methods involve both structures and procedures. Isolation methods are discussed in Chapter 8. This chapter is concerned with the general principles of aseptic and hygienic technique which apply in all hospital wards; the requirements of special departments and some individual procedures are considered in Chapters 16–18. Examples of methods for performing various aseptic procedures are presented in Appendix 7.1, at the end of this chapter.

7.2   The 'Nursing process'

The prevention of infection is the responsibility of all staff, but particularly of those responsible for direct patient care. The 'nursing process' is a system in which a problem-solving approach is applied to individual patient care and is now commonly used in the UK. The basic elements of the 'process' – assessment, planning, implementation and evaluation – are particularly relevant to the prevention of infection and its spread (Bowell 1990).

7.2.1   ASSESSMENT

The patient may have a transmissible infection or be at 'high' risk of acquiring an infection.

7.2.2   PLANNING

Requirements for preventing the spread of infection from the patient or for protecting the patient against infection are incorporated in the care plan. These would include short and long term goals.

7.2.3   IMPLEMENTATION

This should ensure that effective methods, such as handwashing, the wearing of protective clothing etc. are applied to ensure the goals can be attained. It would also include the psychological aspects, for example if the patient is in single-room accommodation.

7.2.4   EVALUATION

The success of the plan and its outcome is assessed. This could be the absence of spread of infection to others, or the absence of acquired infection in a catheterized patient. The probable reasons for any failures should be determined.

The systematic approach to patient care should enable problems to be more readily identified and effective control measures to be introduced.

7.3   Nursing 'models'

A nursing 'model' is a complete framework of all aspects of the care to be delivered to the individual ensuring nothing is missed or overlooked.

When using a nursing model, it must be flexible and take into account the disease process and associated problems, if control or prevention of infection is to be achieved in the ward setting. Infection control can be incorporated into all commonly used nursing models (Worsley *et al.* 1990).

7.4   Ward structure and facilities

Spread of infection (particularly staphylococcal) is more likely to occur in large open wards. Wards should, therefore, be subdivided in units of four to six beds with complete separation from other areas and with adequate single rooms for isolation of infected patients. Although single rooms for 25% of patients have been recommended, a smaller number is probably sufficient (e.g. four single rooms for a 30-bedded adult ward), depending on whether a hospital isolation unit is available. Patients with communicable infections, including staphylococcal sepsis if caused by an epidemic or highly resistant strain, should be given priority for isolation if single room accommodation is limited, but an isolation unit with designated staff is preferred. To further reduce risks of cross-infection, bed centres should be at least eight feet apart and over-crowding with extra beds should be avoided. A day room for walking patients will also reduce the number of patients in the clinical area. Toilet facilities should be adequate and provided with handwashing basins. Since patients today are allowed out of bed much earlier than formerly, washing facilities should be considerably increased. Separate toilet and handwashing facilities should be available for the staff. Showers should be provided whenever possible, in addition to or preferably instead of baths. Handwashing basins for the staff should be readily available in the clinical area and supplied with paper towels of good quality. Hot air hand dryers are slow, often noisy and should be avoided in clinical areas. Sluice rooms should be adequate in size with suitable storage space for bedpans, urinals and cupboards for urine testing and other equipment. Storage areas for cleaning equipment should be provided. Wards should be kept in a good state of repair and provided with readily cleanable surfaces.

7.5   Aseptic techniques

The terms **asepsis** and **aseptic technique** are used to describe methods which have been developed to prevent contamination of wounds or other susceptible sites (e.g. the urinary tract) in the operating theatre, the ward and other treatment areas, by ensuring that only sterile objects and fluids will make contact with these sites and that the risks of airborne contamination are minimized. When first introduced, the term *asepsis* was used to mean the provision of heat-sterilized instruments and equipment in the operating theatre, to supersede *antisepsis* by immersion of instruments etc. in a phenolic solution as previously used by Lister. Today the word asepsis is not used in contrast with antisepsis, but includes antiseptic methods. Antiseptics are solutions used in skin disinfection (e.g. chlorhexidine, povidone iodine and alcohol). Any procedure which involves penetration of the skin, exposure of wounds or instrumentation (except that of the gastrointestinal tract) should be carried out with sterile instruments and materials supplied by an SSD, using a non-touch technique with forceps or gloves. The details of aseptic technique vary to some extent from hospital to hospital.

7.6 Masks

The principle role of the mask is to protect the patient against organisms dispersed from the upper respiratory tract of the nurse or other attendant. Most of the bacteria dispersed on sneezing or talking come from the mouth and are normally harmless to wounds (though occasionally *Strep. pyogenes* and *Staph. aureus* may be present in the mouth). *Staph. aureus* is commonly present in the nose, but the nose disperses very few bacteria into the air. *Staph. aureus* is commonly shed into the environment on skin scales; a mask will do little to reduce dissemination of these and in fact the rubbing of the mask against the skin of the face may actually increase dispersal.

Experimental studies and trials have indicated that masks contribute little or nothing to the protection of patients in wards against infection, and their routine use for aseptic ward procedures, including postoperative dressings is, therefore, unnecessary (Taylor 1980).

If a mask is thought to be necessary, most of the commercially available types will reduce the risk of impaction of bacteria from the mouth and may be considered satisfactory, but a 'filter' type mask is preferred for barrier nursing if considered necessary to protect the nurse against respiratory pathogens. Masks should be changed when they become moist.

7.7 Protective clothing

Clothing may be of some importance in the contact transfer of *Staph. aureus*. The front of the apron is the area most often contaminated. It is, therefore, rational for the nurse to wear protective clothing while she carries out aseptic procedures, so as to prevent the transfer of bacteria from her uniform to the patients, and also to prevent contamination of her uniform. It is unnecessary to change the apron between patients following routine procedures other than aseptic procedures on infected patients, except in high risk units (see also Chapter 8 for procedures on infected patients).

Cotton is permeable to bacteria and moisture, and a water-repellent apron, impermeable to bacteria, is more appropriate. A single-use plastic apron worn during dressings and other aseptic procedures is cheap and convenient. There is little advantage in wearing a gown rather than a plastic apron because the nurse's shoulders and upper arms are unlikely to become contaminated in normal circumstances (Babb *et al.* 1983); however, a gown may be preferred for lifting infected patients, or for nursing neonates, and should be changed daily or when contaminated.

7.8 Hands

The hands of nurses, doctors, physiotherapists and others who handle patients are probably the most important vehicles of cross-infection, and it is essential that effective methods should be used to minimize this hazard. Handwashing with a good technique covering all surface of the hands at the right time is more important than the agent used or the length of time of handwashing. In tests of handwashing with a dye it was found that over half the nurses did not wash some part of the thumb, and many also missed areas of the finger tips and palm (Taylor 1978). These are the areas most likely to come into contact with patients and equipment and to transfer infection. A standardized technique for handwashing should therefore be used (Chapter 6; Ayliffe *et al.* 1978). A satisfactory handwash or alcoholic rub can be completed by this method in 10–20 seconds. Studies have indicated that handwashing by both nurses and doctors is too infrequent. However, excessive handwashing will damage the skin and increase the likelihood of hand colonization with potential pathogens. Hands should be washed on arrival for duty and on leaving the ward, after attending patients in source isolation, before attending patients in protective isolation and before and after aseptic procedures and attending infants and before handling food.

An unpublished study on hand contamination after various procedures showed the following from 1–10 in order of risk; procedures 1–5 were least likely to be associated with significant hand contamination, whereas procedures 6–10 were most likely and required a handwash:

1. handling sterile or disinfected materials;
2. handling materials not handled by patients, e.g. charts etc;

3. handling items minimally handled by patients, e.g. furniture;
4. handling materials in close contact with bedding of non-infected patients;
5. minimal patient contact, e.g. taking pulse;
6. handling moist objects likely to be contaminated, e.g. cleaning materials;
7. handling bedding from infected patients, bed-bathing of any patient, handling of bedpans and urinals;
8. handling secretions or excretions or body fluids;
9. handling secretions or excretions from infected patients or body fluids;
10. direct contact with infected patients.

It is not possible to lay down absolute rules and the requirement for handwashing must be assessed in the individual circumstance. Where handwashing is difficult or inconvenient, clean, but not necessarily sterile, disposable gloves may be used to prevent gross contamination of the hands; they should be used also for handling highly contaminated objects (e.g. drainage tubes, endotracheal tubes) or patients (e.g. those who are incontinent of faeces). For aseptic procedures, sterile gloves or forceps should be used.

Since the emergence of HIV, gloves are often recommended for the handling of all blood and body fluids (often termed 'universal precautions'). This can be expensive and is often unnecessary in hospitals where the risk is low (see Chapter 10). Organisms are more readily removed from gloves than from hands by washing, but the value of repeatedly washing gloves rather than changing between patients remains controversial (Doebeling *et al.* 1988; Newsom and Rowland 1989) and depends on the purpose. Unless this is carefully carried out organisms may remain on washed gloves (as on hands) and gloves may be damaged on repeated washing. Hands should be washed when gloves are removed after handling an infected patient or potentially contaminated objects. However, this should be unnecessary if a careful removal technique of undamaged gloves is used. A further problem is that even unused gloves may have small defects and may allow penetration of organisms, therefore any cuts or lesions on the hands should be covered.

In the course of their work nurses and doctors will touch many objects contaminated with staphylococci and other organisms capable of causing wound infection; they can easily transfer pathogenic organisms, which have just been picked up from an infected patient, to the next patient whom the nurse or doctor visits in the ward. Such recently acquired contaminants are 'transient' bacteria which are not growing on the skin and which, unlike the 'resident' bacteria, can be greatly reduced in numbers by washing with soap and water (Centers for Disease Control 1981); disinfection with 70% ethanol or isopropanol is more effective (Rotter 1984). Some of these bacteria which remain on the skin may become 'residents'. For most purposes in the ward a thorough wash with soap and water is adequate. Antimicrobial preparations (see Chapter 6) may be indicated in special units such as intensive care, infectious diseases and special care baby units, and in general wards during an outbreak of infection. Some antimicrobial agents, such as chlorhexidine, have a persistent effect which may reduce transient organisms, but the value of this effect in prevention of transfer of infection remains uncertain (Ayliffe *et al*. 1988). The use of 70% alcohol with an emollient, with or without an additional antimicrobial agent, is of particular value in wards lacking convenient handwashing facilities or during dressing or napkin-changing rounds. A suitable routine for a ward would be soap for general handwashing, with an alcoholic or antiseptic detergent preparation available for special procedures. During an outbreak of a non-enveloped virus infection, washing with soap and water before the application of 70% ethanol is advised since some viruses, e.g. enteroviruses, are resistant to isopropanol and relatively resistant to ethanol. However, 70% ethanol is effective against rotaviruses.

Soap containers used on wards may be a source of contamination (see Chapter 6). Containers for bar soap should be easy to clean and regularly cleaned. Liquid soap dispensers should be regularly cleaned and maintained and antimicrobial liquid soap preparations should preferably be wall-mounted and operated by elbow, wrist or foot. A replaceable cartridge or equivalent will reduce risks of contamination when compared with refilling the original container. Paper towels are advised for drying hands and should have good drying properties. If hand taps are used, these can be turned off with a paper towel after the hands have been washed.

7.9 Wound dressings

The place where wounds are dressed will be determined by the structure of the ward and the availability of single rooms and whether the hospital has central treatment rooms. If the design of the dressing room is poor and without mechanical ventilation, dressing all wounds in one small room increases the risk of infection by creating a high level of airborne contamination when the wounds are exposed. A single room, preferably with an extractor fan or other mechanical ventilation, should be used for source isolation of patients with infected wounds, priority being given to those infected or colonized by multiple-resistant strains of *Staph. aureus* or with open wounds (see Chapter 8). These patients may then have their wounds dressed in their own rooms. Dressings of small wounds may reasonably be changed at the bedside in an open ward, if care is taken to avoid dispersal of bacteria from dressings that are being removed; such procedures usually cause little increase in airborne contamination by wound pathogens. For larger wounds and burns it is desirable to change dressings in a mechanically ventilated dressing room or operating theatre, if source isolation of the patient in a mechanically ventilated single room is not available.

If a wound dressing or treatment room is considered necessary, it should be ventilated with eight or more air changes per hour (a burns dressing station should have twenty air changes per hour). The doors should be large enough for a bed to pass through. At least ten minutes should be allowed after use by an infected patient, and the cover on the couch should be changed. The ventilation system should be regularly checked by the engineers (e.g. at least six monthly). Even if the room is adequate in all respects, it may be impracticable and time-consuming to move some patients in their beds to a dressing station (e.g. those in traction beds). In addition, where team nursing or patient allocation to individual nurses is practised, one dressing room may be inadequate.

Since the cost of a correctly ventilated room is high and the evidence of its value (except for burns) is limited, it would seem to be rarely worthwhile incorporating a plenum-ventilated dressing room either in a new general ward or an old, open general surgical ward. However, a small treatment room with a limited ventilation system (e.g. extractor fan) may be useful for preparing trolleys and for carrying out minor procedures on walking patients. This system should be adequate if single rooms or an isolation unit are available for patients with wounds infected by organisms likely to be transmitted in the air (e.g. antibiotic-resistant *Staph. aureus*).

Some new hospitals have central treatment rooms. A suite of ventilated single rooms is available for dressings, and for aseptic and other procedures usually done in the ward, e.g. lumbar puncture and for endoscopies and laser procedures. It has the advantage of a controlled environment, adequate and appropriate supplies, experienced trained staff and is available 24 hours a day for wards, outpatients and day cases. It is convenient to work in and removes the problem of not doing aseptic procedures while cleaning or bed-making is in progress. It has the disadvantage of fragmenting care, but patients do not perceive this to be a problem. There is also a potential risk of transfer of infection between wards, but if techniques are good this should not occur.

7.9.1   DRESSING MATERIALS (*Drug and Therapeutics Bulletin* 1991; *Lancet* 1991)

The main functions of a dressing are to protect the wound from trauma or bacterial contamination, to promote healing and prevent the transfer of organisms from an infected wound to other sites on the same or other patients. It should absorb excess exudate, but maintain warm and moist conditions at the wound surface to improve healing and should allow gaseous exchange. It should be impermeable to bacteria. Gauze swabs are not the most suitable of dressing materials as they tend to adhere to the wound and become soaked through with exudate. The healing process is thus disturbed and once 'strike through' of exudate has occurred there is no barrier to microorganisms to or from the environment.

Dressing materials vary in their properties and require selection appropriate to the nature of the wound. Factors to be considered in the selection of dressings or topical agents are size of wound, site, depth and the presence of slough or infection. The progress of the wound should be accurately recorded. Clean, undrained surgical wounds seldom require dressing if they can be protected against contact and friction. Semi-permeable adhesive films are useful since they are permeable to water vapour but not to bacteria and allow the wound to be observed without removing the dressing. They can be used for clean superficial wounds and for covering intravenous insertion sites. They are also useful for sealing infected lesions during surgery – for example, for enclosing a pressure sore during a hip replacement operation. However, these films would not be appropriate on wounds with excessive exudate, although it is possible to aspirate exudate with a syringe and needle. A wide range of other dressing materials is available, including gel and colloid dressings. These are occlusive or semi-occlusive (Hutchinson and Lawrence 1991), adhere to dry skin and form a gel with moisture on the wound surface. The evidence from good controlled trials on the effectiveness of these dressings is limited and it is difficult to make firm recommendations. These newer products tend to be expensive, but improved healing may reduce time spent in hospital or off work.

Wounds can be conveniently classified as black (necrotic), yellow (infected or containing slough), and red (granulating).

The dressing required differs with each of these categories. Hydrocolloid dressings are useful for necrotic, sloughing or granulating, but not usually for infected wounds. They may also prevent infection. Hydrogels can be used on black necrotic or infected wounds and provide good healing conditions. Alginate dressings are used to remove exudate (e.g. in 'yellow' and infected wounds) and assist wound healing. Dextranomers (e.g. as beads) may be appropriate for sloughing wounds or infected wounds with exudate. Foam dressings (e.g. silicone foam) are slightly absorbent and can be used on deep open granulating wounds.

7.9.2   CLEANING OF WOUNDS AND TOPICAL AGENTS

Clean operation wounds should not require routine cleaning, although the removal of blood or other exudate may reduce the presence of nutrients which may aid bacterial growth. Sterile normal saline is adequate for this purpose. The technique of cleaning is of doubtful relevance and most methods only re-distribute organisms present in the wound and on the adjacent skin. The use of disinfectants is also of doubtful value but some, such as 'Savlon', are effective cleaning agents for dirty wounds. Hypochlorite solutions (e.g. Eusol) are often used as debriding agents, but are toxic to cells and should preferably not be used at all or at least for only a short period. Some dressing materials (see previous section) are preferable for removing necrotic materials and slough and do not impair healing. The disadvantages of hypo-chlorites also apply but to a lesser extent to hydrogen peroxide and iodophors. Chlorhexidine is less toxic to cells and has been shown to reduce the emergence of infection in minor burns. Silver sulphadiazine is commonly used to prevent infections in burns. There is some evidence that the wound exudate contains antibacterial properties and complete removal of all exudate may be undesirable. The role of bacteria in delaying the healing of pressure sores and ulcers is also uncertain and it is generally unnecessary to apply antibacterial agents, although there is some evidence that healing may be delayed in the presence of large numbers of organisms (i.e. over 10^5/gm or sq cm). Systemic anti-biotics may be necessary in the presence of clinical sepsis and the possibility of an anaerobic infection should be considered. Topical anti-biotics, particularly those used for systemic treatment (e.g. gentamicin and fusidic acid), should be avoided as resistance is likely to emerge. However, if topical antibiotics are considered necessary, treatment should be limited to 5–7 days. Aminoglycosides such as neomycin may also be associated with hypersensitivity if used for long periods. The use of mupirocin should also be restricted as resistance may emerge and if used the time of application should be restricted as with other agents.

7.9.3   DRESSING TECHNIQUES

These are described in Appendix 7.1. They may require modification in the light of further studies or under special circumstances (Kelso 1989). Some general principles are considered here.

It is usual to recommend that ward cleaning should cease 30 minutes, and curtains should be drawn 10 minutes, before a dressing is started, but the evidence suggests that the recommended routine cleaning methods (see Chapter 6) do not significantly increase the numbers of airborne organisms. Certain other procedures may disperse much larger numbers of organisms into the air. These include bed-making, high dusting and changing curtains. It is often impractical to stipulate that all these activities must cease while dressings are in progress, particularly on wards where allocation of patients to individual nurses or team nursing is practised, as is now generally the case. Nevertheless, it is clearly desirable that cleaning activities should be avoided if possible during dressing sessions and, if unavoidable, reduced to a minimum. It is more practical to ensure that these procedures do not take place in the immediate vicinity of the bed where the dressing is being done. To reduce opportunities for airborne contamination to a minimum, a wound should be exposed for the minimum time and dressings should be removed carefully and placed quickly in a bag and sealed; a large paper or plastic bag should be available for disposal of large dressings.

Sterile Services Department (SSD) packs should be supplied in dispenser racks or boxes, stored in a preparation room and transferred to the dressing trolley when required. All instruments should be supplied by the SSD and chemical disinfection before use should now be unnecessary. The dressing trolley top should be thoroughly cleaned at the beginning of a dressing round with 70% alcohol or a clear soluble phenolic disinfectant. The top of the trolley must be dry before the sterilized paper pack is placed on it. Repeated cleaning of the trolley top during a dressing round is unnecessary.

An aseptic or non-touch technique is important. Forceps are usually used, but disposable gloves (or a plastic bag, enclosing a hand) could with advantage be used more often, particularly for removing large, contaminated dressings. There is evidence to indicate that ungloved hands, previously disinfected with an alcohol-based hand disinfectant, are more convenient than forceps and do not expose the patient to an increased infection risk (Thomlinson 1987). Dispersal of organisms may be further reduced by inverting the glove (or plastic bag) over the dressing and discarding both together.

The dressing pack should be opened carefully with washed hands as instructed. The paper working surface should lie flat on the trolley top and should never be flattened with the fingers. Forceps used for removal of stitches or for inserting safety-pins in drains should be capable of holding the sutures or the pin firmly; otherwise gloved fingers should be used.

If dressings on clean and dry wounds without drainage are thought to be necessary, they should be left in place until the stitches are removed unless there are signs of infection or leakage. These wounds are unlikely to become infected in the ward, and, depending on surgical approval, may be left after the first 24–48 hours without a covering dressing. Drained wounds should be covered with a dressing until the drainage wound is healed and dry. This may not be necessary with very small drains with a closed drainage system (e.g. 'Redivac') until after removal. Drains should not be used unless absolutely necessary and should be removed as quickly as possible. If required at all, drainage must be adequate and may, therefore, require large drains, but 'Redivac' and other small tube drains are less likely to be associated with acquired infection. Contaminated wounds (e.g. after colectomy, abdominoperineal excision of the rectum, and operations on pelvic abscess), though initially infected with the patient's own sensitive organisms, may acquire antibiotic-resistant hospital strains if care is not taken with aseptic techniques. All discharging wounds should be adequately covered, and dressings must be changed immediately if they are soaked; organisms readily penetrate wet dressings.

Septic wounds and contaminated wounds (e.g. colostomy) should be dressed at the end of the dressing list. Sutures should be removed at the beginning of the list. The use of absorbable sutures may allow a patient to be sent home earlier. Any procedure which reduces the patient's time in hospital, either pre- or postoperatively, will reduce the hazards of infection.

7.10   Injections

Several studies have shown that the risk of infection is minimal following an injection without prior disinfection of the skin. Skin disinfection is often not recommended for insulin injection in diabetics and some hospitals have given up the practice except before intravenous injections. Nevertheless, many hospital patients are particularly susceptible to infection, for example elderly patients in whom heavy skin contamination with Gram-negative bacilli or *Staph. aureus* is possible, particularly in the area of the upper thigh. Since it is difficult to know which patients are at special risk until adequate trials on hospital patients of all age groups have been carried out, it is recommended that the skin of the injection site should be thoroughly cleaned by rubbing with 70% ethanol or isopropanol and allowed to dry. This is relatively inexpensive, and disinfection for some procedures and not others may cause confusion.

7.11 Intravenous infusions

The setting up of intravenous infusions should be carried out with strict aseptic precautions (Greene 1990). The hands of the operator should be disinfected with an antiseptic detergent or preferably with 70% ethanol or 60% isopropanol. The skin of the infusion site should also be thoroughly disinfected with 70% ethanol, or isopropanol, with or without added chlorhexidine, povidone-iodine or triclosan and allowed to dry. The site should not be palpated after disinfection. Shaving of the skin should be avoided if possible. Disposable gloves should be worn by the operator and assistant if contamination of the skin with blood is likely and always if the patient is at increased risk of having HIV or HBV infection. The wearing of a mask is unnecessary but a disposable or other sterilized plastic apron should be worn. For central venous catheterization, sterile gloves should be worn in addition to a disposable gown and, preferably, should be carried out in an operating theatre with full surgical precautions. This is particularly desirable if tunnelling of the catheter under the skin is required.

The infusion container should be inspected for faults, leaks, cloudiness or particulate matter before connecting to the drip set and, if any of these are present, it must be discarded. It should be recognized that the fluid can remain clear despite the presence of significant numbers of organisms (Phillips *et al.* 1976). The rubber plug or diaphragm must be swabbed with 70% alcohol before the cannula is introduced on the infrequent occasions when a bottle rather than a bag is used. When a bottle is used a single-use sterile air inlet is inserted. Check that the cotton wool plug is present in the air inlet and if wet at any time the plug should be changed.

The insertion site should be covered with a sterile dressing. Either a non-woven or a transparent semi-permeable dressing can be used which is changed every 48–72 hours or the life of the catheter after dressing (Maki and Ringer 1987). The semi-permeable dressing allows good observation of the site, but can be associated with an increased growth of organisms on the skin underneath the dressing.

The insertion site must be inspected daily to detect phlebitis or infection. The value of treating the site at the time of a dressing change with an antibacterial agent is uncertain, although colonization of the cannula has been reduced by the use of a neomycin, bacitracin and polymyxin ointment (Maki and Bond 1981). Spraying with povidone-iodine or chlorhexidine or applying a chlorhexidine or povidone-iodine solution or ointment is sometimes recommended. Reduction of colonisation has also been reported with 2% mupirocin applied after skin disinfection and before insertion of the cannula (Hill *et al.* 1990), but selection of resistant organisms could be a problem.

The intravenous line should be securely anchored. The giving set should be changed every 48–72 hours and immediately after giving blood or lipids. The bags or bottles should be changed at least every 24 hours, and preferably every 12 hours. Peripheral cannulae should be re-sited every 48–72 hours if suitable alternative sites are available.

Peripheral cannulae should be removed when the earliest signs of infection or phlebitis are observed and the catheter tip should be cultured. The skin around the catheter site should be disinfected with 70% alcohol before removal. Central venous catheters should similarly be removed if there are signs of infection, although in some instances may be left *in situ* or even replaced in the same site using a guide wire; appropriate antibiotics are given. Blood culture should be taken at another site.

Although infection is usually caused by skin organisms colonizing the outside of the cannula, it can arise from organisms gaining entrance to the system. A closed system should be maintained as carefully as possible. Therapeutic substances should preferably be added to the infusate in the pharmacy in a laminar flow cabinet. Nevertheless, trained medical or nursing staff can often more conveniently carry out this procedure in the ward. Provided the fluid is used immediately, the risk of infection is small. Most intravenous fluids will not support the growth of organisms normally present in the air. The risk of infection is increased by the use of three way taps and injection ports, but the use of protective caps and cleaning with 70% alcohol before injection will reduce the hazard. Multi-lumen catheters are sometimes convenient, but the risk of infection may be slightly increased. There is some evidence that an antiseptic-impregnated cuff (e.g. with silver) may reduce the infection rate in central venous catheters (Maki *et al.* 1988).

In-line filters reduce the incidence of phlebothrombosis and prevent the access of bacteria. However, studies on the prevention of clinical infection have shown variable results (Spencer 1990). Their use may be considered for patients particularly at risk. Parenteral hyperalimentation therapy is now commonly used. The risk of infection is particularly great because of the possibility of bacterial or fungal growth in the fluid. Few organisms grow in saline or dextrose-saline, but Gram-negative bacilli, and especially yeasts, are able to grow in some of these solutions. Prevention of infection depends on scrupulous aseptic techniques both in inserting the cannula and subsequent daily care. Infection can be minimized if central catheters are inserted by an experienced operator and subsequently managed by a trained IV team. The fluid should be used immediately, but if not should be kept at 4°C and should be administered within 24 hours.

7.12 Urinary catheters

7.12.1 MANAGEMENT OF INDWELLING CATHETERS

Bacteria enter the bladder through the lumen of the catheter or between the catheter and wall of the urethra. The latter is the more difficult to prevent (Slade and Gillespie 1985; Glenister 1990). The likelihood of infection increases with length of time of catheterization and catheters should be removed as soon as possible, preferably within a few days following urological surgery. Urethral catheterization may be avoided in some patients by suprapubic drainage, or by the use of absorbent pads to avoid the necessity for artificial drainage.

It has been demonstrated that with closed drainage infection can be prevented for several days. A continuous unbroken connection is required extending from the urethral catheter to the receptacle. However, even this system does not remain closed, since the bag must be drained at intervals, allowing possible entrance of bacteria. It is suggested that silicone catheters are preferable for long term catheterization as they are less irritant. Teflon and polyvinylchloride catheters can be used for intermediate periods (4–6 weeks), but latex catheters are adequate for short term use. Drainage bags with a tap are now most frequently used but great care is necessary in handling and emptying. Most of the so-called non-return valves allow bacteria to ascend into the bag and into the tubing above, particularly if the bag is tipped upside down or sat on by the patient. The bag should be kept below bladder level, but not on the floor; drainage should not be obstructed. Bags vary in design with non-return valves, drip chambers and different type of tap etc., but design improvements may considerably increase the cost without necessarily reducing infection. The addition of a disinfectant to the bag remains of uncertain value and cannot be recommended on available evidence. An experimental study has shown that organisms deposited on the outside of the tap can reach the patient end of the catheter in several days (Bradley *et al.* 1986). Hands should therefore be washed prior to emptying a bag. When emptying the bag, the nurse's hands are often heavily contaminated with Gram-negative bacilli (over 10^6/ml) which may be incompletely removed by handwashing. Wearing of disposable gloves is recommended, one pair for each patient, and the use of alcohol for hand disinfection after emptying each bag. The bag should be emptied into a separate disinfected or disposable container for each patient. Some Gram-negative bacilli, such as *Klebsiella* spp., may survive better than others in a dry environment and on hands (Casewell and Phillips 1977).

Specimens for culture should be collected using a syringe and needle after thoroughly cleaning the sample port with 70% alcohol. The closed system should not be broken to collect samples and samples should not be collected from the bag.

Irrigation of the bladder should be avoided if possible. There is little evidence that irrigation with an antiseptic is of value in preventing or treating an infection. If irrigation is necessary to remove or prevent blood clots postoperatively, it should be carried out as part of the closed drainage system using a three-way Foley catheter.

Infection in catheterized patients mainly occurs by the spread of organisms along the outside of the catheter. Applications of disinfectants or topical antibiotics to the catheter-meatal junction has had limited success in preventing infection by this route (Classon *et al*. 1991). However, daily catheter care with sterile saline would seem to be a reasonable hygienic measure. The incorporation of an antimicrobial (e.g. silver compounds or antibiotics) into the catheter material would seem to be a promising approach as suggested for central venous catheters (Maki *et al*. 1988), but as yet a proven method suitable for routine use has not been commercially produced.

The use of systemic prophylactic antibiotics to cover the insertion of the catheter or the period of urological surgery remains controversial. However, patients with infected urine at the time of operation or catheterization should be treated with the appropriate antibiotic.

Urinary tract infection is the commonest cause of hospital-acquired infection and is usually associated with catheterization. Although some patients with in-dwelling catheters remain free from bacteriuria for long periods, a catheter care regime which will consistently prevent infection has not been defined. Nevertheless, the present recommendations should be carefully followed and the catheter removed as soon as possible.

7.13 Collection of clinical specimens for laboratory examination

Hazards of infection, both to patients and staff, occur during collection of specimens, during transport to the laboratory and during examination in the laboratory. The last of these hazards is discussed in Chapter 17 (also Health Advisory Committee, 1991). The following notes are not a guide to techniques for collecting laboratory specimens, but a consideration of infection hazards in the collection and delivery of specimens and ways in which they may be prevented.

Faulty technique during collection may result in inadequate, misleading or delayed laboratory reports which may affect a patient's treatment, including management of infection. During collection, especially of urine specimens, the patient may become infected. The nurse may be infected by contamination of the hands or clothing or by inhalation of infected aerosol material during transfer to the containers. During transit the person carrying the specimen may be infected by contaminants on the outside of the container, or through leakage or breakage of the container. In addition the environment may become contaminated during these procedures and lead to an indirect spread of infection. Laboratory staff receiving unlabelled, potentially hazardous material (e.g. sputum from a patient with suspected pulmonary tuberculosis, or blood from a patient with suspected hepatitis) are also at risk. To ensure correct investigation, specimens should be correctly labelled and accompanying request forms should contain appropriate and adequate clinical details. Specimens should not be collected by inexperienced or untrained staff, unless under close supervision. Specimens should routinely be transported in an upright position in dual compartment plastic bags and should be labelled 'biohazard' if from high risk patients (e.g. with tuberculosis, HIV, HBV, or enteric infections).

7.13.1 SWABS

Swabs collected from infected sites such as the throat, infected surgical wounds or vagina should be transferred carefully to the swab container and inserted slowly to avoid contamination of the rim with infected material. The container should be held as near to the infected site as possible to avoid shaking infected material in the air. If a spatula has been used, this should be discarded unbroken into the waste container; the jerking movements involved in breaking a spatula may cause infected material to be released into the air. The swab should be sent to the laboratory as soon as possible. Where there is a heavy discharge of pus from an infected wound or abscess, it is preferable to send a sample of pus in a sterile universal container, rather than a swab.

7.13.2 FAECAL SPECIMENS

These should be collected from a bedpan with a small applicator or scoop, and sent as soon as possible to the laboratory. A sterile container with an integral scoop is preferred. For bacteriological examination only, a small amount of faeces, approximately the size of a pea, is all that is necessary. There is no need to fill a container. A water-proofed container with a wide mouth and a tight fitting screw cap is essential, so that the specimen can easily be placed in the container and leakage does not occur. Samples of faeces collected on bacteriological swabs (especially rectal swabs) are usually unsuitable, although a sample of liquid faeces may be collected in hospital by this method. If a rectal swab is taken, ensure that faeces are actually sampled; most anal specimens are useless.

7.13.3 URINE SPECIMENS

The organisms which are found in urinary tract infections, apart from renal tuberculosis and typhoid fever, are not usually infective for the person collecting the specimen; faulty collection technique, however, may lead to contamination of the specimen and an erroneous diagnosis of urinary infection when this does not exist. Specimens should be collected with care, following the prescribed technique exactly and sent as soon as possible to the laboratory. Examination of the urine is necessary before contaminating bacteria begin to multiply in it (i.e. within two hours). Alternatively, if delays are unavoidable, the specimen should be placed in a designated refrigerator soon after collection. A dip slide is useful if laboratory facilities are not immediately available, or boric acid can be added to the urine to prevent growth of organisms.

Infection can be transferred to a patient while a specimen is collected from an indwelling catheter, and care must be taken to avoid this.

7.13.4 ASPIRATED FLUIDS (including cerebrospinal fluid)

Equipment used to aspirate fluids from thoracic cavity, joints, cerebrospinal space, facial sinuses etc., must be supplied sterile from the SSD. An effective skin disinfectant, such as 70% ethyl alcohol, is used to prepare the site. Antibacterial agents with a strong residual effect (e.g. chlorhexidine) should preferably not be used if bacteriological examination of the aspirate is required. When cerebrospinal fluid (CSF) is aspirated from patients with certain infectious diseases (e.g. acute poliomyelitis or untreated meningococcal meningitis) a protective mask (see Chapter 9) is probably advisable; the organisms may be highly infectious, and some degree of aerosol production is almost unavoidable when screw caps and syringes are handled, although infection from this procedure is very unusual. It may also be advisable on rare occasions to wear a protective mask when aspirating purulent fluids from other sites, though in general a mask is not essential for these procedures. Wearing of gloves is not essential, but great care must be taken to avoid contamination of the skin with pus. Having collected the fluid, the operator should disconnect the needle (if any) and expel the material gently into the container, avoiding spraying of droplets or release of aerosols.

7.13.5 SPUTUM SPECIMENS

It is often difficult to obtain a specimen of sputum without contamination of the rim and outside wall of the vessel, and contamination will occur even when wide mouthed bottles are used. Some protection to porters and laboratory staff can be given if, after collection of the specimen, the rim and outside of the vessel are wiped with a paper tissue to remove any major contamination before putting on the lid of the container. The tissue should be discarded into a clinical waste bag. Should the patient be suspected of having tuberculosis, gloves should be issued for handling the container, which should be placed in a small plastic bag and sealed before transport to the laboratory.

7.13.6   BLOOD SPECIMENS

In addition to HBV and HIV infection (Chapter 10) several other infections, including typhoid fever, can be acquired from blood specimens. Blood specimens should, therefore, be regarded as potentially infected and care should be taken to avoid the dispersal of droplets which occurs when the blood is squirted vigorously into the container although there is little evidence that aerosols are an infection hazard. Before discharging blood into a container, the needle should be separated from the syringe with care using forceps or gloves. In cases of known HBV or suspected HIV infection some prefer to leave the needle attached; after carefully discharging the contents, the syringe and needle are discarded together into an approved sharps container. Needles should not be recapped unless a safe technique is available. Nozzles of syringes should not be broken before discarding. Blood samples are frequently collected with an evacuated container system rather than a syringe and needle. Blood contamination may occur at the puncture site in the plug of the container on withdrawal of the needle and should be removed with 70% ethanol. If the needle holder is contaminated with blood it should be discarded. The evacuated container should be safer than a syringe if used correctly. The hands should be thoroughly washed after taking a blood sample. Gloves should be worn when taking blood from high risk patients or routinely in high risk wards.

For protection of the patient during collection of blood specimens, only autoclaved or pre-sterilized disposable equipment should be used. When finger prick specimens are taken an individual single-use needle is essential.

7.13.7   BONE MARROW BIOPSY

The biopsy procedure can often be carried out in an open ward without special risk of infection, but the patient (e.g. with leukaemia or aplastic anaemia) is often particularly susceptible to infection, in which case a side room should be used for the procedure (if the patient is not already in protective isolation in a single-bed room). Adequate skin preparation with 70% alcohol, with or without chlorhexidine or povidone-iodine, is essential; prophylactic antibiotic cover is not necessary. Sterile gloves should be worn. A dry dressing should be placed over the puncture wound and left in place for 1–2 days.

Infective agents, including tubercle bacilli and brucella, may be present in the bone marrow; care must therefore be taken to avoid aerosols during preparation of microscope films and on expulsion of the contents of the syringe. Films should be allowed to dry naturally and not waved in the air.

7.13.8   RENAL BIOPSY/LIVER BIOPSY

These procedures are rarely followed by infection if the equipment is properly sterilized and the skin adequately disinfected. In many hospitals they are performed in open wards without hazard. Masks are unnecessary but sterile gloves should be worn. However, care is necessary when taking biopsies from a jaundiced patient (see above on blood specimens for HIV). Tests for HB_sAg in blood should be made before liver biopsy is undertaken.

7.14   Miscellaneous procedures

7.14.1   WARD EQUIPMENT

Cleaning and disinfection of many items of equipment, including nail-brushes, soap dishes, shaving equipment, thermometers, bedpans, urinals, suction, gastric aspiration and rectal equipment, beds, bedding and curtains are considered in Chapter 6.

7.14.2   WASHING AND BATHING

Patients should use wash basins in the washing areas whenever possible and their own soap, hand and bath towels and other toilet requisites. Communal towels should not be available. Bathing or showering in the bathroom is preferred to bed-baths, but if bed-baths are necessary, patients should preferably have their own individual wash bowls. If not possible, bowls should be thoroughly cleaned between use by different patients (Chapter 6). Water from the wash bowls should be emptied into a sink and not into a bucket at the bedside; bathing trolleys should not be used. Bathroom furniture should be simple, easily cleaned and reduced to a minimum and the bathroom should not be used as a store room.

Communal bath mats should not be used; patients should use a towel, unless disposable mats can be supplied. A routine of cleaning baths after each use should be instituted. Instructions as to the correct method of cleaning the bath or wash-basins should be given to staff and also to patients if they are expected to clean their own bath. Cleaning is particularly important before and after a bath if the patient has an open wound; such patients should preferably not use a bath used by pre-operative patients. Showers should overcome this problem to some extent. Salt is still commonly added to the bathwater, but the practice has little if any value as an antimicrobial measure. If a disinfectant is required (e.g. during an outbreak or as part of the treatment of infected patients and carriers) the patient should apply an antiseptic detergent to the skin. This will also disinfect the bath water. Alternatively if activity is required against *Staph. aureus*, a disinfectant may be added to the bath water (e.g. 'Sterzac' or 'Savlon' bath concentrates). Disinfection of the bath before and after use is still necessary, even if a disinfectant is used for bathing.

7.14.3 PRE-OPERATIVE PREPARATION (see Chapter 11)

Patients should be admitted preferably on the day or the day before operation and should have a shower if available rather than a bath. If a bath is required, it should be disinfected before use. Pre-operative shaving should be avoided if possible to reduce risks of infection from small cuts or abrasions. If shaving is required it should be done on the day of operation. Alternatively hair may be removed by clippers; a depilatory cream or with an electric razor. The head of the electric razor (not the motor) should be disinfected by immersion in 70% alcohol for five minutes. Shaving brushes should not be used and only experienced staff should shave patients, so that local trauma can be reduced to a minimum.

Preliminary disinfection of the operation site in the ward is not usually necessary (see also p. 105). The value of repeated bathing with chlorhexidine-detergent before prosthetic hip or cardiac surgery is controversial and is discussed in Chapter 11.

7.14.4 TREATMENT OF PRESSURE AREAS

Staff carrying out these treatments should wash their hands between patients. Patients with bedsores should be treated as infected and may be nursed in isolation, if this is indicated from bacteriological examination (e.g. if multi-resistant organisms, particularly MRSA, are isolated). All breaks in the skin should be treated as wounds. If these patients are bed-bathed, the water should be disposed of carefully without splashing since it may be heavily contaminated. Nurses carrying out these procedures should wear disposable plastic aprons. *Staph.*

aureus are often dispersed in large numbers from healed as well as open pressure sores.

7.14.5   MOUTH-CLEANING AND DENTURES

Mouth care is required to keep the mouth clean, moist and free from infection. The most effective method is to brush the teeth, gums and tongue with a soft toothbrush. Alternatively a sponge stick moistened in a sodium bicarbonate solution (1 in 60) may be used. A mouth pack can often be supplied by the SSD, the contents of which should be discarded after use or returned for processing if appropriate. The use of an antiseptic mouthwash has a limited effect on the mouth organisms and is not required as a routine. Rinsing with water is usually adequate. If glycerine and thymol is also used it should be supplied in small containers and discarded daily, since contamination of the solution is frequent. Dentures may be stored in the patient's own preparation (e.g. 'Steradent'), but if this is not available a weak hypochlorite solution may be used (e.g. 'Milton', 1 in 80). Solutions should be changed daily. Paper bags should be supplied for disposal of foam sticks, paper wipes etc.

7.14.6   RESPIRATORY SUCTION TECHNIQUES

A no-touch technique with non-sterile gloves and a sterile catheter should be used for each suction procedure. The saline solution should be discarded after each use. Suction tubing should be changed daily. In suspected cases of pulmonary or laryngeal tuberculosis, the operator should wear a mask to protect the wearer from direct contamination (see Chapters 8 and 16).

7.14.7   DISPOSAL OF SPUTUM

Sputum containers should be disposable and should be regularly discarded and the responsibility for this task should be clearly defined. Used containers and paper wipes used by patients should be placed in a plastic bag and well sealed (see also the section on secretion and exudate precautions in Chapter 8).

7.14.8   ENTERAL FEEDS

Enteral feeds may be carried out on patients unable to tolerate a normal diet. Feeds can be given as a bolus or a continuous drip monitored by a pump. There is a risk of contamination of feeds during preparation in the hospital or from inadequate refrigeration. Commercially prepared feeds are preferred (Casewell *et al.* 1982; Bastow *et al.* 1982). If special feeds are required, care must be taken to ensure they are prepared using clean equipment and careful hygienic practices. Where liquidizers are used, these must be thoroughly cleaned and dried after use.

7.14.9 EYES

Hands should be thoroughly washed before carrying out any procedures, and a no-touch technique should be used. Non-woven gauze, fluids or ointments should be sterilized (Chapter 16).

7.14.10 DEAD BODIES

Most bodies are not infective and no special care is necessary; washing the body with soap and water is adequate. Bedding can be disposed of in the usual way; mattresses and pillows may be cleaned by the recommended routine. Bed frames do not require routine cleaning. Disinfection of these or other items associated with the patient is not necessary, unless death was due to or associated with a communicable disease. For details of disposal of infected dead bodies see Chapter 9.

Appendix 7.1 Use of packs in surgical procedures

PREPARATION OF TROLLEY AND PATIENT: GENERAL PRINCIPLES

The patient is made comfortable and the screen is drawn and the procedure is explained. The nurse washes her hands or applies 70% alcohol and prepares the trolley. At the beginning of each dressing round the trolley top may be wiped with 70% alcohol and allowed to dry.

The requisite pack, supplementary packs, lotions and non-sterile items such as bandages, adhesive plaster and dressing scissors are placed on the lower shelf of the trolley. Lotions should be kept in small containers and replaced daily or preferably supplied as single use sachets.

The trolley is taken to the bedside and the patient prepared. Bed-clothes and clothing are gently removed to expose the appropriate site and the patient is placed in a suitable position.

The dressing pack is opened and the inner pack is placed in the centre of the trolley top. A bag of adequate size is fixed to the side of the trolley nearest to the patient for soiled dressings, and another bag is fixed to the opposite side for soiled and unused instruments. On completion of the procedure, instruments are placed in one bag (or directly into the used instrument container) and the unused dressings and disposables are rolled up in the paper towel covering the trolley top and placed in the soiled dressings bag.

ROUTINE DRESSING TECHNIQUE

The trolley and patient are prepared as already described. The wound should not be cleaned unnecessarily. Some antiseptics have an adverse effect on wound healing and there is evidence that the cleaning techniques traditionally used are ineffective in removing bacteria.

The inner wrap is opened, handling corners only, and forms the sterile field. Supplementary packs are opened and the contents are gently slid onto the sterile field.

The pack contents are arranged using handling forceps and handles of instruments are placed in a small defined handling area near the edge of the trolley. The lotion, if required, is poured into the gallipot.

The adhesive plaster is loosened and the dressing is removed with handling forceps, or a non-sterile glove or a plastic bag and discarded into the soiled dressing bag. The forceps (if not disposable) are placed in the other bag. The wound is more effectively cleaned with either a gloved or disinfected hand than with forceps. Clips or sutures are removed if necessary and the dressing completed using two pairs of sterile forceps or gloved hands or alcohol-rubbed bare hands (Thomlinson 1987). After securing the dressing, instruments and unused or soiled materials are placed in bags as described. If two nurses are available, the assistant prepares the patient, opens the outer bag of the pack and supplementary packs and pours the lotions. The dresser prepares the trolley and the sterile field and carries out the dressing technique.

URINARY CATHETERIZATION

The patient, trolley and sterile field are prepared as already described. In male patients the penis is held with sterile gauze, the foreskin is retracted if necessary and glans and external meatus are thoroughly cleaned with sterile saline or 'Savlodil' (see p. 70). The local anaesthetic is inserted into the urethra. The nurse opens the catheter packet and the catheter is slid into a sterile receiver. A surgical drape is placed over the patient's thigh and the receiver with the catheter is placed between the patient's thighs. The penis is held with sterile gauze and the catheter is passed into the bladder. Catheters should be handled only with sterile gloves or forceps and should not be touched unless sterile gloves are worn. The catheter on removal is discarded into the soiled dressing bag.

If two nurses are available the assistant prepares the patient, opens the outer bag and supplementary packs and pours the lotion. The assistant also opens the catheter pack and slides the catheter carefully into the sterile receiver.

Similar procedures are used for female catheterization. The vulva and urethral orifice are cleaned thoroughly with sterile saline or 'Savlodil'. The labia are held apart with a gloved hand or with sterile gauze after cleaning and during the insertion of the catheter. A female length catheter is preferred. To further reduce risk of infection the urethra can be disinfected by combining the anaesthetic with an antiseptic, usually chlorhexidine, and 50 ml of 1/5000 aqueous chlorhexidine can be instilled in the bladder before the catheter is removed (Slade and Gillespie 1985).

LUMBAR PUNCTURE

The doctor washes and dries his hands and arranges the pack contents on the sterile field with handling forceps. Sterile gloves may be worn if preferred. The doctor arranges the surgical drapes in position, swabs the lumbar region with a 1% alcoholic solution of iodine or 0.5% solution of chlorhexidine in 70% ethyl or isopropyl alcohol and injects the local anaesthetic from a single-use vial. The manometer is prepared and the lumbar puncture needle inserted. Specimens are collected as required. The nurse applies a dressing after the needle has been removed.

Similar procedures are used for chest and other aspirations.

References and further reading

Ayliffe, G.A.J., Babb, J.R., Davies, J. *et al.* (1988) Hand disinfection and comparison of various agents in laboratory and ward studies. *Journal of Hospital Infection*, **11**, 226.

Ayliffe, G.A.J., Babb, J.R. and Quoraishi, A.H. (1978) A test for hygienic hand disinfection. *Journal of Clinical Pathology*, **31**, 923.

Babb, J.R., Davies, J.G. and Ayliffe, G.A.J. (1983) Contamination of protective clothing and nurses' uniforms in an isolation ward. *Journal of Hospital Infection*, **4**, 149.

Bastow, D., Greaves, P. and Allison, S.P. (1982) Microbial contamination of enteral feeds. *Human Nutrition: Applied Nutrition*, **36a**, 213.

Bowell, E. (1990) Infection control and the nursing process. In *Infection Control. Guidelines for Nursing Care* (ed.) Worsley *et al.*, ICNA, Great Britain.

Bradley, C.R., Babb, J.R., Davies, J. *et al.* (1986) Taking precautions. *Nursing Times*, **82** (70), Supplement.

Casewell, M.W. and Phillips, I. (1977) Hands as a route of transmission of Klebsiella species. *British Medical Journal*, **ii**, 1315.

Casewell, M.W. (1982) Bacteriological hazards of contaminated enteral feeds. *Journal of Hospital Infection*, **3**, 329.

Centers for Disease Control (1981) Guidelines for hospital environmental control. *Infection Control*, **2**, 131.

Classen, D.C., Larsen, R.A., Burke, J.P. *et al.* (1991) Daily meatal care for prevention of catheter-associated bacteriuria. Results using frequent applications of poly antibiotic cream. *Infection Control and Hospital Epidemiology*, **12**, 157.

Crow, S. (1989) *Asepsis, the Right Touch*. Everett Co., Louisiana.

Doebbeling, B.N., Pfaller, M.A., Houston, A.C. *et al.* (1988) 'Removal of' nosocomial pathogens from the contaminated glove: implications for glove re-use and handwashing. *Annals of Internal Medicine*, **109**, 394.

Drug and Therapeutics Bulletin. (1991) Local applications to wounds – II Dressings for wounds and ulcers. **29**, 97

Glenister, H. (1990) The catheterized patient. In *Infection Control. Guidelines for Nursing Care*. (ed.) Worsley *et al.*, ICNA, Great Britain.

Greene, C.M. (1990) Prevention of Infection during intravenous therapy. In *Infection Control. Guidelines for Nursing Care*. (ed.) Worsley *et al.*, ICNA, Great Britain.

Health Services Advisory Committee (1991) Safe working and the prevention of infection in clinical laboratories. HMSO, London.

Hill, R.L.R., Fisher, A.P., Ware, R.S. *et al.* (1990) Mupirocin for the reduction of colonization of internal jugular cannulae – a randomized controlled trial. *Journal of Hospital Infection*, **15**, 311.

Hutchinson, J.J. and Lawrence, J.C. (1991) Wound infection under occlusive dressings. *Journal of Hospital Infection*, **17**, 83.

Kelso, H. (1989) Alternative technique. *Nursing Times*, **85** (no. 23), 68.

Lancet (1991) Leading article: Healing of cavity wounds. **1**, 1010.

Maki, D.G. and Band, J.D. (1981) A comparative study of polyantibiotic and iodophor ointments in prevention of vascular catheter-related infection. *American Journal of Medicine*, **70**, 739.

Maki, D.G. and Ringer, M. (1987) Evaluation of dressing regimes for the prevention of infection with peripheral intravenous catheters. *Journal of American Medical Association*, **258**, 239.

Maki, D.G., Cobb, L. and Garman J. K. *et al.* (1988) An attachable silver-impregnated cuff for prevention of infection with central venous catheters: a prospective randomized multicentre study. *American Journal of Medicine*, **85**, 307.

Newsom, S.W.B. and Rowland, C. (1989) Application of the hygienic hand-disinfection to the gloved hand. *Journal of Hospital Infection*, **14**, 245.

Phillips, I., Meers, P. and D'Arcy, P.F. (1976) *Microbiological Hazards in Infusion Therapy*. MTP Press, Lancaster.

Rotter, M. (1984) Hygienic hand disinfection. *Infection Control*, **5**, 18.

Slade, N. and Gillespie, W.A. (1985) *The Urinary Tract and the Catheter*. John Wiley, Chichester.

Spencer, R.C. (1990) Use of in-line filters for intravenous infusion. *Journal of Hospital Infection*, **16**, 281.

Taylor, L.J. (1978) Evaluation of hand-washing techniques, Parts 1 and 2. *Nursing Times*, **74**, 54 and 108.

Taylor, L.J. (1980) Are masks necessary in operating theatres and wards? *Journal of Hospital Infection*, **1**, 173.

Thomlinson, D. (1987) To clean or not to clean. *Journal of Infection Control Nursing*, **35**, 71.
Worsley, M.A., Ward, K.A., Parker, L. *et al.* (eds) (1990) *Infection Control: Guidelines for Nursing Care*. ICNA, UK.

8 Prevention of infection in wards II: Isolation of patients, management of contacts and infection precautions in ambulances

8.1 Introduction

The spread of infection to patients in hospital can be controlled by physical protection (isolation); the extent of this control varies with the methods used (Bagshawe *et al*. 1978). Isolation for control of infection is applied in two ways:

1. **source (or 'containment') isolation** – the isolation of infected patients to prevent the transfer of their infection to others; and
2. **protective (or 'reverse') isolation** – to prevent the transfer of infective microorganisms to patients at special risk from infection (those with diminished resistance because of their illness or treatment, e.g. patients taking immunosuppressive drugs).

In some patients, for example those with extensive burns, combined source and protective isolation is desirable to protect patients already infected with one pathogen against infection with other pathogens.

8.2 Methods of physical protection

The methods of physical protection are as follows:

1. **Barrier nursing** – special nursing procedures which reduce the risks of transferring infective organisms from person to person, especially by direct contact or by way of fomites.
2. **Segregation** – in single rooms, cubicles or plastic isolators which reduces airborne spread to and from patients, and facilitates nursing techniques.
3. **Mechanical ventilation** – which reduces the risk of airborne spread by removing bacteria from the patient's room and, in protective isolation, by excluding from the room bacteria present in the outside air.

The transfer of infection by the airborne route (e.g. respiratory infections) can be controlled only by confining the patient in a single room or isolator, whether for source or protective isolation. On the other hand, the control of diseases spread by contact (e.g. enteric fever) depends primarily on barrier nursing, including blood/body fluid precautions.

The term isolation is commonly used in the sense of segregation of the patient in a single room; it is used here to include all methods by which the patient may be physically protected, including barrier nursing in an open ward. Barrier nursing, like single room accommodation and mechanical ventilation, is one of the basic components of patient isolation and can be used on its own or together with other components.

8.3   Modes of spread of infection in wards (see Table 8.1)

Direct contact spread means transfer of infection to the patient by direct contact with an infected person or with a healthy carrier of a virulent organism. Indirect contact spread means transfer of such organisms on needles, instruments, bedding and other 'fomites', in food, or on the hands of staff. This includes the transfer of dysentery and other intestinal infections through faecal contamination – the 'faecal-oral' route. Airborne spread refers to spread of infection through the air in small droplets from the mouth, or on skin scales, or in dust particles. Some infections are transmitted by more than one route – for example, staphylococcal infections can be spread by direct and indirect contact and also by airborne transfer, and poliomyelitis may be acquired either by inhalation or ingestion.

8.4   Infections unlikely to spread from person to person in hospital

Actinomycosis, amoebiasis, aspergillosis, brucellosis, cat scratch fever, campylobacter enteritis, cryptococcosis, cryptosporidiosis, gas gangrene, histoplasmosis, infectious mononucleosis (glandular fever), legionellosis, leptospirosis, pneumonia, rabies, rheumatic fever, tetanus, toxocara infections, toxoplasmosis and worm infestations are unlikely to be transmitted in hospital. However, spread can occasionally occur with some of these organisms, e.g. camplyobacter, cryptosporidiosis, and special precautions are necessary for some of these diseases (Chapter 9).

Table 8.1 Mode of person to person spread of transmissible diseases in hospital

Diseases	Routes and possible routes of transfer Airborne	Contact Faecal-oral route	Hands, personal and/or fomites
Anthrax	X		X
AIDS see: Human immunodeficiency Syndrome			
Candidiasis			X
Chickenpox	X		X
Cholera		X	X
Cryptosporidiosis		X	X
Diphtheria	X		X
Eczema vaccinatum	X		X
Fungal infections (skin)			X
Gastroenteritis in babies		X	X
Gonococcal ophthalmia neonatorum			X
Hepatitis A		X	X
Hepatitis B			X*
Herpes simplex			X
Herpes zoster	X		X
Human immunodeficiency syndrome			X*
Influenza	X		X
Measles	X		X
Meningitis			
(a) meningococcal	X		X
(b) viral	X	X	X
Mumps	X		X
Plague	X		X
Pneumonia (viral and some bacterial, e.g. *Staph. aureus*)	X		X
Poliomyelitis	X	X	X
Psittacosis	X		X
Q fever	X	X	X
Rubella	X		X
Salmonella and Shigella infections		X	X
Scabies			X
Staphylococcal disease	X		X
Streptococcal disease	X		X
Syphilis (mucocutaneous)			X
Tuberculosis (open)	X		X
Typhoid and paratyphoid		X	X
Viral haemorrhagic fevers	?	X	X*
Whooping cough	X		X
Wound infection	X		X

* Spread by blood/body fluid route usually percutaneous

Legionnaire's disease and aspergillosis are transmitted by airborne route, but not person to person

8.5 Varieties of accommodation for isolating patients

There are various types of isolation offering different degrees of protection.

8.5.1 HIGH SECURITY INFECTIOUS DISEASES ISOLATION UNITS

These are usually part of an infectious diseases hospital, and have facilities for treating patients with highly communicable viral infections, having a high mortality rate and no or limited definitive treatment (e.g. Lassa, Marburg and Ebola fevers). Total environmental control is usually achieved by the use of negative pressure plastic isolators, although a lesser degree of isolation is probably adequate.

8.5.2 INFECTIOUS DISEASES HOSPITALS

At the present time these units are usually separate from other hospital buildings but may be situated in a general hospital. If so, separate ventilation and nursing staff should be provided. Facilities are available for the treatment of all infections, excluding the African viral haemorrhagic fevers. Patients are admitted both from the community and from other hospitals.

8.5.3 GENERAL HOSPITAL ISOLATION UNITS

These provide source isolation facilities for hospital-acquired infections and for most community-acquired infections. They also provide facilities for protective isolation and for the screening of patients with suspected infections before admission to a general ward or transfer to a communicable diseases unit if necessary.

8.5.4 SINGLE ROOMS OF A GENERAL WARD (WARD SIDE ROOMS)

These provide less secure source isolation than the above methods because of close proximity to other patients and sharing of nursing and domestic staff with a general ward. Their value in protective isolation depends on the types of patient in the general ward, on the thoroughness of barrier nursing, on whether the room is self-contained (with WC) and on the type of ventilation used.

8.5.5 BARRIER NURSING IN OPEN WARD

Can be effective in controlling infections transferred by contact but not by air; single room isolation is preferable.

8.5.6   ISOLATORS IN OPEN WARDS

Plastic enclosures ('isolators') for individual patients have been shown to be of value as a form of protective isolation for high risk patients and of source isolation for infected patients, but are now rarely used.

8.5.7   ULTRA-CLEAN WARDS

Units have been set up in special centres for organ transplantation, treatment of leukaemia, chorion-carcinoma and other diseases associated with extreme susceptibility to infection.

At present very few general hospitals have satisfactory isolation units or even a sufficient number of single rooms for the treatment of patients suffering from, or particularly susceptible to infection. The size of a general hospital isolation unit depends on a number of factors, including availability of single room accommodation in the general wards (which should have not less than two), proximity of a major communicable diseases unit and the size of the hospital. The number of rooms in such a unit might vary from 10 to 20, depending on the above factors. A proportion of these rooms (about one third) should have an appropriate form of mechanical ventilation for the treatment of 'high-risk' patients – those with increased susceptibility to infection (e.g. patients on immunosuppressive therapy or with extensive burns) and those suffering from severe infections which are likely to spread by air. The number of beds required would be greater if paediatric patients are included. Since these wards are likely to contain ill patients from all areas of the hospital and since they are in individual rooms, a much higher nurse/patient ratio (e.g. two nurses to one patient over the 24-hour period) is required than in general wards. A specially trained team of domestic workers should be available for cleaning isolation rooms or units. Most hospitals are unlikely to be able to staff separate isolation wards for source and protective isolation (Rahman 1985). A single unit for both would be appropriate, but requires particular care by the staff to prevent spread of infection (Ayliffe *et al.* 1979).

8.6   Categories of isolation

Various systems for categorizing patients have been proposed. A method widely used is to subdivide patients into categories according to the mode of spread of the organism (e.g. respiratory, enteric, wound, skin and blood) and includes strict isolation for highly transmissible and dangerous infections and protective for highly susceptible patients.

Coloured cards with nursing instructions are attached to the door of the room. A more recently described system is disease-specific isolation in which precautions are decided on the basis of the individual infection rather than the category (Garner and Simmons 1983). The advantages and disadvantages of these systems are discussed by Haley and colleagues (1985). We propose a simplified system consisting of three main categories: standard, protective and strict. Strict isolation (e.g. for viral haemorrhagic fevers and diphtheria) is rarely required and should only be undertaken in the Regional Infectious Diseases Unit.

8.6.1 SUGGESTED LABELS FOR CATEGORIES OF ISOLATION

Adhesive labels are recommended for rooms occupied by patients in isolation. These should be attached to the door of the isolation room and will help to inform staff going into the room of the measures to be taken. Examples of colour codes are as follows:

1. **red** – strict isolation;
2. **white** – protective isolation;
3. **blue** – standard isolation.

VISITORS	PLEASE REPORT TO SISTER'S OFFICE BEFORE ENTERING ROOM
SINGLE ROOM	Necessary for all infections transferred by air, and preferred, when available, for all communicable infections. Door must be kept closed
GOWNS OR PLASTIC APRONS	Must be worn when attending to patients
MASKS	Not necessary
HANDS	Must be washed on leaving room
GLOVES:	Not necessary unless excretion, exudate, secretion or blood precautions are required.
ARTICLES	Normal supplies. Linen and waste disposed of according to guidelines
COMMENTS	BLUE LABEL

Figure 8.1 Standard source isolation.

A yellow card may be used for blood precautions and a brown card for enteric precautions, although a single card for all source isolation may be preferred. An example of a card is shown in Fig. 8.1. The visitor's line only should be translated into other languages as required. If the disease-specific system is used, requirements for gowns, masks, etc. are filled in separately for each patient, depending on the infection. Guidelines are provided to allow ward staff to make the appropriate decision.

In a general isolation unit, instructions for each patient are unnecessary, but an unmarked coloured card is still useful for the staff, particularly for domestic staff when cleaning cubicles in an agreed order; protective isolation cubicles (white label) should be cleaned before source isolation cubicles (blue label). In single rooms in general wards, the instruction to visitors to report to the nurse in charge should be included on the isolation label or card.

8.6.2   STANDARD ISOLATION (see Appendix 8.1)

The main diseases requiring isolation in a general hospital are diarrhoeal infections, e.g. salmonella, shigella, rotavirus infection, also untreated pulmonary tuberculosis and infections caused by highly-resistant *Staph. aureus* (e.g. MRSA). Additional isolation facilities may be required for childhood communicable diseases (e.g. measles, chickenpox, respiratory syncytial virus infection) or their contacts, particularly if there are paediatric wards. Patients infected with antibiotic resistant Gram-negative bacilli can be treated in an open ward with suitable precautions against contact spread, but single-room isolation may be preferred.

Although it is recognized that special precautions may sometimes be necessary, e.g. for enteric infections, the following guidelines are applicable to most patients requiring isolation in a general hospital. These also include protective isolation with some modifications (p. 154). It is easier to maintain strict and minimal practices than to observe a list of rules without defining priorities. Discipline of the staff is of major importance and the three main requirements of standard isolation are:

1. keep the door of the room closed at all times;
2. wash hands after handling the patient or his/her immediate surroundings (and before, if the patient is in protective isolation);
3. wear a disposable apron or gown when handling a patient or his/her immediate surroundings (this may be unnecessary for patients with airborne infections, but removes the necessity for making decisions on individual patients. Many infections spread by the airborne route are also spread by contact).

It is also necessary to ensure that staff of an isolation unit are protected against tuberculosis, measles, rubella, poliomyelitis and hepatitis B. Evidence of a past infection with chickenpox should be recorded and, if uncertain, antibody levels should be measured. Staff with inadequate levels and who are chicken pox contacts should be excluded from nursing patients in protective isolation.

8.7 Accommodation

This can vary from a ward side room to a fully-equipped suite with an airlock. The minimal requirement is a side room of a main ward. It should have a handwash basin and, preferably, a toilet. A ventilation system (consisting of at least an extractor fan) is desirable for patients with a communicable respiratory or airborne infection, especially for chickenpox and untreated pulmonary tuberculosis, and is preferred for heavy staphylococcal dispersers. A positive pressure system (plenum) providing 8–10 air changes per hour is required for patients in protective isolation. If in a unit with mixed source and protective isolation facilities (Ayliffe *et al*. 1979), a room with both systems for positive and negative pressure ventilation can be used for either source or protective isolation, but requires a decision on the direction of airflow required for individual patients. Although an airlock is generally unnecessary, an airlock with an extractor system can be similarly used for both types of patient isolation and avoids the necessity for changing the airflow depending on the type of patient. An airlock requires more space and may reduce contact between staff and patient. A plenum system filtering to a standard of 95% for 5 μm particles is generally adequate, but more efficient filtration may be needed in bone-marrow and liver transplantation units where *aspergillus* infection is a potential hazard (see Chapter 9).

A ventilated room with toilet and shower or bathroom *en suite* and an airlock provides the highest standards of isolation, apart from a plastic isolator or the use of laminar flow ventilation. However, if a toilet or bathroom is not present in the isolation suite, particular care is necessary to prevent contact between patients using the ward facilities and to ensure adequate disinfection of toilet and bath after use.

The isolation room should not contain unnecessary furniture, and surfaces should be washable. Good visibility of the patient is desirable and glass panels in the walls and door are helpful. The room should have talk-through panels, or a good communication system and a television set to lessen the adverse psychological effects of isolation.

8.8 Nursing procedures for standard isolation

8.8.1 HANDS

Hand-washing before and after contact with the patient is the most important measure in preventing the spread of infection. Either a non-medicated soap or an antiseptic-detergent is adequate for routine purposes, but 70% ethanol or isopropanol is more effective in killing transient flora and should be used in high-risk situations. Prior washing is still necessary after handling patients with enterovirus infections and isopropanol should not be used in this situation.

Disposable gloves which need not be sterilized are used when directly handling contaminated materials and for enteric and blood precautions.

8.8.2 GOWNS AND APRONS

Disposable plastic aprons are preferred. Aprons with a different colour on each side are more expensive, but can be re-used with less potential risk of contamination to the wearer. Cotton gowns provide limited protection, but are acceptable in most circumstances. Gowns may be required for lifting of patients. If aprons are used for this purpose, arms should be kept bare to the elbows and should be washed after handling the patient. Gowns made of water-repellant materials (e.g. ventile or suitable non-woven materials) which have a low permeability to bacteria, give better protection but, as with disposable gowns, can be expensive. The gown or apron should be left hanging inside the room and changed daily, although evidence exists that contamination does not increase if the gown is used over longer periods (Babb *et al.* 1983).

8.8.3 MASK AND EYE-PROTECTION

Masks are rarely necessary and are of doubtful value in protecting against organisms spread in the air. However, if used, they should be of the filter type. Goggles or spectacles may sometimes be required, e.g. for procedures involving possible splashing of blood from patients with HBV or HIV infection.

8.8.4 CAPS AND OVERSHOES

These are not required.

8.8.5   MEDICAL EQUIPMENT

Disposable or autoclavable equipment should be used whenever possible. Equipment such as stethoscopes, sphygmomanometers and thermometers should preferably be left in the room and terminally disinfected on discharge of the patient.

8.8.6   OTHER EQUIPMENT

A bedpan washer and dishwashing machine heating to 80°C for one minute or an equivalent time/temperature relationship should be available in the isolation ward. The temperature profile of the cycle should be monitored regularly.

8.8.7   LAUNDRY

Linen from patients with open pulmonary tuberculosis, salmonella and shigella infections, HBV and HIV (if bloodstained) and others specified by the infection control doctor should be sealed in water soluble bags and enclosed in a red outer bag (HC (87) 30) (Chapter 12). Linen from other patients can be treated routinely as 'used' linen, although it may be convenient to classify linen from all patients in source isolation as infected.

8.8.8   WASTE

Waste contaminated with body fluids or secretions from patients listed above should be sealed in a yellow plastic bag for incineration. Fluids should be disposed of by carefully pouring into a sluice. Prior disinfection before disposal is rarely necessary.

8.8.9   CHARTS

Patient's charts should be kept outside the contaminated areas, if only to discourage frequent visits to the room. The infective hazard of contamination from charts is small.

8.8.10   TRANSPORTING PATIENTS

Patients should be sent to other departments only if it is essential to do so. The department in question should be notified in advance, so that it may make arrangements to prevent possible spread of infection. It may be advisable for the order in which patients visit other departments to be arranged in advance.

8.8.11   SECRETION, EXCRETION AND EXUDATE PRECAUTIONS

(Precautions against infected oral or other secretions, or against pus and other infected exudates)
Oral Secretions   Patients should be encouraged to cough or spit into paper tissue and then discard this into a plastic bag.

Exudate   A 'non-touch' technique using forceps or disposable gloves should be used and contaminated material should be placed in sealed paper or plastic bags. Bags containing contaminated materials should be placed in sealed paper or plastic bags. These should be placed in a pedal-bin lined with a plastic bag and disposed of as hazardous clinical waste.

Excretion   For patients with enteric fever, dysentery, cholera and other infections spread by urine or faeces, disposable gloves should be worn to take the bedpan from the patient to the disposal area; it is necessary for the nurse to put on a plastic gown to prevent contamination of the uniform. The pan should be covered with a disposable paper bag before transport. Gloves should be placed in a plastic bag for disposal after use. Disposable gloves and a plastic apron or gown should be worn to handle contaminated equipment or linen, and when cleaning the perineal areas (see Chapter 7 for disinfection of bedpans, etc).

8.8.12   BLOOD PRECAUTIONS

See Chapters 7 and 10.

8.8.13   DISPOSAL OF PERSONAL CLOTHING

Used clothing requires no special treatment unless from patients with infection potentially hazardous to staff. Infected clothing should be transferred to the hospital laundry in a sealed water-soluble or alginate-stitched bag and treated by the routine method used for this category of linen (see Chapter 12). Rarely other methods of disinfection (chemical or low temperature steam) or incineration may be necessary for heat-sensitive materials. Articles from patients with anthrax and viral haemorrhagic fevers should be autoclaved.

8.8.14   DISPOSAL OF THE DEAD

When death of a person suffering from a Notifiable Disease takes place in a hospital, provision is made under the Public Health Act (1936. S. 163 164) to prohibit the removal of the body from the hospital except for the purpose of being taken direct to a mortuary or being forthwith buried or cremated. Under the Act, every person having charge or control of premises where such a body may be lying must take such steps as may be practicable to prevent persons coming unnecessarily into contact with or proximity to it. Wakes over such bodies are prohibited. Furthermore, a Justice of the Peace has the power to order the removal or burial of such a body subject to a medical certificate issued by the Consultant in Communicable Disease Control (CCDC) (or other registered practitioner on his staff) that the body constitutes a risk of spread of infection. In practice the above powers are not generally enforced today. Cremation is perhaps the safest method of disposal of the infected dead: relatives should be encouraged to agree to this method, but it cannot be legally enforced.

Death may occur from infectious diseases which are not notifiable and the corpse may remain infectious to those who handle it. The precautions already described for handling infected patients do not become unnecessary with the patient's death. The isolation category should be stated on a card attached to the body. Porters, mortuary attendants, pathologists and funeral undertakers must be informed of the possible danger in order that appropriate precautions may be taken. Bodies of patients with infections potentially transmissible to personnel (e.g. typhoid and other enteric infections, open tuberculosis, HBV, or HIV infections) should be sealed in a leak proof cadaver plastic bag, labelled as above. However, it should be possible to arrange for the face of these patients to be seen by relatives if required provided suitable precautions against spread are taken.

8.8.15 TERMINAL DISINFECTION OF ISOLATION ROOMS

All surfaces, including beds, other furniture, wash-basins etc. and the floor should be washed. The necessity to use a disinfectant is doubtful, but may be advisable if there is visible contamination or following the presence of infections transferred by contact (e.g. MRSA) or hazardous to personnel (e.g. untreated tuberculosis) (see Chapters 5 and 6). It is unnecessary to wash walls and ceilings unless they are visibly contaminated. The room may be occupied when the surfaces are dry.

8.9 Strict isolation techniques (in addition to the standard)

If the infection is likely to be airborne and the personnel are non-immune, masks protective to the wearer (of a recommended filter type stored outside the room) should be put on before entering the room and discarded into a pedal bin before leaving. Disposable water-impermeable gowns, with a low permeability to bacteria, are preferred to aprons. Clean gowns should be stored outside the room and discarded into a pedal bin on leaving. Patients with a suspected or confirmed viral haemorrhagic fever must be transferred between hospitals in specially equipped ambulances with crews wearing protective clothing. Disposable gloves should be worn when handling the patient or his immediate surroundings. (See also p. 145 and 186.)

8.10 Protective isolation

This is required for diseases, lesions or therapy associated with an increased susceptibility to infection and in which patients need special protection from the hospital environment. The type of infection (bacterial, viral and fungal) and the risks of infection vary with the condition and procedure. Precautions are required to prevent the acquisition of exogenous organisms which may be more hazardous to immunosuppressed than to healthy persons. Isolation requirements vary with the degree of immunodeficiency which is ill-defined (Hart 1990). These requirements are usually minimal but more intensive measures are included here as they may be preferred in some hospitals. Isolation measures are usually maximal for liver and bone-marrow transplantation and minimal for kidney transplantation patients. Most infections acquired by immunosuppressed patients are endogenous and isolation in a single room is of doubtful value (Nausef and Maki 1981). However, cross-infection can be a hazard and single rooms, preferably in a self-contained unit (with shower and toilet) and a positive pressure ventilation system (8–10 air changes per hour) are preferred at the present time for highly immunosuppressed patients (e.g. with very low level neutrophil counts). High standards of hygiene to prevent contact spread of infection, for example by handwashing and wearing plastic aprons, are probably of greater importance (see standard isolation techniques). Masks and gloves are rarely required. No special precautions are required for the disposal of waste and linen, and terminal disinfection is not necessary. Filtration of air with HEPA filters to reduce airborne aspergilli is also advisable for nursing highly susceptible patients, particularly in liver and bone-marrow transplant units. The cost of a laminar flow air system would appear to be unwarranted and a failure in filtration of the recirculated air could represent a greater hazard. Positive pressure plastic isolators are sometimes used for bone-marrow and cardiac transplant patients, but their use is decreasing. Other measures may sometimes be recommended – for example, sterile linen, sterile food and other supplies, decontamination of mouth or other orifices, gut and skin, and prophylactic systemic antimicrobial agents such as co-trimoxazole. The evidence of effectiveness of these procedures is conflicting and they are not routinely recommended, although some measures may be of value (e.g. prophylactic co-trimoxazole in the prevention of pneumocystis infection in bone-marrow or liver transplant patients). Uncooked food, particularly salads, may be contaminated with Gram-negative bacilli or listeria and should generally be avoided in highly immunosuppressed patients. Similarly, the value of routine screening of nose, throat, faeces and skin of immunosuppressed patients, although frequently recommended, is of uncertain predictive value.

8.11 Management of contacts of infected patients in hospital
(Brewer and Jeffries 1990 for viral infections)

8.11.1 CHICKENPOX

If indicated, an injection of human specific immunoglobulin may be given to patients suffering from, or contacts of, chickenpox who are on steroid therapy or receiving cytotoxic or immunosuppressive drugs (e.g. patients with leukaemia). Non-immune contacts should be sent home or isolated from seven days after contact if the ward is not closed.

8.11.2 CYTOMEGALOVIRUS INFECTION

Children excreting cytomegalovirus are not normally a hazard to pregnant women, provided the usual hygienic precautions are taken, especially handwashing.

8.11.3 DIPHTHERIA

Throat and nasal swabs should be taken from all close contacts of patients who develop diphtheria while in hospital; they should be given prophylactic erythromycin (2 g daily for seven days); swabs should be taken from carriers on completion of treatment. The Consultant in Communicable Disease Control (CCDC) should be informed. Active immunization of contacts if not known to be immune should be started (see also Chapter 13). All contacts should be kept under surveillance, and if any develop sore throat or nasal discharge, antitoxin should be given.

8.11.4   INFANTILE GASTROENTERITIS

If an outbreak of gastroenteritis due to enteropathogenic or toxigenic *E. coli* occurs, stools should be cultured from all contacts, and admissions to the ward must be suspended. Children who are well enough to go home should be discharged as soon as possible. The isolation of a gastroenteritis serotype of *E. coli* in the laboratory from a child without symptoms should not cause alarm, but is an indication that this child should be kept away from any susceptible children (under two years old) in the ward. Nurses working in a ward where cases of gastroenteritis are present should not be transferred to other wards. Infantile gastroenteritis is also commonly caused by viruses, especially rotaviruses.

8.11.5   INTESTINAL INFECTIONS (including typhoid fever, other salmonellosis, cholera and bacillary dysentery)

Other patients and staff in the ward should be kept under surveillance and stool samples should be obtained from those developing signs of the disease. Under certain circumstances it may be necessary to close a ward or unit. When typhoid contacts, in whom the incubation period may be prolonged to three weeks, are discharged from hospital, the general practitioner should be made aware of the contact so that cases are not missed. The Occupational Health Department should be informed of contacts among members of staff.

8.11.6   MEASLES

Contacts under two years of age and other children in whom measles might be particularly dangerous (e.g. those suffering from chronic or debilitating diseases such as leukaemia, or receiving corticosteroid drugs) should be given an injection of human normal immunoglobulin as soon as possible after contact. It may be necessary to close a children's surgical ward because operations on children with measles can be dangerous. Admissions should be limited to children who have had a definite attack of measles or have been immunized.

8.11.7   MENINGOCOCCAEMIA

Household contacts should be kept under surveillance and throat swabs should be taken: a prophylactic course of rifampicin should be given to close family contacts or staff contacts if they have given mouth to mouth respiration. Only use sulphonamide if the organism is known to be sensitive.

8.11.8   POLIOMYELITIS

All contacts, staff and patients, should be offered oral poliomyelitis vaccine.

8.11.9   HAEMOPHILUS MENINGITIS

A prophylactic course of rifampicin for close family contacts (children only).

8.11.10   RUBELLA

Rubella is generally a benign disease, but infection during the first four months of pregnancy is associated with a significant incidence of abnormal fetuses. Estimation of the antibody titres in the blood of contacts in early pregnancy can be helpful and should be done without delay. Immunoglobulin is not recommended.

8.11.11   SCABIES

When scabies is diagnosed in a patient admitted to hospital, arrangements must be made for all home contacts to be treated.

8.11.12   TUBERCULOSIS (open pulmonary)

The names of all close patient contacts of a case of sputum-positive tuberculosis should be notified to the appropriate Consultant in Communicable Disease Control (CCDC) and the general practitioner. Staff contacts are reported to the hospital control of infection or occupational health departments and immune status checked. Tuberculin tests and chest x-rays should be carried out immediately on close contacts in long-stay wards or at 6 weeks depending on time of contact, also in neonatal, paediatric (under 3 months) or in immunocompromised close contacts.

8.11.13   VIRAL HEPATITIS

Human normal immunoglobulin gives protection against hepatitis A, but not against hepatitis B: 500 mg should be given to debilitated contacts and pregnant women. Human specific immunoglobulin, conferring protection against HBV, is available for those at risk by reason of accidental exposure to infection, and hepatitis B vaccine should be given (see Chapter 10).

8.12   Visiting of patients in isolation hospitals

8.12.1   INFECTED PATIENTS

In general, patients in hospital suffering from infection should be allowed visitors in the normal way, and daily visiting of small children by their parents is encouraged. However, under certain circumstances, some restrictions may have to be imposed for the protection of visitors or to prevent the spread of disease. It is sometimes necessary for the visitor to wear a gown or plastic apron (e.g. if handling a child with an intestinal infection) and instruction must be given on handwashing. Language and cultural difficulties may have to be considered in some cases. Visitors must not visit patients other than those whom they have come to see. It is unwise to allow children to visit patients in isolation or communicable disease units, and adults who are not considered to be immune to a particular infection should be excluded from contact with that disease. Pregnant women must not visit patients suffering from rubella.

8.12.2   PATIENTS IN PROTECTIVE ISOLATION

Parents may visit children, but contacts should be restricted, especially in visiting immunosuppressed patients. If the intending visitor has an infection of the respiratory or intestinal tract, boils or other septic lesions, the visit should be postponed.

8.13   Ambulance services: general procedures for control of infection

Many diseases are infectious before symptoms appear and contact with a sick person before a final diagnosis is made will always carry some risks of infection. Most infections (e.g. bronchitis, pneumonia, abscesses, and urinary tract infections) will not be transferred to normal healthy staff and the risk of acquiring infection is minimal. The inanimate environment within the ambulance is unlikely to be an infection hazard and the risk of transfer of infection from one occupant to the next is remote.

The minimal measures required are:

1. immunization of ambulance staff (if not already immune) against poliomyelitis, tuberculosis and tetanus;
2. handwashing after a patient and his belongings have been removed from the ambulance. Bedding (blankets, sheets and bedcovers), should be sealed in a plastic bag and laundered after use by a patient

with a notifiable or other communicable disease, or if soiled with blood, secretions or excreta whether the patient has a known infection or not. Spillage should be removed with disposable wipes, which should be sealed in plastic bags for incineration.

Disposable plastic aprons and gloves should be available for handling contaminated patients (e.g. with diarrhoea and vomiting) or cleaning up contaminated surfaces. A phenolic disinfectant may be used for cleaning contaminated surfaces.

8.13.1   ADDITIONAL PROCEDURES FOR SPECIAL INFECTIONS

A few infections are potentially dangerous to staff as well as to patients and require special care. These include typhoid, dysentery, HBV, and HIV infections, diphtheria and open tuberculosis. For potentially dangerous infections (e.g. Lassa and other haemorrhagic fevers and rabies) see Chapter 9.

8.13.2   SUGGESTED PROCEDURES

Typhoid, dysentery and other gastrointestinal infections   Bedpans, urinals, vomit bowls, etc., should be either washed in a bedpan washer with a steam disinfection cycle or washed in a phenolic disinfectant. Disposable cups should be used. If surfaces are extensively contaminated the ambulance should be taken out of service and all surfaces cleaned with a phenolic disinfectant. Surfaces should be dry before the ambulance is re-used. Fumigation with formaldehyde is unnecessary.

HBV and HIV infections   As above, but disinfect with 1% hypochlorite or other chlorine-releasing agents (containing 0.1% available chlorine). Rinse to reduce corrosion of fixtures and fittings after a short exposure (e.g. one minute) to the hypochlorite solution.

Tuberculosis (open untreated pulmonary)   As above. Sputum containers and wipes used for removing secretions from patients should be sealed in a plastic bag and incinerated. Disinfect contaminated surfaces with a phenolic solution.

Diphtheria   As for typhoid, dysentery etc. above. Prophylactic antibiotics may be recommended by the CCDC.

Methicillin-resistant *Staph. aureus*   Infection caused by these organisms is no special hazard to personnel or their relatives. Lesions should be sealed if possible (Chapter 9).

To reduce risks of transfer to another patient, ambulance staff should wear a plastic apron when in contact with a patient. Hands should be washed (an alcoholic preparation is convenient for hand disinfection in an ambulance). The patient should be given clean clothing and local areas of contact with the patient can be disinfected with a phenolic solution or, for small areas, with an alcohol wipe.

8.13.3   AMBULANCE

If an ambulance is specially designated for transport of infected patients it is advisable:

1. to remove any equipment not considered necessary (e.g. spare stretcher);
2. to seal equipment locker with adhesive tape (terminal cleaning of inside will not then be necessary);
3. to seal clean blankets and bedding in a plastic bag and carry in bag, and to seal the box containing resuscitation equipment so that only the outside of the box will require cleaning or disinfection.

Respiratory resuscitation equipment should be returned to a hospital SSD or equipment cleaning and disinfection department for processing.

Appendix 8.1   Isolation methods for individual diseases

Isolation for infections
This section lists diseases in alphabetical order, the category of isolation and special nursing procedure, if any required. Abbreviations used:

HIU	Hospital Isolation Unit
HSIU	High Security Isolation Unit
IDH	Infectious Diseases Hospital
SR	Single-bedded Sideroom
CCDC	Consultant in Communicable Disease Control

Actinomycosis	Isolation unnecessary
	Exudate precautions
Acquired immunodeficiency syndrome (AIDS)	See Human immunodeficiency virus infection
Amoebiasis	Isolation unnecessary
	Excretion precautions
Anthrax	
Category of isolation	Strict (pulmonary or systemic); standard (cutaneous)
Period of isolation	Length of illness (e.g. until completion of successful chemotherapy)

Place of isolation	HIU, IDH, or SR, for cutaneous infection
	HSIU, or IDH for pulmonary infection
Comments	Laboratory must be warned of any specimens sent for examination. Notify CCDC

Aspergillosis No special precautions (see Chapter 9)

Brucellosis Exudate precautions only if a draining lesion

Campylobacter enteritis
Category of isolation Standard
Period of isolation Until diarrhoea stops
Excretion precautions without single-room isolation usually adequate

Candidiasis (moniliasis, thrush) Exudate precautions
Category of isolation Standard isolation in neonatal wards

Cat scratch fever No special precautions

Chickenpox
Category of isolation Standard (in room with extractor fan)
Period of isolation Seven days from start of eruption
Place of isolation HIU or IDH
Comments Take precautions with secretions. Isolate non immune contacts from 7 days after exposure. Staff who have not had the disease must be excluded. Visitors who have not had the disease must be warned of the risks

Cholera
Category of isolation Standard
Period of isolation Length of illness
Place of isolation IDH
Comments Excretion precautions. Notify CCDC

Common cold See influenza

Conjunctivitis (gonococcal) See Ophthalmia neonatorum and Venereal diseases

Cryptosporidiosis Excretion precautions

Diarrhoeal disease of unknown origin
Category of isolation Standard
Period of isolation Duration of illness
Place of isolation SR or HIU
Comments Excretion precautions

Diphtheria
Category of isolation Strict
Period of isolation Until bacteriologically negative
Place of isolation IDH
Comments See section on Contacts
Notify CCDC

(continued)

Appendix 8.1   *Continued*

Dysentery, bacillary (Shigellosis)
Category of isolation   Standard
Period of isolation   Until three consecutive negative stools after
                             acute phase, whenever possible
Place of isolation   HIU or IDH
Comments   Notify CCDC
                             Excretion precautions

Dysentery, amoebic   Isolation unnecessary
                             Excretion precautions for stools
Comment   Notify CCDC

Ebola virus disease   See viral haemorrhagic fevers

Food poisoning
Staphylococcal and clostridial   No special precautions
                                 Notify CCDC
Salmonella   See p. 178

Fungal infections
Systemic, e.g.   No special precautions
  cryptococcosis,
  histoplasmosis
Ringworm   Precautions against contact transfer
                             Isolation in a cubicle may be advisable,
                                 especially in children's wards

Gastroenteritis in babies
Category of isolation   Standard
Period of isolation   Length of illness or until stools are negative
Place of isolation   HIU, or IDH, or SR
Comments   Excretion precautions are important
                             Notify CCDC in Northern Ireland only

Gas gangrene   No special precautions

Gonorrhoea   See Venereal diseases

Herpes simplex
Category of isolation   Standard (children's wards only)
Period of isolation   Length of illness
Place of isolation   SR or HIU
Comments   Staff with infection should be excluded from
                                 neonatal, maternity or children's wards
                                 and should cover cuts or abrasions on
                                 fingers if in contact with infected child

Herpes zoster
Category of isolation   Standard
Period of isolation   Length of acute illness (when lesions stop
                                 discharging)
Place of isolation   SR or HIU
Comments   Staff who have not had chicken-pox must be
                                 excluded. Visitors who have not had the
                                 infection should be warned of the risk

Hepatitis A
Category of isolation	Standard
Period of isolation	Isolation probably not required once jaundice has developed. However, patients are infectious in early febrile phase of illness
Place of isolation	SR or HIU
Comments	Excretion precautions Notify CCDC

Hepatitis, B, C, & δ   Isolation not required
Blood and body fluid precautions

Human immunodeficiency virus infections   Isolation only required in special circumstances (e.g. superadded TB or salmonellosis)
Blood and body fluid precautions

Infectious mononucleosis   Oral secretion precautions

Influenza
Category of isolation	Standard (if admitted with disease)
Period of isolation	Length of illness
Comments	Isolation of doubtful value if acquired in hospital or if other patients with the disease are in the ward

Lassa fever   See Viral haemorrhagic fevers

Legionnaire's disease   Isolation unnecessary
Oral secretion precautions

Leprosy
Category of isolation	Standard
Period of isolation	Length of hospital stay
Place of isolation	HIU or IDH
Comments	Not infectious following adequate treatment Exudate and secretion precautions Notify CCDC

Leptospirosis   Isolation unnecessary
Notify CCDC
Excretion precautions (urine)

Listeriosis   Person to person spread rare: isolation unnecessary apart from neonates
No special precautions

Malaria   Isolation unnecessary
Notify CCDC

Marburg disease   See Viral haemorrhagic fevers

Measles
Category of isolation	Standard (preferably in room with extractor fan)
Period of isolation	Five days from onset of rash

(continued)

Appendix 8.1   *Continued*

Place of isolation   SR, HIU, IDH
Comments   Secretion precautions
                                      Notify CCDC
                                      If outbreak in paediatric ward, do not admit
                                          children who are not immune until 14 days
                                          after the last contact has gone home (see
                                          section on Contacts)

Meningitis (meningococcal)
Category of isolation   Standard
Period of isolation   48 hours after onset of treatment
Place of isolation   SR, HIU or IDH
Comments   Secretion precautions. See section on Contacts
                                      Notify CCDC

Meningitis (tuberculous)   See Tuberculosis, p. 157

*Meningitis (viral) and meningo-
encephalitis*
Category of isolation   Standard
Period of isolation   Length of acute illness
Place of isolation   SR, HIU or IDH
Comments   Excretion precautions
                                      Notify CCDC

Meningitis (pneumococcal,   No isolation required
haemophilus, coliform and other   Notify CCDC
causes)

Mumps
Category of isolation   Standard
Period of isolation   Nine days after onset of parotid swelling
Place of isolation   SR, HIU, or IDH
Comments   Secretion precautions
                                      Exclude staff who are not immune
                                      Warn visitors who are not immune

Nocardiosis   No isolation required unless
                                          immunosuppressed patients are in the
                                          ward
                                      Exudate and secretion precautions

*Ophthalmia neonatorum (see
also Venereal diseases)*
Category of isolation   Standard
Period of isolation   Length of illness (24 hours after start of
                                          chemotherapy)
Place of isolation   SR
Comments   Secretion precautions
                                      Notify CCDC

Orf   No isolation required
                                      Exudate precautions

Paratyphoid fever   See Typhoid and paratyphoid

Plague
Category of isolation   Strict
Period of isolation   Until bacteriologically negative
Place of isolation   IDH or HSIU
Comments   Secretion and exudate precautions
                                 No visitors if pneumonic
                                 Notify CCDC

Pneumonia   No isolation or special precautions required
                                     for lobar (unless due to antibiotic-resistant
                                     strains of *Strep. pneumoniae*) or evidence of
                                     transmissible strain or primary atypical
                                     (mycoplasma) pneumonia. For other causes
                                     see staphylococcal infection, plague and
                                     psittacosis, Legionnaire's disease

Poliomyelitis
Category of isolation   Standard
Period of isolation   Until stools negative for poliovirus (or 7 days
                                     from onset)
Place of isolation   IDH
Comments   Excretion precautions. Visitors and staff
                                     should be immunized
                                 Notify CCDC

Psittacosis
Category of isolation   Standard
Period of isolation   For 7 days after onset
Place of isolation   SR, HIU or IDH
Comments   Secretion precautions
                                 Notify CCDC

Puerperal sepsis
Category of isolation   Standard
Period of isolation   Until bacteriologically negative (48 hours or
                                     longer)
Place of isolation   SR or HIU
Comments   Exudate precautions
                                 Notify CCDC

Q fever   As for psittacosis

Rabies
Category of isolation   Strict (though person-to-person transfer is
                                     unlikely) (see Chapter 9)
Period of isolation   Length of illness
Place of isolation   IDH or SR in Intensive Care Unit
Comments   Secretion precautions
                                 Immunize staff in close contact
                                 Notify CCDC

Rheumatic fever   No isolation or special precautions required

Ringworm   See fungal infections

(continued)

Appendix 8.1   *Continued*

Rubella
Category of isolation   Standard
Period of isolation   Five days from onset of rash
Place of isolation   SR or HIU
Comments   Secretion precautions
Exclude young women staff or visitors who
    may be pregnant unless they are immune.
    The congenital rubella syndrome is highly
    infectious
See section on Contacts

*Salmonella infections (food
poisoning)*
Category of isolation   Standard
Period of isolation   Until three stools negative, whenever possible
    or cessation of symptoms
Place of isolation   SR, HIU, or IDH
Comments   Excretion precautions
Visitors avoid close contact with patients
Notify CCDC
Carriers: send home and inform CCDC

Scabies
Category of isolation   Standard until successfully treated
Comments   See sections on Contacts, and on Human
    infestation (p. 190)

Scarlet fever   See streptococcal infections

Schistosomiasis   No isolation or special precautions

Shigellosis   See dysentery

*Staphylococcal infection
(epidemic or highly resistant
strains) including pneumonia*
Category of isolation   Standard
Period of isolation   Until the organism is no longer isolated from
    the lesion
Place of isolation   SR or HIU
Comments   Exudate and secretion precautions
    (see Chapter 9)

*Staphylococcal infection
(sensitive, or resistant only to
penicillin)*   No isolation needed, unless in maternity and
    neonatal wards or evidence of epidermic
    strain

*Streptococcal infection
(including scarlet fever and
erysipelas)*
Category of isolation   Standard
Period of isolation   Until organism no longer isolated, following
    chemotherapy (or not less than 3 days)
Place of isolation   SR or HIU

Comments	Exudate and secretion precautions (see Chapter 9)
	Notify CCDC for scarlet fever and in Scotland, erysipelas
Syphilis	See Venereal diseases
Tapeworm	No isolation needed
	Excretion precautions
Tetanus	No special source isolation precautions, but patient should be in SR, for medical reasons
	Notify CCDC
Threadworms	No isolation needed
	Excretion precautions
Tonsillitis	See streptococcal infection
Toxocara	No isolation needed
	Excretion precautions
Toxoplasmosis	No isolation or special precautions
Trichomoniasis	No isolation needed
	Exudate precautions
Tuberculosis (open, including pulmonary, urinary or draining lesions)	
Category of isolation	Standard
Period of isolation	Two weeks after beginning effective treatment (or 4 weeks in neonatal and paediatric wards or if immunosuppressed patients are present)
Place of isolation	IDH (or special hospital) or HIU
Comments	Secretion and exudate precautions
	Staff and visitors who are not immune should be warned of risk and given suitable protection
	See section on Contacts
	Notify CCDC
Tuberculosis (closed)	Isolation and special precautions not needed
	Notify CCDC
Typhoid and paratyphoid fever (and carriers)	
Category of isolation	Standard
Period of isolation	Until six negative stools, and urines if applicable
Place of isolation	IDH, HIU
Comments	Excretion precautions
	Notify CCDC
	It is not necessary to keep the patient in hospital until he is no longer excreting typhoid bacilli

(continued)

Appendix 8.1   *Continued*

Venereal diseases (syphilis (muco-cutaneous) and gonorrhoea)

Category of isolation	Standard
Period of isolation	Until bacteriologically negative; this will occur after 48 hours in syphilis, and after 24 hours in gonorrhoea unless the strain is resistant to the antibiotic
Place of isolation	SR or HIU
Comments	Use of gloves for handling secretions or infected sites

Varicose ulcers (with sepsis)   See wounds

Viral haemorrhagic fevers

Category of isolation	Strict
Period of isolation	Until virus no longer isolated
Place of isolation	HSIU
Comments	See Chapter 9 Notify CCDC

Whooping cough

Category of isolation	Standard
Period of isolation	Three weeks after onset of paroxysmal cough, or 7 days after appropriate chemotherapy (e.g. erythromycin or amoxycillin)
Comments	Secretion precautions Notify CCDC

Wounds   See Chapter 9

1. Extensive wounds (with sepsis caused by epidemic or highly antibiotic-resistant *Staph. aureus* or Gram-negative bacilli)

Category of isolation	Standard
Period of isolation	Until wound is healed or organism eliminated
Place of isolation	SR or HIU
Comments	Exudate precautions

Worm infestations (see also tape-worm, threadworm and toxocara)   Isolation not necessary
Excretion precautions only

Isolation for susceptible patients

Neutropenic, leukaemic and immunosuppressed patients

Category of isolation	Protective
Period of isolation	Duration of illness or period of immunosuppression
Place of isolation	SR, HIU
Comments	See p. 153

Burns

Category of isolation	Combined protective and standard source
Period of isolation	Duration of hospital stay for larger burns (see p. 181)

References

Ayliffe, G.A.J., Babb, J.R., Taylor, L. *et al.* (1979) A unit for source and protective isolation in a general hospital. *British Medical Journal*, **2**, 461.

Babb, J.R., Davies, J.G. and Ayliffe, G.A.J. (1983) Contamination of protective clothing and nurses' uniforms in an isolation ward. *Journal of Hospital Infection*, **4**, 149–57.

Bagshawe, K.D., Blowers, R. and Lidwell, O.M. (1978) Isolating patients in hospital to control infection. *British Medical Journal*, **ii**, 609, 684, 744, 808, 879.

Brewer, J. and Jeffries, D.J. (1990) Control of viral infections in hospitals. *Journal of Hospital Infection*, **16**, 191.

Garner, J.S. and Simmons, B.P. (1983) CDC guidelines for isolation precautions in hospitals. *Infection Control*, **4**, (Supplement), 245.

Haley, R.W., Garner, J.S. and Simmons, B.P. (1985) A new approach to the isolation of hospitalized patients with infectious diseases: alternative systems. *Journal of Hospital Infection*, **6**, 128.

Hart, S. (1990) The immunosuppressed patient. In *Infection Control: Guidelines for Nursing Care*, Worsley, M.A., Ward, K.A., Parker, L., Ayliffe, G.A.J., Sedgewick, J.A. (eds.) ICNA, Great Britain.

Nauseef, W.M. and Maki, D.G. (1981) A study of simple protective isolation in patients with granulocytopenia. *New England Journal of Medicine*, **304**, 448.

Rahman, M. (1985) Commissioning a new hospital isolation unit and assessment of its use over five years. *Journal of Hospital Infection*, **6**, 65.

9 Special problems of miscellaneous infections and human infestation I

9.1 Outbreaks of infection with *Staph. aureus* in general hospital wards

Staph. aureus is one of the commonest causes of wound infection. Many of these infections are endogenous in origin and major outbreaks are now uncommon in UK hospitals. However, methicillin-resistant strains (MRSA) are a major problem in some hospitals in the UK and are endemic in hospitals in many countries.

Strains of *Staph. aureus* which have a propensity for spreading and causing sepsis in a ward are known as 'epidemic strains'. These are usually resistant to two or more antibiotics; not all multiple-resistant strains, however, spread readily to other patients. Antibiotic-sensitive strains (or strains resistant to penicillin only) rarely spread in wards (apart from neonatal units), but may be responsible for infection in the operating theatre or for self-infection of the patient. People are the most important source of infection; staphylococci multiply in noses, on the skin (e.g. the perineum) and in lesions, but not in the inanimate environment. Nevertheless, staphylococci, which can survive for some time outside the body, especially in dry conditions, may spread from the inanimate environment – for example bedding and baths are sometimes important reservoirs. Some infected patients, and occasionally healthy people who may be carriers, are responsible for heavy environmental contamination; they are known as 'dispersers' and are a special hazard in a ward or operating theatre.

Staphylococci may be transferred by direct (i.e. personal) or indirect (i.e. fomite-borne) contact, or through the air. Transfer of organisms from an infected patient on the hands or clothing of members of staff is an important mode of transmission. Strains carried in the noses of staff are rarely responsible for wound infection acquired in the ward, but nasal carriers of epidemic strains of MRSA are potentially hazardous. People with concealed lesions, such as a boil in the axilla or on the buttock, may be an important source of infection.

9.1.1 CONTROL OF INFECTION

Control of infection is based on a good reporting system, high standards of aseptic technique and immediate isolation or removal from the open ward of any patient with a potentially epidemic strain (Report 1990).

9.1.2 ISOLATION

All patients with an infection due to a highly resistant strain, especially if resistant to fusidic acid, gentamicin or methicillin, should, if possible, be transferred to the hospital isolation unit, or to a single room (preferably equipped with appropriate mechanical ventilation) or, if clinically feasible, sent home. The doors of cubicles or side wards should be kept closed. Isolation should include precautions against contact transfer as well as against airborne transfer.

Priority of isolation Since isolation facilities are limited in most hospitals, priority for isolation is given to patients with the following lesions: major open staphylococcal sepsis (e.g. generalized eczema, chest infection, urinary tract infection, profusely discharging wounds, generalized furunculosis or skin sepsis, burns, enterocolitis, bed-sores) due to multiple-resistant (especially epidemic) strains; in particular, strains resistant to methicillin, clindamycin, fusidic acid, gentamicin or mupirocin. Priority of single rooms is not always given to infected patients; too frequently they are used for difficult patients, for private patients, or for social or ill-defined medical reasons, while infected patients are nursed in open wards. Patients with major open sepsis caused by a highly resistant or epidemic resistant strain should be isolated in single rooms, since barrier nursing measures in an open ward are of limited value in reducing the spread of infection (especially staphylococcal infection) from such patients. Although side wards on general wards are preferable to open wards, the isolated patients are still nursed by the same staff; an isolation unit with designated staff is preferred.

9.1.3 OTHER MEASURES IF NO ISOLATION FACILITIES ARE AVAILABLE

If no isolation facilities are available or single-bed wards are already occupied with high priority patients, some measures may help to limit the spread of infection. Topical chemoprophylaxis of burns with an effective agent contributes much more to the exclusion of hospital infection in a burns unit than isolation methods (see Chapter 16). In the absence of an outbreak (i.e. more than two or three infections due to the same phage type), a good aseptic technique and adequate covering of a wound may be sufficient for preventing spread of infection from patients with minor sepsis. Infection can be spread from a patient with a small septic lesion (e.g. a bedsore); even a healed lesion, or a healthy nasal or skin carrier of a multiple-resistant strain, can sometimes disperse large numbers of staphylococci. However, 'source isolation' cannot be used for all potential sources of infection since there are rarely enough single rooms available.

Additional measures which can be used for treating patients with sepsis or dispersing epidemic strains in the open ward (or in isolation) are as follows.

1. Treatment of nasal carriers   Apply a cream containing neomycin and chlorhexidine ('Naseptin' or one of equal effectiveness) to the anterior nares four times a day for two weeks or until the staphylococcus is removed. If neomycin-resistant staphylococci are present in the hospital, 1% chlorhexidine or 0.5% bacitracin cream or ointment may be used, but 2% mupirocin 'Bactroban' is more effective (see MRSA).

2. Skin treatment   An effective antiseptic detergent preparation (e.g. 4% chlorhexidine-detergent solution) should be used for bathing and washing. One oz of 2% triclosan or 'Savlon' concentrate added to bath water reduces the hazard of transfer of infection through contamination of the bath. Patients who are perineal carriers should wash the perineum and 'bathing-trunk area' daily with an effective detergent antiseptic preparation such as chlorhexidine-detergent (Chapter 7).

3. Open wounds and lesions (excluding burns)   Open and drained wounds, ulcers of the skin and pressure sores should be dusted with chlorhexidine (1%) powder or covered with dressings impregnated with chlorhexidine (e.g. 'Bactigras'). These may be effective against *Staph. aureus* but not against many Gram-negative rods. (It should be noted that hexachlorophane and chlorhexidine ('Hibitane') are different compounds: hexachlorophane has toxic properties and must **not** be applied to open wounds. An iodophor spray may also be used. Open or drained wounds and lesions should be covered with bacteria-proof dressings.

4. General measures   Careful handling and disposal of bedding and dressings is important.

Bedding and clothing should be changed daily if possible, or every two days. Bedding should be carefully removed and transferred at the bedside to a container or bag which is immediately closed and sealed.

Contaminated dressings must not be handled with fingers but should be placed with forceps, or gloves, immediately into a bag and sealed. Large dressings are best handled with disposable gloves. Contaminated instruments should be placed into a sealed bag or container immediately after use and returned to the SSD.

Urine bottles used by patients with staphylococcal urinary infection should be handled carefully with gloves and the bottles should be disinfected after use, preferably by heat.

Wash-bowls, bedpans, baths and the barber's razor should be disinfected after use by an infected patient (see Chapter 7). The infected patient should preferably retain his own wash-bowl which is terminally disinfected on discharge from hospital.

5. Special prophylactic measures

(a) Patients   In the presence of a severe outbreak of staphylococcal infection it may be advisable to treat prophylactically the noses of all patients in the ward twice daily with the special antibiotic cream or ointment (see above); all patients should also use antiseptic soap and take antiseptic baths. Hexachlorophane powder should be applied daily to the groins, trunk, buttocks and upper thighs of bed-ridden or long-stay patients; hexachlorophane must not be applied to open lesions. Lesions and open wounds, whether infected or not, should be treated as described in the previous section.

(b) Staff handwashing   All staff working in the ward (including physiotherapists, radiographers and laboratory technicians) should wash their hands with a chlorhexidine-detergent solution, or povidone-iodine detergent or disinfect with a solution of 70% ethanol or 60% isopropanol rubbed on until hands are dry, before and after handling any patient or his immediate environment (Chapters 6 and 7).

9.1.4   SEPSIS AND NASAL CARRIERS IN HOSPITAL STAFF

Members of staff carrying an epidemic strain of *Staph. aureus* in the nose or on the skin, especially if dispersers or with a septic lesion caused by any strain of *Staph. aureus*, require treatment. This should be controlled by the staff medical officer and the microbiologist. It is not necessary to treat a nasal carrier of a strain which has not caused an infection or an epidemic of MRSA colonization or infection. A member of the staff with a septic lesion should be excluded from the wards until this is healed. Minor cuts and abrasions should be covered with a waterproof dressing. Prophylactic nasal treatment of staff is rarely required. Nasal carriers requiring treatment should be treated with nasal cream and antiseptic soap (see section on treatment of nasal carriers. If there is evidence of skin carriage of an epidemic strain or repeated septic lesions, daily baths with chlorhexidine-detergent solution or another recommended antiseptic detergent preparation should be taken for one week, and the hair should be washed twice weekly with chlorhexidine-detergent, or povidone-iodine or cetrimide shampoo in addition to the routine treatment. If the staphylococci are not removed after two weeks, a further course of nasal treatment should be given and bathing with chlorhexidine or other antiseptic detergent solution should be continued. If eradication proves difficult it may be necessary to continue treatment for long periods (e.g. 3–6 months). Changing to a different antiseptic-detergent preparation may sometimes be effective.

9.1.5   CLOSURE OF WARDS

If there are many infections and carriers of an epidemic strain in a ward, and if measures have failed to control an epidemic, it may be necessary to close a ward. The ward should be cleaned, and when it is re-opened patients should be screened for the presence of the epidemic strain before they are admitted to the clean ward. Screening is particularly important if patients are transferred to the clean ward from another hospital or from another ward in the same hospital. Unless required for aesthetic reasons, cleaning of walls and ceilings is unnecessary.

9.1.6   NEONATAL UNITS

Staphylococci are particularly likely to be transferred on the hands of staff. A baby with any staphylococcal infection, however small, irrespective of the antibiotic sensitivity pattern, should be isolated in a single room with full precautions against airborne and contact spread. If an outbreak occurs, all babies should be treated with hexachlorophane powder (e.g. 'Ster-Zac') at each napkin change or twice daily (if this is not already routine procedure). The buttocks, groins, lower abdomen, umbilicus and axilla should be powdered. Infected babies should be bathed daily with chlorhexidine-detergent solution. A 4% chlorhexidine-detergent solution, or 70% alcohol solution rubbed to dryness should be used for all handwashing by the staff. Hexachlorophane detergent or liquid soap may still be used for staff handwashing, but not for bathing babies. If a nursery has an outbreak involving more than two or three babies, no new babies should be admitted until all occupants are discharged and the room and equipment have been cleaned (see also Chapter 16). Routine screening of staff for *Staph. aureus* is not necessary, but in an outbreak carriers of the epidemic strains should be treated.

9.1.7 EPIDEMIC METHICILLIN-RESISTANT *STAPHYLOCOCCUS AUREUS* (EMRSA)

An increase in the number of outbreaks of methicillin-resistant staphylococcal infection has been reported in Australia, USA, Eire, South Africa, and more recently in certain areas of the UK. The strains causing these infections are usually resistant to penicillin, tetracycline, erythromycin, clindamycin, trimethoprim, often to gentamicin and sometimes to other antibiotics such as neomycin, chloramphenicol, fusidic acid, ciprofloxacin. Many methicillin-resistant *Staph. aureus* (MRSA) are not epidemic strains, but there is no laboratory test available to differentiate them rapidly from epidemic strains. However, experimental phages which can differentiate strains of known epidemicity and other techniques are available for use in specialist centres (Marples *et al.* 1986, Mulligan and Arbeit 1991). Some precautions must therefore be taken with all MRSA. Infections with EMRSA have often been severe and the outbreaks difficult to control. Most of the measures already described for prevention of spread of *Staph. aureus* are appropriate, but additional measures to prevent inter-ward and inter-hospital spread are required (Report 1990).

A known infected patient or carrier of EMRSA, or a patient admitted from a hospital or unit in which the strain is endemic, should be admitted directly to an isolation room and screened. The transferring hospital should inform the receiving hospital and this is the responsibility of the infection control team. On discharge, infected or colonized patients should be identified by marking their medical records, or be given cards so that necessary action can be taken if they are admitted to another hospital. Staff transferred from wards or hospitals with this strain should also be screened. Care is particularly required with agency staff, who preferably should not work in wards containing MRSA infected or colonized patients.

If a strain is first identified when the patient is in a ward, particularly if it is a surgical or intensive care ward, or if immunocompromised patients are present, the patient should be immediately isolated, preferably in a special unit. Isolation in side wards is often ineffective. If more than one patient is found to be carrying the strain, all patients and staff should be screened and appropriate action taken.

Screening should involve swabs from the nose, throat, axillae, perineum and any lesions. In elderly bedridden patients, the buttocks and other pressure areas should be sampled irrespective of the presence of an actual lesion. EMRSA may also be found in the sputum, faeces, urine, and in association with indwelling lines, catheters and tracheostomies when present. Contact or sweep-plates from bedding are useful for identifying new infections or colonized patients and reduce the number of screening samples required. Contact plates taken from the floor are also helpful in determining whether a ward is clear of the organism, but will not necessarily detect the presence of non-dispersers.

Eradication of the strain from a patient is often difficult, since the organisms are usually resistant to neomycin, and nasal carriage often responds poorly to chlorhexidine cream. Mupirocin 2% in a paraffin base and applied three times daily for five days is usually effective, or if applied in a polyethylene glycol base may also remove the organisms from superficial lesions, but treatment should be limited to seven days because of the possible emergence of resistance. Nasal carriers on the staff can be returned to duty in a non-high risk area before a negative swab is obtained after two day's treatment with mupirocin but not other topical agents. As already discussed, nasal treatment should be associated with bathing, washing and shampooing with antiseptic detergents such as chlorhexidine, povidone-iodine or triclosan, and similar agents should be used by staff for handwashing. Systemic agents for a short period, for example a combination of fusidic acid and rifampicin (not more than seven days) have been used to treat resistant nasal or throat carriers, but this should not be a routine since resistance to these agents can emerge rapidly.

Transferring infected or colonized patients to an isolation unit may abort an epidemic, but if such a unit is not available it may be necessary to convert an existing ward to an isolation ward and provide it with its own nursing staff. This can be very expensive.

Although most MRSA strains are unlikely to spread, it may be advisable to treat patients colonized with any strain, epidemic or not, with a nasal ointment and skin antiseptics and isolate particularly if in a surgical or high risk unit, but treatment without isolation should be considered even in geriatric wards.

Three successive negative swabs from nose, and any other colonized sites are necessary before a patient is considered clear of MRSA, but even then late recurrence up to 12 months can occur.

9.2   Infections due to Gram-negative bacilli (other than intestinal pathogens)

Gram-negative infection is often due to self-infection from the patient's own bowel flora but cross-infection is also common (including infections first acquired by the patient's intestinal flora from hospital food). Gram-negative bacilli are usually transferred by contact; airborne spread is rare. Transfer on the hands of staff is probably the main route of spread, although contaminated solutions or equipment are sometimes responsible for infection. Precautions against contact transfer should be taken for all infections, but for patients infected with Gram-negative bacilli (with the exception of some severe *Ps. aeruginosa* infections and highly resistant strains) isolation in a single room should be given a lower priority than patients with staphylococcal infection; combined infection of wounds with staphylococci and Gram-negative bacilli are common, but *Ps. aeruginosa* is less likely to spread by air then *Staph. aureus*. Patients infected with gentamicin-resistant pseudomonas, and other highly resistant Gram-negative bacilli in special units – such as neonatal or intensive care units (especially in the presence of patients on mechanical ventilation), ophthalmic and neurosurgical units, or areas where patients are treated with immunosuppressive drugs – should be isolated in single rooms because of the difficulty of preventing the spread of infection and the high susceptibility of the patients. If infection occurs in a ward where patients are particularly susceptible, staff should use povidone-iodine, chlorhexidine detergent, or 70% ethanol preparation for hand disinfection and if it is necessary to bathe patients with discharging wounds, povidone-iodine detergent should be used for bathing.

9.3   Infections due to Lancefield Group A, β haemolytic streptococci (*Streptococcus pyogenes*)

The organisms can spread both by contact and through the air. All patients with infections in maternity units should be isolated in a hospital isolation unit or in single rooms, and treated with an appropriate antibiotic (e.g. benzyl penicillin or penicillin V for mild infections for seven days) except for those with burns – see below. In an outbreak (two or more cases), staff and patients should be screened (nose, throat and lesion swabs) and staff carriers should be excluded from duty and treated. Other sources in patients may also be sought (e.g. vaginal, rectal lesions, and umbilical lesions in neonates). Staff carriers should be kept off duty for at least three days after commencing treatment. The ward should be closed to new admissions and staff not transferred to other wards unless swabs are clear. If the outbreak is not controlled, repeat swabbing is required and prophylactic treatment of all patients and staff should be considered. Patients in other wards, particularly surgical wards, with profusely discharging wounds or extensive skin sepsis due to this organism should be given a high priority for isolation. Failures of treatment with penicillin should be treated with erythromycin and patients with colonized burns should initially be treated with flucloxacillin or erythromycin. All colonized burns patients (throat and burn) should be isolated and treated.

9.4   Infections due to Lancefield Group B streptococci

Outbreaks occasionally occur in neonatal wards. Early onset infections are usually acquired from the mother, whereas late onset may be acquired by cross-infection. In an outbreak, infected babies are isolated and treated with benzyl penicillin for seven days. Swabs are taken from throat and the umbilicus of all babies, and carriers are treated with penicillin. Umbilici of all babies are treated with alcoholic chlorhexidine and the babies are bathed with chlorhexidine-detergent.

9.5   Outbreaks of diarrhoea and/or vomiting

The outbreak is commonly due to bacterial infection or intoxication, viral infection, or rarely to chemical intoxication. The source may be food or an infected patient.

9.5.1   INCUBATION PERIODS

Food poisoning

Staphylococcus aureus	2–4 hours
Bacillus cereus	1–2 hours or 10–12 hours
Vibrio parahaemolyticus	8–16 hours
Clostridium perfringens	12–24 hours
Salmonella spp	12–48 hours
Campylobacter spp	3–5 days

Other organisms

Shigella spp	**3–5** days
Enteropathogenic *Escherichia coli*	2–3 days
Rotaviruses	1–2 days

Salmonella infections are particularly hazardous in neonatal, geriatric and psychiatric units. Campylobacter infections are now as or more common than salmonella, but infrequently cause hospital outbreaks. Rotavirus infections are the commonest cause of intestinal infection in neonatal nurseries, but also occur in paediatric and geriatric wards. Enteropathogenic *E. coli* infections also occur in infant nurseries but are now infrequent. Small outbreaks of diarrhoea, probably of viral origin, are common in geriatric and psychiatric wards.

9.5.2 INVESTIGATION

1. Arrangements should be made to ensure that ward staff immediately report possible outbreaks to the infection control team and send specimens of faeces and/or vomit to the laboratory.
2. Infection control staff should visit wards and collect epidemiological data on onset of infection (e.g. whether one or more wards are involved, whether staff are affected and what food was eaten by infected patients). If food poisoning is suspected a dietary history of infected patients and staff and of non-infected controls should also be investigated.
3. Arrangements should be made for isolation of infected patients (salmonella) or closing the ward. Staff should be instructed in hygienic techniques.
4. If food-poisoning is suspected, samples of suspected food should be collected from the kitchen. Catering staff should be questioned for symptoms and samples of faeces collected if necessary. Hygienic practices in the kitchens should be investigated.
5. The Consultant in Communicable Disease Control (CCDC) should be notified if a notifiable disease or food poisoning is involved and the environmental health officer if food poisoning is suspected.

Most outbreaks in hospitals will be small and can be managed by the infection control team without additional resources. Often no causative organism will be isolated and no further case will occur. If the outbreak is large, or particularly severe (e.g. responsible for deaths in patients), the emergencies committee should be assembled and procedures outlined on page 20 should be adopted where applicable. It is particularly important to appoint a spokesman to keep the media informed, to ensure adequate staff and materials are available to treat infected patients and to consider whether assistance is necessary for investigations (e.g. PHLS Laboratory, Communicable Disease Surveillance Centre). A daily meeting of the emergencies committee may be necessary in the early stages of the outbreak.

A particular problem may occur if staff are also infected. Nursing staff can be allowed to return to work when symptoms have ceased. Instructions on hygienic precautions should be given. Catering staff who have been infected should not handle food until three negative faecal samples are obtained. In the event of prolonged carriage, a discussion between occupational health, infection control departments and the manager involved may be necessary to determine the future of the individual.

9.6　Pseudomembranous colitis

This is an infection caused by *Clostridium difficile* which is a toxin-producing organism, carried in the intestinal tract. It is usually associated with antibiotic therapy, particularly clindamycin and to a lesser extent with β lactam antibiotics. Infection occurs most frequently in neonates or the elderly. The spores survive well in the environment and have been isolated from floors, bedpans and hands of staff. The infection usually occurs sporadically, but probable outbreaks have been reported. Transfer on instruments such as sigmoidoscopes has been suggested. Infected patients should be treated with vancomycin or appropriate alternatives (e.g. metronidazole) and nursed with excretion precautions. During a possible outbreak, infected patients should be isolated if possible, or the ward should be closed. Thorough cleaning of the ward is recommended before re-opening. *Cl. difficile* is resistant to most disinfectants, but is killed by 2% glutaraldehyde in 10 minutes (see p. 72). However, single-use or autoclaved instruments should preferably be used on infected patients.

9.7　Enteroccal infections

Outbreaks of enterococcal infections have been increasingly reported in recent years (Terpenning *et al.* 1988). Some strains show increased resistance to aminoglycosides, may produce β lactamase and, less frequently, are resistant to vancomycin. Enterococci are part of the normal flora of the gastrointestinal tract and may be selected by the use of third generation cephalosporins or quinolones. Infection with resistant strains tends to occur in long standing intra-abdominal or urinary tract infections, neurological diseases in severely ill or in immunosuppressed patients, after repeated courses of antibiotics. Rapid identification of an epidemic strain is important. Spread is believed to be mainly on the hands of staff, but adequate decontamination of bedpans and urine bottles and effective care of indwelling catheters are important. Patients infected or colonized with resistant strains should preferably be isolated and excessive use of aminoglycosides, third generation cephalosporins and quinolones should be avoided.

9.8　Infections due to *Clostridium perfringens* and other gas gangrene bacilli

Hospital-acquired infection with *Cl. perfringens* is almost always postoperative and derived from the patient's own bowel flora. Gas gangrene is rare, but it occasionally follows orthopaedic operations on the leg (especially above the knee) when the arterial blood supply is defective, and may occur after certain abdominal operations.

Because gas gangrene bacilli which are no different from those that cause infection are carried in abundance by most healthy people in their bowel flora, and are also commonly found in the environmental air and dust, there is no reason to close a theatre after operations on patients with clostridial infection; all that is needed is a thorough routine cleaning of the theatre after the operation. Though, for the same reason, isolation to prevent cross-infection with *Cl. perfringens* is unnecessary, a patient with gas gangrene should preferably be nursed in an isolation room because he is dangerously ill, and requires special nursing care.

9.9   Isolation of patients with burns (Symposium 1985)

Patients with burns are commonly thought to require protective isolation before the burns become infected, and to require source isolation if they do become infected. In practice, the burns are infected for at least 24 hours before this state can be recognized by bacterial cultures. Moreover, a patient may be infected with one pathogen (e.g. *Staph. aureus*) but for the moment free from other pathogens (e.g. *Ps. aeruginosa*) from which he should be protected. For these reasons it is logical to use combined source and protective isolation for extensive burns.

Many burns, especially those of small or moderate extent, can be kept free from bacterial colonization for long periods by topical chemoprophylaxis (e.g. with 0.5% silver nitrate solution or silver sulphadiazine cream) (see Chapter 16). Segregation in cubicles, even with mechanical ventilation, has been shown to have little protective value for burned patients in a burns unit. Good barrier nursing techniques (especially the use of gloves for handling the patient) and topical chemoprophylaxis are of particular importance for such patients. Isolation in single bed rooms facilitates the aseptic handling of extensively burned patients and should be adopted. Such single bed rooms should, ideally, have plenum ventilation and an exhaust ventilated air-lock; if no air-lock is provided, the extracted air should not be discharged into the ward. For smaller burns, given effective local chemoprophylaxis, barrier nursing in an open ward with exudate precautions is acceptable, provided the dressings can be changed in a mechanically ventilated dressing room.

If a patient with burns, whether small or extensive, is in a general surgical ward, it is of the greatest importance that he should be source-isolated in a single bed room. If a patient is nursed in such a room, it should be remembered that while staphylococci are commonly transferred by air, Gram-negative infections of burns, when not acquired from the patient's faecal flora, are more often acquired by contact. Barrier nursing techniques are more effective in preventing cross-infection of the patient than physical segregation by the walls that surround him, though this will facilitate barrier nursing and reduce the risk of cross-infection by discouraging unnecessary visits.

9.10   Legionnaire's disease (*Legionella pneumonia*)

This is a potentially severe respiratory infection which was first recognised in 1976; it is caused by a Gram-negative bacillus, *Legionella pneumophila*, and several other related species. The organism is widely distributed in nature and is commonly found in soil and surface waters. It multiplies over a temperature range varying from 20°C to over 40°. Colonization of static water is likely, and the organism may commonly be found in the hot water systems of large buildings such as hospitals, hotels and offices, usually without any evidence of infection amongst staff or patients. Outbreaks have originated from air conditioning systems, particularly their associated cooling towers; hot water systems and showers have also been recognized as sources of infection (Bartlett *et al.* 1986; Edelstein 1986). However, the exact source of the outbreak is often far from easy to establish. Outbreaks in the UK have been reported in hospitals, usually new ones, and occasionally in hotels and other large buildings with cooling towers. Sporadic cases also occur in the community with no recognizable source. Although some aspects of the epidemiology of the disease remain obscure, there is no evidence of person-to-person spread, nor is infection thought to be acquired by ingestion. It is believed that the pneumonia is acquired by inhaling fine aerosols – legionella-containing particles of about 5 μ in diameter – which are able to find their way into the lung alveoli. From this belief it also follows that some mechanism for making a fine spray of legionella contaminated water should be sought as a possible source of any outbreak (e.g. cooling tower drift, showers, 'whirlpools' etc). The elderly, especially with pre-existing chronic respiratory tract disease, and the immunosuppressed are particularly susceptible but the disease can occur at any age. The organism has probably been one of the causes of pneumonia, particularly in the elderly, for many years and the risk of acquiring legionella, as distinct from other pneumonias (e.g. pneumococcal), has been exaggerated. Legionella is responsible for about 2% of community acquired pneumonia.

Early detection of cases of infection is of major importance and is usually based initially on clinical suspicion by the clinician or microbiologist. Sputum, if obtainable, is usually mucoid and shows scanty neutrophils and no predominant organism. Legionella can sometimes be identified by direct immunofluorescence and by culture of sputum, but usually additional techniques such as trans-tracheal or bronchial aspiration, or lung biopsy are required. Antibody levels in the acutely ill are often of little help, but diagnosis can be made at a later stage if a fourfold increase is obtained, or a single high titre (> 128), particularly if specific IgM is detected. Serotyping of the legionella strain may be useful if an epidemiological investigation is required. Isolation of the patient is unnecessary, but source isolation may be indicated because of the severity of the established disease and the untoward publicity associated with it.

If the patient has been in hospital for 10 days or more, it is likely that infection was acquired in hospital and enquiries may reveal other possible cases, confirmed by antibody tests. However, further investigation is not usually warranted following a sporadic case, since legionellas are commonly found in hospital water supplies and control measures could be excessive and unnecessarily expensive.

Two or more cases warrant further investigation, which would include case control studies, antibody testing and sampling of possible environmental sources. If there is evidence of a community acquired outbreak or if an extensive investigation is likely, the Public Health Laboratory Service should be asked for assistance as soon as possible. The emergencies committee should be convened and the hospital engineer should be co-opted.

If environmental sampling is required this should be done before any control measures are instituted.

Five litre samples of water should be collected from all known potential sources (e.g. hot and cold water systems, and cooling towers). Samples should be taken from the mains supplies, holding tanks, calorifiers, hot and cold taps and showers. Temperatures should be recorded at hot water taps at the time of sampling and three minutes later. If a cooling tower is a possible source, samples should be taken from various points in the pipe-work, the cooling water return at the top and from the pond.

Routine sampling of the water supplies is not recommended, except possibly in wards for immunosuppressed patients, but a follow-up for a limited period is advisable after measures have been introduced to control an outbreak.

The elimination of legionellas from a water supply depends on chlorination or raising the temperature.

Chlorination of a cooling tower may be achieved by addition of a hypochlorite solution or tablets to give a level of available chlorine of 5 mg/l (ppm) for a period of several hours followed by cleaning and rechlorination. Higher levels of available chlorine (e.g. up to 50 mg/l) have been recommended. Levels of 50 mg/1 are also suggested in header tanks for disinfection of hot or cold water supply systems. Continuous chlorination to give levels of 1–2 mg/l available chlorine is an expensive alternative. Metal corrosion may be a long-term consequence of continuous or repeated chlorination.

It is also recommended that hot water should be stored in tanks (calorifiers at 60°C and distributed to taps at 52°C + 2°C). These temperatures are not always easy to achieve in practice, nor can they be relied upon to destroy the organism; in addition, patients, particularly the elderly and confused, must be protected from accidental scalding.

Good maintenance of equipment is the main preventative measure (DHSS 1988, 1989).

Hospital engineers should ensure that water systems are correctly designed and adequately maintained; for example storage tanks should have an adequate flow rate and have well-fitted covers, calorifiers should have facilities for easy drainage and cleaning and stratification should be minimized, 'dead legs' should be avoided, water pipes should be lagged to prevent incidental heating of cold water pipes and loss of temperature from hot water pipes, washers should be replaced as necessary with approved types which do not support the growth of legionella; cooling towers should be cleaned at least twice yearly and treated with appropriate biocides and corrosion inhibitors. Cold water supplies should be maintained at 20°C or less.

Legionnaire's disease can also be transmitted by whirlpools, humidifiers and nebulizers. This equipment should be treated with hypochlorites, or if nebulizers are used for respiratory therapy they can either be disposable or disinfected by heat (e.g. low temperature steam), although occasionally chemical disinfection may be required.

Legionella are widely distributed and the reason why infection occurs on some occasions and not others is unknown. In the absence of infection it is not recommended that expensive additional measures are introduced. However, careful surveillance of patients to detect cases is necessary in hospitals, particularly in units for immunosuppressed patients.

9.11   Aspergillus infections

Invasive aspergillus infections occur mainly in highly immunocompromised patients and particularly in liver and bone-marrow transplant patients. Prolonged neutropenia and use of high dose steroids are important risk factors (Rogers and Barnes 1988).

Aspergilli (*A. fumigatus*, *A. niger*, and *A. flavus*) are always present in air, dust, soil etc., and infection mainly occurs through inhalation of airborne spores (Walsh and Dixon 1989). Most outbreaks have been associated with demolition and renovation of adjacent buildings, presumably associated with the release of an unusually large number of spores. Occasional outbreaks have been associated with the release of spores within the hospital, for example from service ducts and contaminated filters in ventilation systems.

9.11.1 PREVENTION (Rhame 1991)

High risk units (e.g. liver and bone-marrow transplantation units) should be provided with filtered air. The filters should be capable of removing spores (diameter 2–3 μ). High efficiency particulate air (HEPA) filters are commonly recommended and remove 99.97% of particles 0.3 μ in diameter. Laminar flow is not required.

The effectiveness of conventional filters of operating room type removing 90% of particles 5 μ in diameter is uncertain, but these are probably adequate for most leukaemia units. If adjacent building operations are in progress, it is important to ensure that all windows are sealed. Service ducts passing through high risk wards should be sealed. If an outbreak has occurred, the ward surfaces should be thoroughly cleaned with a solution of a chlorine-releasing agent (1000 ppm av Cl_2), service ducts and windows should be sealed and a portable HEPA filtering unit should be introduced. A window unit introducing some external filtered air (e.g. 20%), in addition to recirculated filtered air, has the advantage of providing a positive pressure in the room. During an outbreak prophylaxis with an antifungal agent, such as amphotericin B or itraconazole may also be considered.

9.12 Cryptosporidiosis

Cryptosporidiosis is a diarrhoeal disease caused by protozoa of the *Cryptosporidium* spp. Infection is commonly acquired from water supplies and is a common complication of HIV infection. Spread of infection in hospital has been rarely reported (Lettau 1991a). Cryptosporidium oocysts are resistant to 70% ethanol, iodophors, chlorine-releasing agents, quaternary ammonium compounds and aldehydes in practicable exposure times; high concentrations of chlorine dioxide, ozone, hydrogen peroxide and ammonia may be effective, but further tests are necessary under practical conditions (Department of Environment and Health 1990). There is no effective treatment of clinical infections, but thorough cleaning of contaminated equipment should minimize the possibility of spread.

9.13   African viral haemorrhagic fevers (VHF)

These virus infections (Lassa fever, Marburg disease and Ebola virus diseases) are endemic in West and Central Africa. All have a significant mortality and there is no vaccine available. Treatment with tribavirin is effective in Lassa fever, the commonest of these infections. Lassa fever is contracted by man from a rodent, *Mastomys natalensis*, which is widely distributed in Africa but not in Europe. Human-to-human transmission of infection is probably uncommon and has never been known to occur outside Africa. The incubation period of these infections is usually 7–10 days with a range of 3–17 days. For control purposes, if no infection has occurred in a period of up to 21 days from exposure, a contact is usually taken to be free from infection.

9.13.1   EARLY IDENTIFICATION OF KNOWN OR SUSPECTED CASES

A medical practitioner suspecting that a patient might be suffering from a viral haemorrhagic fever (pyrexial illness, occupation and residence in endemic area) should **not** refer the patient to hospital but should immediately seek the advice of a consultant in communicable or tropical diseases. If the patient is already in hospital he should be confined in a single room until seen by the consultant. If a suspected case arrives in a casualty department, the infection control doctor should be informed, and the patient placed in a room specially designated for this purpose, where a box containing special protective clothing is available. There is considerable urgency in making contact with the appropriate expert not only for epidemiological purposes, but also to exclude *Plasmodium falciparum* malaria, which can be rapidly fatal, as a cause of the illness. Typhoid fever should also be excluded.

In practical terms, the above advice applies to any patient with a pyrexia of unknown origin during a period of 21 days after arrival from West or Central Africa. It is the duty of the medical practitioner who first sees the patient and/or the second opinion to notify the CCDC at the earliest possible opportunity.

The Memorandum on the Control of Viral Haemorrhagic Fevers (DHSS 1986) recommends that suspect patients should be graded according to the degree of suspicion (strong, moderate or minimal). Although these guidelines should generally be followed, recent evidence suggests that spread will not occur if adequate blood and body fluid precautions are taken. In countries without a high security infectious diseases unit, patients may be isolated in a single room with blood and body fluid precautions (Holmes *et al.* 1990).

9.13.2 GRADES OF SUSPICION

Strong A patient from a known endemic area (particularly health-care staff from a rural area), a contact of a confirmed case or a laboratory worker working with a VHF virus.

Moderate A patient from a rural area or small town, not usually considered to be an endemic area but where the onset and course of fever are consistent with VHF.

Minimal A patient from a major city where the risk is negligible.

A history of malaria prophylaxis should also be considered when grading the degree of suspicion.

9.13.3 ACTION

Strong suspicion Admit to high security infectious diseases unit, carry out surveillance of close contacts for 21 days.

Moderate suspicion Admit to a regional infectious diseases unit for strict isolation. Review level of suspicion if illness proves more consistent with VHF, and if malaria and other infections have been excluded.

Minimal suspicion Admit to a regional infectious diseases unit or a district general hospital isolation unit with blood/body fluid precautions. A consultant in infectious diseases should review the case.

With all grades of suspicion, patients must be transported using specific ambulance precautions and laboratory specimens should be examined in a high security (Category 4) laboratory. If the suspicion is high, and the patient is seen in the accident department or has been admitted to a ward, the hospital emergencies committee should be convened to decide the action required.

Names and addresses of close contacts should be obtained. If the patient is in a ward he/she should be transferred to a side room of the same ward and strict isolation precautions instituted involving a minimal number of staff (e.g. the doctor making the diagnosis and one nurse).

9.13.4 NOTES

1. Protective clothing (cap, gown, mask, gloves and overshoes) and a disposable urinal and bed-pan should be available in a box in the

emergency department. This box can be taken to a ward if necessary or provided for the ambulance service.

2. Particular care is required in the disposal of urine and faeces. The viruses are susceptible to the usual antiviral disinfectants. Autoclaving in the laboratory is preferred, but a hypochlorite solution would be appropriate, prior to incineration.

   The CCDC is responsible for surveillance of contacts, terminal disinfection of wards, departments or ambulances, but advice on disinfection should be obtained from the infection control doctor, who will usually be responsible for these procedures within the hospital.

3. Although all laboratory samples should be examined in a secure containment laboratory, films for malaria, rendered microbiologically safe (e.g. with formaldehyde) can be examined in the routine hospital laboratory, since this is an urgent investigation.

More detailed information on surveillance of contacts, terminal disinfection and disposal of corpses etc. can be found in the Memorandum and the US guidelines (Centers for Disease Control 1988).

9.14   Rabies

Human-to-human transmission of rabies has never been reported and the strict precautions recommended for the prevention of transmission are therefore unnecessary. However, the disease has emotive connotations for hospital staff, while the intensive medical and nursing care which is essential if the patient is to have any chance of survival increase the possibility of exposure to infection.

The following precautions are recommended:
1. the patient should be isolated in a single room, preferably in an intensive therapy unit;
2. attendant staff and other close contacts (e.g. anaesthetists) should be offered immunization with human diploid cell vaccine (4 intradermal injections of 0.1 ml given on the same day);
3. staff should wear protective clothing including goggles, mask and gloves;
4. mouth-to-mouth resuscitation should not be used;
5. pregnant female staff should not attend the patient;
6. specimens from the patient should not be sent to routine diagnostic laboratories but only to Category A pathogen laboratories;
7. equipment soiled by secretions or excretions must be destroyed or autoclaved.

Further information is contained in the *Memorandum on Rabies* (DHSS 1977).

9.15   Human infestation

Biting insects and burrowing mites may cause irritation and scratching may lead to infections such as impetigo. Although insects and mites are unlikely to be a major source of infection in hospitals in the UK, the problem of infestation is often referred to infection control staff (Lettau 1991b).

Lists of insecticides and acaricides suitable for treatment of the skin can be found in the *British Pharmacopoeia* or *British National Formulary*. These include dosages, methods of application and contraindications. Most health districts operate a rotating policy for the treatment of head lice to suppress the emergence of resistant strains. Details of the drugs currently recommended should be available from your District pharmaceutical officer.

9.15.1   LICE

All three species of human lice are blood sucking insects which are host-specific. The head and crab (pubic) lice are usually found in specific areas (e.g. scalp and pubic hair) but can also occur in the axillae, chest, legs, beard, and eyebrows; the nits (eggs) are firmly attached to hair and not easily removed. Body lice are found mainly in clothing, but also on the body surface, especially in axillae and around the waist. Superficial skin infection due to scratching is common.

Control measures
1. Carefully remove all clothing of patients with body or pubic lice and seal in a bag. Disposable gloves and a plastic apron should be worn.
2. Process linen in the laundry in a washing machine using conventional heat treatment.
3. In infestation with head or crab lice, treat the specific hairy areas of the host with an appropriate insecticidal lotion, such as 0.5% carbaryl or malathion, and repeat within 7–10 days. Patients with body lice do not require specific treatment but should be bathed.
4. No special treatment of the environment is required as spread is by personal contact. Body lice are, however, capable of surviving for a limited time in stored clothing, but head and pubic lice rapidly die when detached from their host.

9.15.2   ITCH MITES (scabies)

Scabies is an allergic reaction to the presence of a small mite (0.3–0.4 mm) which burrows into the top layer of skin. Patient symptoms are intense itching which may persist for some time after effective treatment, and the appearance of a hypersensitive rash. Burrows may occur anywhere, but are mainly on the hands, and arms, and particularly finger-webs. The associated rash is usually on the groins, elbows, inside thighs and around the wrists and waist. Transmission is by person-to-person contact and is usually assumed to require fairly prolonged and intimate contact. Hand-holding or patient support for long periods is probably responsible for most hospital-acquired scabies. Spread from bedding, clothing or fomites is unlikely. However, in elderly or immunosuppressed patients the mites multiply rapidly and large numbers of the parasites are present. This form of scabies is often known as 'crusty' or 'Norwegian' scabies and is far more readily transmissible.

Control measures
1. Apply a suitable acaricide such as 1% lindane or 0.5% malathion to all areas of the skin below the chin. A bath is not necessary prior to treatment but if a bath is given the skin must be thoroughly dry before applying the acaricide and it should not be washed off for 24 hours. If a second treatment is necessary repeat after 7–10 days.
2. Treat bedding and clothing as described for lice.
3. No special environmental control measures are necessary.
4. Refer members of the family and those in close physical contact to their general practitioner so that they can be treated if necessary.

9.15.3   FLEAS

Infestation is usually with dog, cat or bird fleas which will bite humans in the absence of the preferred host. The human flea is more likely to be introduced from outside the hospital, but it is now fortunately rare. Fleas are able to survive for some months in the environment without feeding. Elimination of the host or treatment of pets and the use of suitable insecticides on environmental surfaces is therefore essential if control is to be effective (see also p. 244).

Control measures (patient admitted with fleas)
1. Remove all clothing and bedding and seal in a bag. Whenever possible, process linen in the laundry in a washing machine using conventional heat treatment. A hot water-soluble plastic bag will allow transfer to the machine without handling. Clothing not suitable for washing may be sealed in a laundry bag and treated with low temperature steam. Autoclaving at higher temperatures is satisfactory

but is likely to damage some fabrics. This is the process commonly used by health authorities.
2. Use aerosol dispensers containing insecticide to kill fleas and arrange with your pest control operative to treat surfaces in the environment concerned.

Control measures (infestation in a hospital ward)
1. Identify the flea, and if possible, treat or remove the host. If it is a cat flea, take steps to exclude feral cats from the site.
2. Heat treat clothing and bedding as described above.
3. Vacuum clean floors, carpets, upholstery, fabrics, etc.
4. Contact your pest control operative to treat the environment e.g. ducting, hard surfaces, and under fixtures, with a residual insecticide.

For further advice on control management of lice, scabies and human infestations contact the Medical Entomology Centre at the University of Cambridge, Department of Applied Biology, Pembroke Street, Cambridge. (For Pharaoh's ants, see p. 244).

References and further reading

Bartlett, C.L.R., Macrae, A.D. and Macfarlane, J.D. (1986) *Legionella Infections*. Edward Arnold, London.

Brewer, J. and Jeffries, D.J. (1990) Control of viral infections in hospitals. *Journal of Hospital Infection*, **16**, 191.

Centers for Disease Control (1988) Management of patients with suspected viral haemorrhagic fever. *MMWR*, **37**, (Supplement S3).

Department of Health and Social Security (1986) *Memorandum on the Control of Viral Haemorrhagic Fevers*. HMSO, London.

Department of Health and Social Security (1977) *Memorandum on Rabies*. HMSO, London.

Department of Health and Social Security (1988) *The Control of Legionellae in Health Care Premises. A Code of Practice*. HMSO, London.

Department of Health and Social Security (1989) *Report of the Expert Advisory Committee on Biocides*. HMSO, London.

Department of the Environment and Health (1990) Report of the Group of Experts, *Cryptosporidium in Water Supplies*. HMSO, London.

Edelstein, P.H. (1986) Control of Legionella in hospitals. *Journal of Hospital Infection*, **8**, 109.

Holmes, G.P., McCormick, J.B., Trock, C.C. *et al.* (1990) Lassa fever in the United States. Investigation of a case and new guidelines for management. *New England Journal of Medicine*, **323**, 1120.

Lettau, L.A. (1991a) Nosocomial transmission and infection control aspects of parasitic and ectoparasitic disease, Part 1. *Infection Control and Hospital Epidemiology*, **12**, 59.

Lettau, L.A. (1991b) Nosocomial transmission and infection control aspects of parasitic and ectoparasitic diseases, Part 3. *Infection Control and Hospital Epidemiology*, **12**, 179.

Marples, R.R., Richardson, J.F. and de Saxe, M.J. (1986) Bacteriological characters of strains of *Staphylococcus aureus* submitted to a reference laboratory related to methicillin resistance. *Journal of Hygiene* (Camb), **96**, 217.

Mulligan, M.F., Arbeit, R.D. (1991) Epidemiologic and clinical utility of typing systems for differentiating among strains of methicillin-resistant *Staphylococcus aureus*. *Infection Control and Hospital Epidemiology*, **12**, 20.

Rhame, F.S. (1991) Prevention of nosocomial aspergillosis. *Journal of Hospital Infection*, **18** (Supplement), 466.

Report (1990) Report of a combined working party of the Hospital Infection Society and the British Society of Antimicrobial Chemotherapy. Revised guidelines for the control of epidemic methicillin-resistant *Staphylococcus aureus*. *Journal of Hospital Infection*, **16**, 351.

Rogers, T.R. and Barnes, R.A. (1988) Prevention of airborne fungal infection in immunocompromised patients. *Journal of Hospital Infection*, **ii** (Supplement A), 15.

Symposium on Infection Control in Burns (1985) *Journal of Hospital Infection*. **6** (Supplement B).

Terpenning, M.S., Zervos, M.J., Schaberg, D.R. *et al.* (1988) Enterococcal infections: an increasing problem in hospitalized patients. *Infection Control and Hospital Epidemiology*, **9**, 457.

Walsh, T.J. and Dixon, G.M. (1989) Nosocomial aspergillus: environmental microbiology, hospital epidemiology, diagnosis and treatment. *European Journal of Epidemiology*, **5**, 131.

Wenzel, R.P. (1987) Epidemics – identification and management. In *Prevention and Control of Nosocomial Infections*, Wenzel, R.P. (ed.) Williams and Wilkins, Baltimore.

10 *Special problems of miscellaneous infections II: Control of viral hepatitis and human immunodeficiency virus (HIV) infection*

10.1 Viral hepatitis

Several viruses may attack the human liver, but five are relevant here:

1. hepatitis A virus;
2. hepatitis B virus;
3. hepatitis C virus;
4. hepatitis D virus (delta);
5. hepatitis E virus (enterically transmitted non-A, non-B).

10.2 Hepatitis A (infectious hepatitis)

The infective agent is a small RNA virus about 26 nm in diameter. Infection is contracted by swallowing the virus. After an incubation period of about three weeks, a febrile, undifferentiated disease develops. During this stage, virus is excreted in the faeces in quantity. After a few days of this illness, jaundice appears; by that time virus excretion in the faeces is either undetectable or at a very low level. By the time patients have been admitted to hospital, they are usually no longer infectious. At this stage, antibodies are present in their blood. A transient viraemia occurs in the pre-icteric stage of the disease, but this is of such short duration that infection is not likely to be transmitted parenterally by injection of blood or blood products.

10.2.1 LABORATORY DIAGNOSIS

This can be made by radioimmunoassay of IgM (macroglobulin) antibodies to the virus in a single sample of serum taken in the acute phase of disease. Virus can be detected in the faeces, especially in the prodromal stage of the illness, by electron microscopy of faeces, but this is not as sensitive nor as reliable a technique as the radioimmunoassay for IgM antibodies which appear by the time the patient is in hospital with jaundice. IgG antibodies can also be determined; their presence without IgM antibodies indicates not a recent but an earlier infection by the virus. There is only one serological variety of the virus, and the presence of antibodies indicates full immunity.

10.2.2   PROTECTION AGAINST HEPATITIS A

About 30% of the population of the UK appear to have some antibody to hepatitis A virus in the circulation; gammaglobulin extracted from pooled donors' serum therefore confers good protection upon those who are likely to be exposed, as are, for example, travellers to tropical countries where the standards of hygiene are low and the chances of infection are considerable. Particularly at risk are those who work in the countryside, while undertaking voluntary service overseas. The globulin, present in the blood after infection, decays with a half-life of about a month, so that one injection will not confer protection for more than about 3–4 months, after which the subject can again become susceptible. To confer continuing protection, an injection of gamma-globulin is needed about every three months. Gammaglobulin can also be used to protect close contacts of a patient suffering from hepatitis A. It is usually only indicated for debilitated contacts or those suffering from serious diseases such as leukaemia.

10.3   Hepatitis B

This disease has an incubation period of about 40–160 days, often about 90 days. It is usually transmitted by the parenteral route, but can be transmitted in other ways. The disease is often subclinical; it is usually a relatively mild infection, but is generally more severe than hepatitis A. Individual cases of hepatitis B cannot be distinguished from hepatitis A on clinical grounds alone, though associated arthritis suggests hepatitis B. A chronic virus carrier state may follow acute hepatitis B and lead to chronic liver disease.

10.3.1   LABORATORY DIAGNOSIS

Different serotypes of hepatitis B virus (HBV) occur. At least 10 antigenic determinants on the hepatitis B surface antigen (HB_sAg) particles are known, and the antigens can be typed. Typing is of value in epidemiological studies. Subtype *ay* has caused most incidents of hospital-transmitted infection, but blood containing any subtype must be regarded as potentially dangerous. Another antigen known as '*e*' is often found in the blood of HB$_s$Ag carriers. There is some evidence that the presence of this *e* antigen indicates that the blood is more likely to be infectious than the blood of carriers whose serum does not contain it; but the distinction is not absolute, and blood which does not contain *e* antigen may also be infectious. All blood donations in the UK are nowadays tested for HB$_s$Ag. Because the virus cannot be grown in tissue culture, its presence is detected by finding virus antigens or DNA in blood or tissues. For screening blood donations the test almost universally used now is a radioimmunoassay. ELISA tests have improved in sensitivity and reliability in recent years and are preferred in many countries. Their sensitivity is almost equal to that of radioimmunoassay. Hepatitis is a potential hazard in general wards, especially when patients with the disease are being treated, or in operations upon immunosuppressed patients who are known carriers; but provided the rules of safe working are observed (see below, and Chapter 19) the risk is small.

10.3.2 CARRIERS OF HEPATITIS B VIRUS

About 1:800 of the population in the UK continuously carry HBV virus in their blood. In many other parts of the world (e.g. China) the proportion of the population who carry the virus is much higher; the nearer they live to the equator and the humbler their status in the social scale, the more likely people are to carry the virus. Men are more likely to be carriers than women. High carrier rates are found among certain members of the community, in the UK especially among inmates of prisons, drug addicts, mental defectives (in institutions rather than those living at home) and immigrants from tropical countries. Healthy carriers in the general population usually carry virus in comparatively low titre in their blood, but certain patients, if infected, may carry the virus in very high titre and for that reason their blood is much more likely to transmit infection than blood from most carriers. The patients who, if infected, constitute a special hazard, are those who are immunosuppressed through their illness or as a result of treatment, for example patients with chronic renal failure (this condition is immunosuppressive), and those with inborn immunodeficiency and patients immunosuppressed as part of the treatment (e.g. after kidney grafting or for certain diseases such as leukaemia). Before blood from these patients is put through other laboratory investigations, it is advisable to test it to make sure that it does not contain HB$_s$Ag.

Because the damage to the liver in hepatitis B patients is immunologically mediated, those with chronic renal failure and those who are immunosuppressed when they become infected usually do not show characteristic features of the disease; if they are in dialysis units, however, they may very easily transmit infection to other patients or to the staff of the unit. In the past infection has entered dialysis units by transfusion of blood from a carrier and has been spread from patient-to-patient by shared dialysis machines or possibly by other mechanisms also. Infection may be spread to staff by spilt blood getting into a scratch, or into the eye, or by a prick from a contaminated needle. It may be transmitted by acupuncture. Patients with hepatitis B and patients who are carriers, even high titre carriers, do not transmit the infection as an aerosol. To acquire infection from them one has to get their blood or possibly other tissue fluids under one's skin. Medical procedures are by no means the only, or even the most important, ways of acquiring serum hepatitis; it may be transmitted by sexual intercourse, by sharing a razor with a carrier or by tattooists.

10.3.3   AVOIDANCE OF HEPATITIS B TRANSMISSION

The main hazards are due to contamination of small skin wounds, conjunctiva or mucous membranes with blood from patients with serum hepatitis or from immunosuppressed carriers of hepatitis B virus (e.g. those with chronic renal failure or grafted kidneys), in which, if infected, it is likely to be present in high titre. Healthy carriers usually have a relatively low titre and therefore present a much smaller hazard.

The main risks of infection with the virus obviously are in hospital departments where blood is handled, especially in accident departments, operating theatres, maternity departments, dental departments, laboratories and mortuaries. Special units, such as isolation wards and those treating drug addicts, haemophiliacs and patients with liver or renal diseases are also high risk. Recommendations for protection of patients in these areas are presented in this chapter and Chapter 19 (Renal units). Although the same basic principles apply wherever a special hazard exists, there are practical features peculiar to each area.

10.4   Hepatitis C

Hepatitis C is a recently described RNA virus which is transmitted in similar ways to hepatitis B. It therefore causes infection in drug addicts and blood and blood product recipients. The infection can also be transmitted sexually and may be contracted during occupational exposure to blood in hospital. Measures designed to prevent accidental transmission of hepatitis B (see below) should be successful in preventing accidental transmission of hepatitis C.

There is no available vaccine against hepatitis C.

10.5   Hepatitis D (delta agent)

This virus requires the presence of the hepatitis B virus for successful infection which usually occurs in drug addicts but can also be acquired sexually.

10.6   Hepatitis E

Otherwise referred to as 'enterically transmitted non-A, non-B hepatitis', this infection is common in the developing world where sanitation is poor, and waterborne outbreaks occur. It has a high mortality in pregnancy.

10.7   Human immunodeficency virus (HIV) infection

The occurrence in 1981 of severe and often fatal pneumonia caused by the opportunistic pathogen *Pneumocystis carinii* in apparently healthy male homosexuals in the United States led to the recognition of the acquired immunodeficiency syndrome (AIDS). Two years later the infectious agent causing this apparently new disease was identified as a previously unknown retrovirus which was initially called the human T-cell lymphotropic virus (HTLV3) or lymphadenopathy associated virus (LAV). It is now known as the human immunodeficiency virus (HIV). This virus has a particular tropism for thymus derived lymphocytes, particularly T4 (helper) cells which play a crucial role in regulating the immune system. Damage to or destruction of T4 lymphocytes leads to the development of a cellular immunodeficiency disease rendering the patient susceptible to a wide variety of infections, but particularly to those caused by viruses, protozoa, fungi and intracellular bacteria. Patients suffering from AIDS also develop various malignancies, most notably Kaposi's sarcoma (a skin tumour) and also lymphomas.

HIV infection is most commonly a sexually transmitted disease amongst homosexual males in Europe and the US, although heterosexual spread is increasing. Heterosexual spread is the most common mode of transmission in some parts of central Africa. Blood and blood products such as Factor VIII have been responsible for transmission in the past but this route has been almost eliminated by routine screening. The routes of transmission are therefore similar to those of hepatitis B virus and infected persons also include drug addicts and haemophiliacs. The virus may be present in blood, tissues, semen, vaginal secretions and saliva (very small amounts only). There is evidence that HIV is less infectious than the hepatitis B virus. The risk of infection from an HIV contaminated needle-stick injury has been calculated as 0.4%, whereas from an HBV contaminated needle-stick injury it is about 20%.

Infection with HIV is usually sub-clinical, although a very small number of patients can develop a mononucleosis-like illness with fever, lymphadenopathy and rash within two to three weeks of infection. The majority, however, initially remain symptom-free. After a long and variable incubation period the majority of these and possibly all will develop one (or more) of the following syndromes.

1. The acquired immunodeficiency syndrome (AIDS) associated with profound cellular immunodeficiency, major opportunistic infections, especially *Pneumocystis carinii* pneumonia, and Kaposi's sarcoma. Present evidence suggests that most, if not all of HIV infected persons will eventually develop AIDS.
2. Persistent generalized lymphadenopathy (PGL) or AIDS-related complex (ARC) which is often referred to as 'prodromal AIDS'. Patients with ARC are always symptomatic and may have weight loss, diarrhoea, oral candidiasis and fever along with leucopenia and T4 depletion. They have a high probability of the early development of AIDS.
3. Idiopathic thrombocytopenic purpura.
4. Nervous system involvement, including psychotic illnesses and neurological disorders.

The diagnosis of HIV infection is confirmed by the demonstration of serum antibodies to the virus. Current knowledge suggests that the virus persists in the body for life and a patient who is HIV antibody positive must therefore be considered to be permanently infectious.

HIV antibody takes a variable time to develop, but will usually be positive within 2–3 months after infection but can take longer. It is, therefore, unwise to rely on a negative antibody test, particularly in a 'high risk' subject.

Tests for antibody should only be carried out with patient's agreement, and pre-test counselling should be given to ensure the patient is aware of the consequences of a positive result. Exceptions may rarely be necessary, for example, in very ill patients and to exclude HIV infection as part of the differential diagnosis of an unknown infection in low risk patients. The clinician is responsible for making this decision. Screening of high risk patients before major surgery (e.g. cardiac) may be considered but is unlikely to be accepted as a routine procedure until the social consequences of a positive result are alleviated.

Arrangements should be made for further counselling in the event of a positive result.

There is as yet no cure for HIV infection although certain anti-viral drugs such as zidovudine (Retrovir) will suppress the virus and slow the progress of the infection; side-effects, however, are common and sometimes serious. The management of AIDS therefore depends primarily on supportive therapy and the prevention and treatment of opportunistic infection such as pneumonia. HIV is readily inactivated by heat and by disinfectants such as glutaraldehyde, chlorine-releasing agents and formaldehyde (see Chapter 5).

Prevention of transmission of infection depends on modification of sexual practices, particularly the avoidance of promiscuity and unprotected sexual intercourse in high risk groups, screening of donated blood and of blood products for HIV antibody, and the counselling of persons found to be antibody positive. HIV infection has been acquired by a small number of health care workers from patients in the course of their work. There have been a number of reports of HIV seroconversion following needle-stick injuries and rarely, following contamination of skin and mucous membranes with HIV positive blood in the ward or in the laboratory. There is no available vaccine.

The problem arises as to whether to treat all patients as potential sources of HIV infection or to introduce special precautions for known infected or 'high risk' patients. The use of a single tier or double tier level of prevention depends mainly on the population to which it would apply (Jenner 1990). In most hospitals with a very low incidence of HIV antibody-positive patients, special arrangements can be introduced for known positive or high risk patients only. However, the detection of 'high risk' patients is often difficult and care is still necessary in handling any blood – for example, cover lesions on hands, avoid as much as possible splashing, skin contamination and needle-stick injuries. The requirement to wear gloves and possibly a disposable apron when taking blood samples for all patients is probably excessive at this time and in view of the low risk in the general population is unnecessarily expensive, but an increasing incidence, as in some cities in the US, may require a change in policy in the future. In the USA, 'Universal Blood and Body Fluid Precautions' are recommended (Centers for Disease Control 1988). These apply mainly to blood or other body fluids containing visible blood, but also include semen, vaginal secretions, CSF, synovial fluid, peritoneal fluid, pericardial and amniotic fluid, but not faeces, nasal secretions, saliva, sputum, urine and vomitus unless they contain visible blood. The precautions include wearing gloves, masks, gowns and protective eye-cover and taking care with sharps. The cost of 'Universal Precautions' is high and there is as yet no evidence that they are effective. Effective handwashing after handling a patient would in most instances prevent the spread of infection (apart from sharps injuries).

High risk patient groups include the following:
1. homosexual/bisexual men;
2. haemophiliacs;
3. intravenous drug addicts;
4. male prisoners;
5. heterosexual partners of above and subsequent children of HIV infected mothers;
6. patients (male or female) from sub-Sahara Africa who have had sexual relations with potentially infected persons.

Patients in hospital who are HIV antibody positive or 'high-risk' should be managed in the same way as those who are carriers of hepatitis B. The use of the term 'inoculation risk' rather than 'high risk' is preferred by some.

There are many codes of practice available and recommendations are often variable. The report of the Working Party of the Hospital Infection Society (1990) provides practical guidance. The following basic rules may be observed.

1. Venepuncture and other invasive procedures must only be carried out when absolutely necessary.
2. Laboratory specimens should be clearly labelled with 'Biohazard' stickers of the same type as are used for hepatitis B.
3. Staff attending to patients and handling specimens should wear disposable gloves. Plastic aprons should also be worn during invasive procedures and eye protection if there is any possibility of aerosol formation (e.g. during surgery).
4. Disposable equipment should be used whenever possible. If any item of equipment is not disposable it should be decontaminated after cleaning by autoclaving or exposure to 2% glutaraldehyde. Special equipment reserved for AIDS patients is not essential for their clinical care nor for the processing of laboratory specimens from these patients.
5. Blood spillage should be treated with sodium hypochlorite or another chlorine-releasing agent either in solution or as a powder or granules (10 000 ppm chlorine).
6. Crockery and cutlery do not require disinfection but should be thoroughly washed and dried.
7. Antibody-positive patients can be nursed in an open ward unless they are bleeding, have diarrhoea, are psychotic or require isolation for other reasons (e.g. open tuberculosis) when single room accommodation is indicated.
8. Brook or similar airways should be used for resuscitation of HIV positive patients.

For more detailed recommendations for:

laboratory staff	see below;
surgical operations	see p. 202;
maternity departments	see p. 203;
dental departments	see p. 204;
mortuary and postmortem staff	see p. 205;
renal units	see p. 357.

10.8   Prevention of infection with HBV and HIV and specific personnel/departments

10.8.1   LABORATORY STAFF

1. General precautions (Health Services Advisory Committee, 1991; see also page 347).
2. Staff must be trained to work safely. This is the responsibility of the director of the laboratory usually exercised through the safety officer or a senior member of the technical staff.
3. Specimens from **high risk** patients must be marked to indicate that they may carry a hazard, and handled with surgical or disposable gloves. Blood must be sent in screw-topped rubber-washered glass bottles (bijous, McCartneys, universal containers) and specimens must be transported in sealed impermeable plastic bags. Blood specimens must either be discarded into a strong hypochlorite solution or, preferably, placed in a bucket and autoclaved. The time and temperature reached by the autoclave must be carefully checked.
4. Specimens of blood and serum should be centrifuged in sealed cups.
5. Auto-analyzers – surgical or disposable plastic gloves must be worn when changing dialysers or tubing. Plastic cup trays should be disinfected in a solution of a chlorine-releasing agent.
6. Work surfaces should be disinfected after use with hypochlorites or other chlorine-releasing agents (1000 ppm av Cl_2).
7. Laboratory equipment should be decontaminated before service or repair.
8. Blood or serum specimens should be tested for presence of HB_sAg or HIV antibody before being included in the 'laboratory pool' of test sera. Staff collecting blood from HB_sAg or HIV antibody positive or known high risk patients must wear gloves and a disposable plastic apron and the patient's arm should be placed on a piece of disposable plastic sheeting before collecting the specimen. It is commonly recommended that containers should be filled from the syringe with the needle still attached; some prefer to separate the needle carefully

with forceps or disposable gloves before discharging the contents. Syringes and needles must be disposed of by placing them in a puncture-proof box with a lid (DHSS 1982), which must be available on the ward. Needles should not be re-sheathed unless a safe method is available.

10.8.2   SURGICAL OPERATIONS

These precautions are required for 'high-risk' and known HIV antibody or HB_sAg positive patients (Hospital Infection Society 1990).

1. It is unnecessary to place patients last on the operating list.
2. Unnecessary equipment should be removed from the zone of contamination in the theatre in order to reduce the amount of decontamination required after the operation. Disposable drapes should be used and the mattress wrapped in a plastic sheet.
3. Pre-operative shaving should be avoided. Wound drainage should be avoided if possible. If drainage is considered necessary closed rather than open wound drainage is recommended. Blood should be cleaned off the patient's skin as far as possible at the end of the operation, and a wound dressing used that will contain exudate within an impervious outer covering.
4. A disposable plastic apron should be worn under the gown or a water impermeable gown should be worn by the scrubbed team. If a plastic apron is used, a gown with water impermeable sleeves should be worn if gross contamination of sleeves with blood is likely.
5. The surgical team should wear two pairs of gloves, and unhealed cuts or lesions should be covered with a waterproof dressing.
6. Spectacles preferably with side pieces, goggles or a visor should be worn to avoid conjunctival contamination or splashing.
7. Needles, syringes and disposable sharp instruments must be discarded into approved containers (DHSS 1982). Syringe needles should not be recapped.
8. Surgical instruments and other tools should be handled with care during and after the operation. After use they should be sealed, unwashed, in a plastic bag, labelled 'Biohazard' and returned to the sterile services department (SSD). If no SSD is available, instruments should be washed carefully and then autoclaved or disinfected.
9. Linen and theatre clothing should be sealed in a water-soluble plastic bag and sent to the laundry for treatment as 'infected' linen.
10. Theatre cleaning of floors and surfaces within the contamination zone should be cleaned with a chlorine-releasing agent (1000 ppm

av Cl$_2$). Walls and other surfaces do not require cleaning unless contaminated with blood. Large volumes of fluid should be used for cleaning, gloves and a plastic apron should be worn by the operator. Definite blood spillage should be treated with a chlorine releasing agent (10 000 ppm av Cl$_2$) before cleaning. Thorough rinsing is necessary after cleaning with a chlorine-releasing agent. The theatre can be used for the next patient immediately after cleaning.

11. Waste materials should be sealed in a plastic bag and incinerated. Used swabs do not present an airborne hazard but should be handled with gloves.
12. Injuries caused by sharp instruments (see p. 207).
13. Blood or organ donors should be screened for HB$_s$Ag and HIV antibody, before a transplant is carried out.
14. The nurse handling the patient in the recovery room should wear gloves and a plastic apron.

10.8.3   MATERNITY DEPARTMENT

The same precautions for known and infected or high risk patients are necessary for a delivery or caesarean section as described for surgical operations (i.e. gloves, plastic apron and eye protection). The labour room may be used provided it is adequately cleaned with a hypochlorite or similar solution afterwards. The placenta and any bloodstained materials should be sealed in a plastic bag and incinerated. Stillborn babies should be enclosed in a plastic bag, secured and appropriately labelled.

Antenatal   The hands should be thoroughly washed after examining the patient during the antenatal period and blood should be taken by an experienced person wearing gloves.

Postnatal   Although the risk of transmission of infection to other patients is small, it is advisable to provide mother and child with a single room. The mother should be reassured that she is not a hazard to her child and can be allowed normal visits. Care is necessary with bloodstained secretions (i.e. handling with gloves, disposal of dressings and cleaning up spillages). The mother may use communal toilet facilities. If a bedpan is used, it is important that it is adequately disinfected by heat or, if disposable, the support is disinfected with a hypochlorite solution. The patient may use a bath provided it is disinfected with a non-abrasive chlorine-releasing powder. The patient may use communal rooms. If possible, blood should be cleaned from the baby while still in the labour room. A plastic apron and gloves should be worn when bathing the baby initially, but afterwards normal procedures are adequate.

Although the risk from breast milk is small, mothers should not breastfeed the infant. Donors to milk banks should be tested and all milk should be pasteurized.

10.8.4 DENTAL DEPARTMENTS

Dentists are exposed to the same risk of infection as their medical and nursing colleagues although there is no evidence of acquisition of HIV. All patients should be handled with care, as described below.

1. Wear gloves when working in the presence of blood or blood-stained instruments and surfaces. Most dentists now wear gloves for all procedures.
2. Cover cuts and abrasions with a waterproof dressing.
3. Heat-disinfect instruments, preferably autoclave, but boiling water for 5–10 mins is an alternative for instruments not used for surgical procedures, provided it is correctly carried out.
4. Whenever there is a need for high-speed or ultrasonic instrumentation, high velocity suction should be used and eye protection should be worn.
5. Use a fresh local anaesthetic cartridge and disposable needle for each patient.
6. Work surfaces should be cleaned with hypochlorite or similar chlorine-releasing solution (1000 ppm av Cl_2) or 70% ethanol, after treating each patient.

'High-risk patients' or known carriers (British Dental Association 1987)

1. Patient should be last on list.
2. Gloves, plastic apron and eye-protection should be worn by dentist and assistant.
3. A high-volume aspirator should be used on all occasions. Where possible, use conventional low-speed hand-pieces of a sterilizable type and the traditional methods of scaling.
4. Patient should wear a disposable bib. Mouthwashes should be dispensed in disposable cups.
5. Cleaning and treatment of instruments should be as described above and waste should be discarded in an appropriate plastic bag for incineration. Needles should be disposed of in a puncture-proof carrier and should be incinerated.
6. For impressions, use a polymer material instead of alginate and immerse in 2% glutaraldehyde or 1000 ppm hypochlorite for at least 10 minutes before sending to technician.

7. If hepatitis B infection or carriage is suspected, the dentist should preferably have been immunized or known to have a protective antibody level.

10.8.5 MORTUARY STAFF – POSTMORTEM EXAMINATION (see also Chapter 16)

Unless there is a particular interest, a full postmortem examination should not be carried out on patients who are known to be infected with HIV. A limited autopsy will often suffice to provide the information required. When a full autopsy is required the pathologist should wear a complete enclosing boiler suit, waterproof boots, and a disposable plastic gown or long apron. A mask, gloves and plastic arm extension pieces should also be worn, and goggles or visor to prevent splash-contamination of the eyes. Any assistant must be similarly clad. If the glove is punctured or the skin broken, the glove must be removed immediately and the injury cleansed; anti-HB$_s$Ag gammaglobulin should be made available where appropriate. After completion of the postmortem the room must be decontaminated by washing down with hypochlorite or another chlorine-releasing solution. Instruments, bowls and trays should be washed and disinfected by boiling, autoclaving or immersion in 2% glutaraldehyde for at least 10 minutes. If available, a pathologist known to be HB$_s$Ag positive or who has been immunized should carry out postmortem examinations on patients known to be HB$_s$Ag positive. Postmortem room staff should be vaccinated against hepatitis B.

10.9 Immunization against hepatitis B infection

Hepatitis B immune globulin, prepared from blood donors' plasma which has been found to contain an adequate level of antibody, is given to persons exposed to hepatitis B by accidental inoculation (e.g. needle-stick injury). It prevents hepatitis B developing in most of those who would otherwise have been infected, but is not 100% effective. In recent years, it has been the custom to give two doses, one as soon as possible after the episode, and another one month later. It is doubtful whether the second dose confers any extra protection. Hepatitis B vaccine is now commercially available from several companies, and two are licensed in the UK. One of these is plasma-derived and the other genetically engineered in yeast. They are almost completely free of side-effects and perfectly safe in that there is no contamination by any other infectious agent. Three 20 µg doses are given to adults. Good protection of babies born to carrier mothers has been achieved by four doses of 10 µg; the first given immediately after birth, the second and third at one month intervals, and the fourth at six months.

Hepatitis B vaccine is moderately expensive and should be offered initially to 'high risk' groups of hospital staff. Doctors, dentists, nurses, midwives and others including students who have direct contact with patients or their body fluids, or are likely to experience frequent parenteral exposure to blood or blood-contaminated secretions and excretions should be considered for immunization (DHSS 1990; Centers for Disease Control 1990). Groups at the highest risk are as follows:

1. health care workers and others who are directly involved over a period of six months in patient care institutions or units for the mentally handicapped and particularly in units with a known high prevalence of hepatitis B;
2. staff directly involved in patient care over a period of six months or more and working in units giving treatment to known carriers of hepatitis B;
3. laboratory staff working with clinical specimens, and mortuary technicians.
4. health care workers seconded to areas of the world with a high prevalence of infection, if directly involved in patient care.

10.9.1   OTHER INDICATIONS FOR IMMUNIZATION

Patients on entry to institutions with a known high prevalence of hepatitis B, patients undergoing haemodialysis or preferably patients with early renal disease who may later require dialysis, recipients of blood products, sexually active homosexuals, inmates of long-term custodial institutions, users of illicit drugs, adoptees from countries of high HBV endemicity, spouses of hepatitis B carriers and infants born to mothers who are persistent carriers of HB_sAg, particularly if HB_sAg is detected. These infants should be given the first dose of vaccine (0.5 ml IM) at birth or as soon as possible, preferably within 12 hours. Hepatitis B immunoglobulin (200 i.u., IM) should be given at a contralateral site at the same time (DHSS 1988).

It should be the eventual aim of a policy to include all health workers with patient and/or blood/body fluid contact to receive the vaccine, including certain SSD, ambulance and laundry workers. However, it must be recognized that the evidence that most of these are at increased risk is small and that immunization takes up to six months for protection.

Vaccine-induced antibody levels decline steadily with time. Booster doses are suggested at intervals of five years, but it is possible that this could be extended to seven years, depending on results of future studies.

10.10 HIV infected health-care workers

Although infection of a patient from an HIV positive health-care worker (HCW) has not been reported, with the exception of transmission from a dentist to several patients in the US, even the remote risk causes considerable public concern. (AIDS – HIV Infected Health Care Workers.)

For infection to occur blood-tissue contact is necessary and this usually involves an invasive surgical procedure (as with hepatitis B). The risk is obviously low with an injection or venepuncture, but greater with surgical procedures involving cutting and suturing. The likelihood of blood being shed by the health-care worker in any quantity is low. The very small risk can be reduced further by routine hygienic procedures (e.g. covering cuts or lesions with a waterproof dressing and wearing gloves) and by the use of modified surgical techniques which reduces the use of sharp instruments.

Nevertheless, a remote risk remains and a health-care worker with known or suspected HIV infection who performs or assists with surgical invasive procedures must seek specialist advice on whether to limit his/her work practice. In general, health service workers need not be restricted in their practice. It is likely that HIV-infected workers will be required to stop undertaking invasive surgical procedures, although there is as yet no evidence of transmission to a patient except in dental surgery.

The health-care worker's physician should obtain broad-based advice, and in the UK it is recommended that a joint advisory panel from professional organizations should be set up for this purpose. Confidentiality is an absolute requirement if workers are expected to seek advice.

There may also be an increased risk to the health-care worker of acquiring certain infections (e.g. salmonellosis or tuberculosis), or of mental impairment. Regular medical supervision is essential.

10.10.1 EXPOSURE TO HBV OR HIV INFECTION

Following accidental percutaneous exposure (needle-stick or other sharp instrument), ocular or mucous membrane exposure, contact with damaged skin (abraded or with dermatitis), from a known HIV antibody positive or high risk patient (or cultures or suspensions of HIV), the HCW should stop work, encourage bleeding and wash the contaminated site thoroughly with soap and running water. If blood is splashed on to the skin or into the eyes wash off with large volumes of water.

The accident should be reported to the senior person present and to the Occupational Health, Infection Control or Accident and Emergency Department.

Blood samples should be collected from the source patient if known and also the exposed HCW. Tests for HB$_s$Ag and anti-HIV should be carried out after obtaining consent from both patient and HCW and arranging for the necessary pre-test counselling. The following data should be obtained:

1. the date and time of exposure;
2. duty being performed at the time of exposure;
3. details of exposure including amount of fluid, depth and extent of injury, damage to skin, source of exposure and whether the source individual was HB$_s$Ag or anti-HIV positive;
4. the HBV vaccination status of the exposed person.

10.10.2   PROCEDURE

The source patient is HB$_s$Ag positive

1. If the exposed person has not been vaccinated, give HBIG (500 i.u.) as soon as possible, preferably within 24 hours (or at least within seven days), and the first dose of hepatitis B vaccine at the same time but in a different site.
2. If the exposed person has been vaccinated and their antibody titre is less than 100 m.i.u./ml, give a booster dose, and if a known non-responder also give two doses of HBIG. If antibody level is more than 100 m.i.u./ml no further action is required.

The source patient is HB$_s$Ag negative   If the exposed person has not been vaccinated commence vaccine schedule.

The HB$_s$Ag state of the source patient is unknown   If the exposed person has been vaccinated and has an adequate level of antibody, no further treatment is required. If the antibody level is low or absent commence vaccination.

Exposure to HIV infection   If the source individual has AIDS, is known to be HIV positive or has refused testing, blood from the exposed person should be tested as soon as possible after exposure and repeated at time intervals of twelve weeks and six months. The initial sample may be stored and only tested if subsequent samples are positive.

If the source person is seronegative and is not in a 'risk' group or has not recently been exposed to infection, no further follow-up is necessary.

References and further reading   209

If the HIV antibody state of the source person is unknown, the necessity to follow up the exposed individual should be decided on the likelihood of a possible HIV infection amongst the potential sources in the patient population.

The value of prophylactic zidovudine in preventing infections is unknown. The decision to give it should be based on the type of exposure and the likely risk of infection. The risk of transmission from a contaminated needle-stick or sharps injury is about 0.4% and is less following mucous membrane or skin exposure. In view of the uncertainty regarding its efficacy, zidovudine should probably only be advised following a significant exposure to blood or body fluids from a known HIV-positive patient (e.g. transfusion, deep penetrating injury, or contamination with laboratory culture of HIV). The response to a lesser exposure should be considered in individual instances. Animal studies suggest that prophylaxis against certain retroviral infections is more effective if started within hours after exposure. The current schedule is 1000 mg in the first four hours and 200 mg 4–6 times daily for 4–6 weeks. Zidovudine is potentially toxic and the risks should be discussed with the individual concerned, as well as the potential risk of acquiring infection. Written informed consent for zidovudine prophylaxis should be obtained.

References and further reading

Advisory Committee on Dangerous Pathogens (ACDP) (1990) *HIV – the Causative Agent of AIDS and Related Conditions*, 2nd revision of guidelines.
AIDS:HIV – Infected Health Care Workers (1988) *Report of the Expert Advisory Group on AIDS*. HMSO, London.
British Dental Association (1987) *Guide to Blood Borne Virus and Control of Cross Infection in Dentistry*. British Dental Association, London.
British Medical Association (1989) *A Code of Practice for Sterilization of Instruments and Control of Cross-Infection*. BMA, London.
British Medical Association (1990) *A Code of Practice for the Safe Use and Disposal of Sharps*. BMA, London.
Centers for Disease Control. (1988) Update: Universal precautions for prevention of transmission of human immunodeficency virus, hepatitis B virus and other blood-borne pathogens in health care settings. *Morbidity & Mortality Weekly Report*, **37**, No. 24.
Centers for Disease Control. (1990) Public Health Service Statement on Management of exposure to human immunodeficiency virus, including considerations regarding zidovudine post-exposure use. *Morbidity & Mortality*, **39**, (RR–1).
Department of Health and Social Security (1982) *Specification for Containers for Disposal of Needles and Sharp Instruments*, TSS/S./330.015. HMSO, London.
Department of Health and Social Security (1990) *Guidance for Clinical Health Care Workers. Protection against Infection with HIV and Hepatitis Viruses*. Recommendations of the Expert Advisory Group on AIDS. HMSO, London.

Health Services Advisory Committee (1991) Safe working and the prevention of infection in clinical laboratories. HMSO, London.

Hospital Infection Society (1990) Acquired immunodeficiency syndrome. Recommendations of a Working Party of the Hospital Infection Society. *Journal of Hospital Infection*, **15**, 7.

Jenner, E. (1990) Seeking a rationale for glove use. *Journal of Infection Control Nursing; Nursing Times*, **86**, (37) 73.

11 *Asepsis in operating theatres*

11.1 Postoperative infection

Clinical wound infection (sepsis) occurs in a small proportion of patients – often 1–5% – (Cruse and Foord 1973) having operations on 'clean' areas such as soft tissues, muscle or bone. Such infections are often exogenous, i.e. acquired from extraneous sources by cross-infection or, more rarely, due to contamination with bacteria from the inanimate environment; many are caused by *Staph. aureus* and other skin bacteria, though other organisms, including Gram-negative bacilli, may be involved, sometimes in mixed infections with staphylococci. Operations on hollow viscera, especially the colon and rectum which contain enormous numbers of bacteria, have a higher incidence (commonly 10–20%) of postoperative infection; most infections following such operations are endogenous and caused by the patient's intestinal flora, the predominant species present being the anaerobic non-sporing bacillus, *Bacteroides fragilis*; *Escherichia coli* and other aerobic Gram-negative bacilli are also abundant. If operation is delayed, some of the intestinal organisms are likely to be strains acquired in hospital and commonly resistant to antibiotics which are usually active against similar organisms found in the intestines of persons outside hospital.

In immunodeficient patients and at operation sites with poor antimicrobial defences (e.g. total joint replacements), microorganisms which have weak pathogenicity and were formerly regarded as non-pathogens (e.g. *Staph. epidermidis* and *Propionibacterium* spp.) may cause clinical infection. After heart transplant operations, the immunosuppressed patient is at risk from toxoplasmas and cytomegalovirus present in some implanted hearts, and in liver transplant operations from inhaled aspergilli if the air of the recovery ward is often unfiltered.

Special forms of postoperative infection are pseudomembranous enterocolitis, gas gangrene and tetanus. It has been shown that pseudomembranous enterocolitis is caused by the toxins of *Clostridium difficile*, an organism sometimes present in normal faeces (George *et al.* 1978). Its proliferation in the gut is apparently promoted by oral administration of certain antibiotics, especially clindamycin and ampicillin. Postoperative gas gangrene is a special hazard after orthopaedic operations or amputations on ischaemic lower limbs. Infection is usually endogenous, arising from contamination of the skin with faecal *Cl. perfringens* which is resistant to standard skin antisepsis and readily transferred to the wound at operation. Postoperative tetanus, by contrast, is more often exogenous, a rare and sometimes epidemic consequence of heavy airborne contamination (e.g. during building works) or of the use of contaminated materials; in former times, catgut was a well recognized source.

In addition to these endemic infections, which are caused by a variety of organisms, outbreaks of epidemic infection occur from time to time due to the presence of a particular strain of a virulent organism carried by some member of the staff (e.g. a staphylococcal disperser) or present in materials (e.g. eyedrops) that should be sterile. Established aseptic methods have been shown to reduce these hazards, but the common development of sepsis after clean operations shows the limitations of aseptic methods and the need for meticulous standards. An 'epidemic' increase in the incidence of postoperative wound sepsis may also be caused by some failure in aseptic technique or sterilization; such outbreaks are associated with an increased incidence of sepsis caused by different types of bacteria, not by one epidemic strain.

The protection of patients in the operating theatre against hazards of exogenous infection involves the application of a large number of methods to prevent the contamination of wounds (asepsis) and to enhance the patient's resistance. Some of the methods are described in the chapters on sterilization and disinfection in this handbook. Protection of patients against endogenous infection with bacteria normally resident in the hollow viscera and in the upper respiratory tract, when indicated (e.g. in resections of colon or rectum), requires the administration, for short periods, of antibiotics or other antimicrobial chemotherapeutic agents by the systemic route, or by mouth, or by both routes. The antimicrobials are selected for their activity against the organisms likely to infect – for example *Bact. fragilis* and miscellaneous Gram-negative bacilli, also *Cl. perfringens* in patients having orthopaedic operations on ischaemic lower limbs (p. 227). Infection of operation wounds with bacteria that happen to be present on the skin of the operation or infusion site can also be regarded as endogenous; protection against this hazard involves effective pre-operative skin disinfection, and asepsis of the infusion site.

Respiratory and, rarely, gastrointestinal infection may be acquired at operation. Prevention of respiratory infection involves avoidance of elective surgery and of inhalation anaesthesia in patients with acute upper respiratory infection. Inhalation anaesthesia may also exacerbate lower respiratory infection in patients with chronic obstructive pulmonary disease, through inhalation of mucous secretions and the development of atelectasis; the latter can be combatted by relief of pain, breathing exercises, suction, humidification of air and other supportive measures after operation. Resistance to infection is lowered by general anaesthesia in patients with systemic disease. For limb operations in such patients regional block anaesthesia, which avoids endotracheal manipulation, has been recommended (Altemeier *et al.* 1984). Cross-infection through the use of contaminated anaesthetic and endoscopic equipment (including gastroscopes) must be prevented by effective disinfection (see Chapter 6).

Methods of preventing infection in the operating suite can be considered under the following sub-headings (Medical Research Council 1968):

1. the operating suite and equipment;
2. preparation of the surgical team;
3. preparation and protection of the patient.

11.2   The operating suite and equipment

11.2.1   DESIGN

A report to the Medical Research Council (1962) recommended six basic design requirements for control of infection in operating suites:

1. separation from the general traffic and air movement of the hospital;
2. a sequence of increasingly clean zones from the entrance to the operating and sterilizing areas;
3. easy movement of staff from one clean area to another without passing through 'dirty' areas;
4. removal of dirty materials from the suite without passing through clean areas;
5. airflow from clean to less clean areas;
6. heating and ventilation to ensure safe and comfortable conditions for patients and staff.

These conditions are best achieved by having the theatres in an operating suite, with a number of operating rooms sufficient to allow adequate time for cleaning (e.g. one theatre for 25–30 surgical beds), and with protective, clean, aseptic and disposal zones. Some of these recommendations are more important than others – for example, a disposal zone is unnecessary if dirty items are removed from the suite in sealed impervious bags.

11.2.2 VENTILATION

Ventilation should remove airborne bacteria released in the theatre suite and prevent the entry of bacteria, especially from the corridors and other indoor areas, but also from outside the hospital. It should provide comfortable conditions, and control the humidity to reduce the risk of electrostatic sparks. Recommended ventilation systems for standard operating theatres are plenum ventilation at 1000–1500 ft³/min in the aseptic area and sterile supply room (or 20 air changes per hour), with lower input into anaesthetic and scrub-up rooms, and no input (or low input) in the entrance lobby, changing rooms and recovery rooms. The efficiency of the ventilation system should, when possible, be monitored daily by use of an airflow switch, which indicates on the theatre panel whether the correct volume of air is being supplied by the plant. When this equipment is not present, measurement of airflow at grilles (by an anemometer) and of room pressure at test points is desirable, and should be recorded in a log book. Measurements of ventilation rate should be made periodically by an engineer; a reduced pressure and air turnover indicate probable blockage of the filters, which require immediate replacement if blocked. A hygrometer in the theatre should be read daily to ensure that the relative humidity does not fall to levels of electrostatic spark hazard (below 55%). Discomfort should be recorded. If an operating suite is not used overnight or during a weekend, the ventilation system can be switched off, provided it is switched on again for one hour before subsequent use.

At total hip or knee joint replacement operations (and possibly at other operations in which exogenous infection presents a special hazard), there is a strong case for the use of theatres or enclosures where the wound is protected against airborne infection by the provision of ultra-clean air. This was made possible by the development of unidirectional ('laminar') airflow at about 300 air changes per hour, recirculated through high efficiency particulate air ('Hepa') filters, and by the development of surgical isolators. Charnley (1979) developed an ultraclean air system for total hip replacement in which the operation was performed in an enclosure ventilated by a large turnover of filtered recirculated air, the operating team inside the enclosure wearing exhaust-ventilated bacteria-proof operating suits. Over a period of years, in which the system was progressively improved, there was a progressive reduction in postoperative joint sepsis rate from about 10% to under 1%, a reduction due, in Charnley's opinion, to the use of ultraclean air.

Charnley's claim was disputed because, during the same period, he had introduced a number of other improvements which might have affected the sepsis rates, and because some other surgeons who did not use ultraclean air reported joint infection rates no higher than

Charnley's (Fitzgerald *et al.* 1977). These uncertainties were resolved by the results of a multi-hospital prospective controlled trial conducted by a Medical Research Council team, which showed that the incidence of both wound sepsis and deep joint sepsis was significantly lower in patients whose operations had been performed in ultraclean air than it was in those who had their operations done by the same teams but in conventional plenum-ventilated operating rooms. The operations which showed the greatest reduction in joint sepsis rate (about 4.5-fold) were those performed in theatres showing the greatest reduction in numbers of airborne bacteria and in the numbers of bacteria present in washings from the operation wounds. These greatest reductions were obtained with unidirectional airflow plus the use of bacteria-proof body-exhaust-ventilated clothing, and also by the use of surgical isolators (Lidwell *et al.* 1982, 1987; see also Salvati *et al.* 1982).

Similar reductions in joint sepsis rates have been obtained by the use of peri-operative antibiotic prophylaxis (Hill *et al.* 1981; Lidwell *et al.* 1982). When antibiotic prophylaxis and ultraclean air were used in combination their effects were additive, leading (with the best ultraclean air systems) to a reduction in joint sepsis rate from 3.4% to 0.19%. Charnley did not use prophylactic antibiotics as did the surgeons whose results were as good as Charnley's without use of ultraclean air. These studies showed that in conventional theatres about 95% of the bacteria that contaminate operation wounds are acquired from the air of the operating room, but in other types of clean surgery a higher proportion of bacteria may originate from the patient's skin.

A cost-benefit analysis has supported the use of ultraclean air on economic as well as clinical grounds (Lidwell 1984). The role of ultra-clean air in other types of clean surgery remains uncertain.

11.2.3 STORAGE OF EQUIPMENT

The amount of equipment should be kept to a minimum, including operating table, lights, conduits for anaesthetic gases, diathermy and suction; an instrument table and trolley are included if there is no setting-up room. Articles needed for servicing a list of operations are kept in the anaesthetic room, the scrub-up annexe and setting-up room. Stored items are arranged to require minimum movement by staff.

Maintenance of sterility of sterile supplies depends on adequate wrapping of packs and on the minimum exposure. Double-wrapping prevents contamination during opening of packs, which must also be protected against moisture; if not used promptly, packs should be kept in a cabinet or box with a well-fitting lid. Instruments should not be kept in disinfectant solutions. Items of equipment (x-ray, diathermy, etc.)

must be stored under clean conditions and be cleaned or disinfected regularly.

Laying-up of trolleys in advance of the operation involves some risk of contamination. When instruments are arranged for individual operations on pre-set trays, wrapping can be removed in the operating room immediately before use.

11.2.4 STERILIZATION OF INSTRUMENTS

The methods of sterilizing instruments are described in Chapter 4. Certain single-use items supplied by the sterile services department (SSD) are obtained pre-sterilized from commercial sources (e.g. suture materials, syringes, needles, catheters and drip sets).

11.2.5 CLEANING OF THE OPERATING SUITE

Principles of cleaning and disinfection are given in Chapter 6. Surfaces should be kept free from visible dirt, and special attention should be given to areas which are likely to become heavily contaminated (i.e. upward facing surfaces). It is advisable to clean the floor of theatres after each operating session. A disinfectant should be used after known contamination of floors with material from infected patients, but for routine cleaning, mopping with water and a detergent is satisfactory. Floors should be rinsed occasionally with clean water after washing or disinfection, otherwise deposit may build up and reduce antistatic properties. A suitable floor-scrubbing machine may be used at the end of the day (see Chapter 6). For other surfaces, normal housekeeping methods are adequate (e.g. daily damp cleaning of ledges and shelves). Walls with intact surfaces acquire very few bacteria even if left unwashed for long periods; they must not, however, be allowed to grow visibly dirty, and washing at least every 3–6 months should be adequate for this purpose. If areas of paint peel off, the wall must be repainted or covered with a new wall finish. The operating lamp should be cleaned daily; oiling is unnecessary.

11.2.6 DISINFECTION OF ANAESTHETIC APPARATUS AND MECHANICAL VENTILATORS

Items which enter or come near to the patient's respiratory tract (e.g. endotracheal tubes, airways, and face pieces) should be disinfected after every use. Anaesthetic circuits, e.g. re-breathing bags and tubing, can be changed after each session. These items should be disinfected in a hospital sterilizing and disinfecting unit (HSDU), or in a special department with technical staff appointed for this work under the supervision of the superintendent of the HSDU. Care must be taken to avoid contaminating the anaesthetic trolley, which should have a discard receptacle.

For details of disinfection of anaesthetic and respiratory ventilating equipment and of methods for preventing contamination of respirators and ventilators, see Chapter 6.

11.2.7 OPERATING ROOMS FOR 'CLEAN' AND 'SEPTIC' CASES: ORDER OF OPERATION

When there is no proper ventilation system in the theatre suite, operation on septic cases should preferably be performed in a separate operating theatre, though the risk of transfer from one patient to the next in a general surgical list is small. In conventional theatre suites with plenum ventilation at 1000–1500 ft³/min, an interval of five minutes, during which the room is thoroughly cleaned, should make it safe for the next patient; no special 'septic' theatre is required. No special cleaning precautions are required after operations on patients with gas gangrene, since these do not contaminate the theatre any more than operations in which the intestine is opened. Septic patients should, when possible, and particularly if infected with MRSA, be placed at the end of an operating list.

11.2.8 SUCTION APPARATUS (see also Chapter 6)

In free-standing units, a filter (British Standards Institute 1967) for electrically driven apparatus should be fitted between the collection bottle and the pump; this will prevent froth and spray contaminated by infective aspirates from being dispersed into the theatre. The filter should not be in the outlet to the atmosphere, because the pump may become clogged with coagulated protein if not protected by a filter.

If piped suction is installed, a filter at each peripheral suction point is required to prevent contamination of the pipeline and the exhaust discharge. Venturi suction units powered by piped oxygen also need protection by a filter between the collection jar and the suction pump.

11.2.9 CONTAMINATION OF FLUIDS

To prevent contamination of fluids with *Ps. aeruginosa*, *Serratia* spp. or other Gram-negative bacilli, aqueous solutions of cetrimide and chlorhexidine should be stocked in the pharmacy in concentrated solutions and diluted for issue with fresh distilled or sterilized water, with the addition of isopropyl alcohol as a preservative. If the solutions will withstand heat, the provision of sterilized antiseptic solutions is desirable. Stock and issue bottles should be covered with a screw cap without cork liners; corks must never be used. Once open, a bottle should be in use for no longer than one day. All bottles should be sterilized or adequately disinfected before being refilled (unless disposable containers are used). Aqueous antiseptics are commonly supplied ready for use in sterile plastic packs. Fluids used in ophthalmic surgery should be supplied, when possible, autoclaved in their final containers and in small volumes, so that none are stored in bottles that have been opened for use. Heat-labile solutions should be sterilized by filtration.

Sterile water for topical use should be supplied autoclaved in bottles. Tank water sterilizers and piped systems are liable to contamination and should be avoided.

Water-baths used in cardiothoracic operating theatres for thawing of blood products have been found responsible for postoperative pseudomonas endocarditis. To prevent this lethal hazard, it has been recommended that water-baths should be effectively disinfected after use, changed 4-hourly, and monitored for counts of bacteria; also that blood products to be thawed should be double-bagged (Casewell *et al.* 1981).

11.2.10 INFECTION TRANSMITTED BY BLOOD

See notes on serum hepatitis and acquired immune deficiency syndrome (AIDS) in Chapter 10.

11.3 Preparation of the surgical team

Under this heading it is usual to consider only those measures which are taken to prevent the transfer of organisms from members of the surgical team to the wounds of patients in the operating room. But it is increasingly seen to be important to consider also those measures by which the surgeon and his assistants can be protected against pathogens carried by the patient, including HIV, HBV and other severe or dangerous infections. This subject is considered in Chapter 10.

11.3.1 DEFINITION OF TEAM; MOVEMENTS

All persons – surgeons, anaesthetists, operating theatre nurses, and others – who enter the aseptic zone of the theatre during an operation, are described as members of the team. They are divided into 'scrubbed' and 'unscrubbed' members.

To reduce the hazard of contamination from dispersers of virulent staphylococci, the team should be kept as small as possible; no one whose presence is not essential should be admitted to the operating room.

Movements in the theatre should be reduced to a minimum; in particular, it should be unnecessary to fetch materials from outside the theatre or to remove instruments for resterilization before the end of an operation. Doors should be kept closed during the operation.

11.3.2 FITNESS OF THE MEMBERS OF THE TEAM FOR DUTY

No one with a boil or septic lesion of the skin or eczema colonized with *Staph. aureus* should remain at work in an operating theatre. Protection cannot be achieved by covering the lesion with an adhesive dressing. When the lesion is cured, it is desirable to use an antiseptic detergent preparation or soap for all ablutions, so that the staphylococci which caused the lesion can be removed from the skin.

When there has been an outbreak of infection with a particular phage-type of *Staph. aureus*, and there is evidence to suggest that the infection was probably acquired in the theatre, nasal or lesion carriers should be sought and treated, nasal carriers with nasal antibacterial creams (containing mupirocin, neomycin or other agent or combination of agents shown to be effective, see Chapter 9).

Respiratory infections in the team may cause respiratory infection in the patient at a time when he is particularly susceptible, and it is preferable for persons with such infection to be excluded from the team; the hazard from respiratory infection applies especially to anaesthetists. A surgeon infected with *Strep. pyogenes* (e.g. streptococcal tonsillitis) must not operate.

11.3.3 BATHING AND SHOWERS

It has been shown that showers tend to increase rather than reduce the number of bacteria-carrying particles dispersed from the skin. Staff should therefore not take showers immediately before operations.

11.3.4 REMOVAL OF EVERYDAY CLOTHES

It is rational to remove the outer clothes before putting on operating room clothes. There is no evidence, however, that the removal of under-clothes reduces the amount of contamination from the body, and this may be left to the discretion of the individual.

11.3.5 OPERATING ROOM CLOTHES

Operating suits (Hambraeus and Laurell 1980). Conventional operating clothes give some protection against contact contamination (if dry), but do not reduce the amount of airborne contamination with bacteria from the wearer's skin. Bacteria escape through pores in the fabric and, if trousers are worn, at the ankles; few escape from the openings at the neck, waist and sleeves. The use of an operating suit made of a woven fabric with pore size of 7–10 μm (e.g. Ventile), and the securing of trousers around the ankles, greatly reduces the dispersal of bacteria. Gowns made of Ventile or similar closely woven fabric are available. In addition to preventing the transfer of bacteria, this type of fabric resists wetting. To retain non-wetting properties, the fabric must be reproofed after about 30 launderings. Wearers have found these fabrics uncomfortable. A more comfortable disposable type of operating clothes has been developed from unwoven cellulose fibre or ceramic polyester. Washable fabrics which allow the passage of moisture and air (e.g. Goretex) are available but are more expensive (Whyte 1988). With the Charnley-Howorth ultraclean air enclosure, a body exhaust ventilated operating suite made of a small-pore woven fabric has been used by the operating team and found comfortable. When ordinary cotton gowns are used, they must be changed if they become soaked with blood or other liquids.

The reduction of airborne bacterial contamination is greater when both scrubbed and unscrubbed staff wear special operating clothes which reduce the dispersal of bacteria than when these are worn only by the operating team. However, the necessity for such special operating clothing in routine general surgery is uncertain, but should be introduced if comfortable and cost-effective.

11.3.6 FOOTWEAR

Footwear with impervious soles (e.g. rubber or plastic boots, or over-shoes made of waterproof material) should be worn in the aseptic zone; the shoes should fit, so that bellows action may be avoided. Overshoes are unnecessary for visiting staff not entering the aseptic area (Marshall *et al*. 1991).

11.3.7 'TACKY' MATS

Mats with tacky or disinfectant surfaces at the entrance to theatres are not recommended, as they have been found to offer little protection against bacterial contamination of operating room floors. If not regularly changed, they may increase the numbers of organisms transferred into the theatre.

11.3.8   HEADGEAR

The hair should be completely covered by a close-fitting cap (preferably made of an impervious plastic, paper or woollen material).

11.3.9   MASKS

To prevent the impaction of large numbers of droplets from the mouth into the operation field, it is the usual practice to wear a mask; formerly it was recommended that an impervious 'deflector' type of mask should be worn, but current practice is to use a disposable mask that acts as a filter and, to some extent, as a deflector. Some disposable paper masks offer poor protection. A fresh mask should be worn for each operation, and masks that become damp should be replaced. Special masks with an aspirator to draw off expired air are appropriate for use in operations on high risk patients. A mask does not reduce airborne contamination and some surgeons do not wear them for general surgery. In one study (Orr 1981) there was no increase in infection rate when masks were not worn for general surgery.

11.3.10   HANDS AND GLOVES

Details on pre-operative cleaning and disinfection of the hands are given in Chapter 7. An antiseptic soap or detergent preparation such as 4% chlorhexidine detergent solution ('Hibiscrub') or povidone-iodine 'surgical scrub' (e.g. 'Betadine', 'Disadine'), should be used. For physically clean hands, an alternative method, which is more effective and less expensive, is to rub 10 ml (in two applications of 5 ml) of 0.5% chlorhexidine in 70–95% ethyl or isopropyl alcohol with 1% glycerol (or 'Hibisol') into the skin of hands and forearms until evaporated to dryness; Ethyl or isopropyl alcohol with 1% glycerol is also very effective, but does not have the possible advantage of residual action by deposited chlorhexidine. A two minute scrub, with a detergent antiseptic preparation and a sterile brush, is recommended for the first operation on the list, and detergents must be used to remove visible dirt or blood. The disinfection must be systematic and cover all areas of hands and forearms.

A metal scraper may be used to remove dirt from under finger nails. Care must be taken to avoid contaminating the contents of soap or detergent dispensers (e.g. by the use of a foot-operated dispenser).

The scrubbed team should wear new gloves which have been sterilized once only. On the appearance of a visible tear, they must be removed and replaced with new gloves after washing the hands with an antiseptic detergent or alcoholic preparation; a fresh gown must also be put on, because the sleeves become contaminated on changing the gloves. If it is necessary for gloves to be resterilized and used again, they must first be tested for invisible holes by inflation with a foot-pump and immersion under water, or by inflation with water. It is desirable to remove rings before putting on surgical gloves. Double gloving and gowns with waterproofed sleeves are often recommended for operations on patients with HIV infection.

11.4   Preparation of the patient and performance of the operation

11.4.1   FITNESS OF THE PATIENT FOR OPERATION: SUSCEPTIBILITY TO INFECTION

Risks of infection vary with the operation and with certain general factors. For example, there is a greater risk in the obese, cachectic, or elderly, in those who spend a long time in hospital before operation, in patients with uncontrolled diabetes (especially in operating on limbs, because of impaired circulation), and in those treated with corticosteroids or immunosuppressive drugs. The chances of contamination are also greater in patients with existing infection. For such 'high risk' patients, additional aseptic precautions are advisable, such as segregation and treatment for staphylococcal carriage before operation, the use of specially ventilated operating enclosures and, in some circumstances, chemoprophylaxis. Other factors such as type and site of operation, length of operation and presence of drains influence the risk and have been incorporated into risk formulae (see Chapter 3). Indices measuring the state of the patient are also available and should be incorporated into any formula used for risk assessment.

11.4.2   PROTECTION AGAINST 'SELF-INFECTION'

An operation wound may become infected with bacteria carried by the patient in his nose, gut or skin; for example, gas gangrene in patients having amputation of a leg with poor arterial blood supply is usually caused by faecal organisms present on the skin. Urinary infections and wound infections in bowel surgery are often due to coliform bacilli from the gut (see, under Chemoprophylaxis, p. 226).

There is a particular hazard if the patient has an active staphylococcal infection, especially if it is near the operation site. In these circumstances, the patient's operation should, if possible, be delayed until the infection is over, or, if this cannot be done, an appropriate antibiotic should be used for prophylaxis (see below). Other measures, such as covering the lesions with a bacteria-impermeable dressing and disinfecting the surrounding skin, may also be helpful. Protection against staphylococci carried by patients who have no infection is unnecessary except during an outbreak of staphylococcal sepsis caused by an epidemic strain, when a nasal antibacterial cream and a disinfectant detergent should be used for a few days before operation.

11.4.3 PROTECTION OF THE OPERATION SITE

Methods of cleansing and disinfection of the skin are described in Chapter 7. The agents recommended for routine use on skin are 0.5% chlorhexidine or 1% iodine in 70% alcohol or alcoholic povidone-iodine applied with friction for at least two minutes. Alcoholic solutions are more effective and rapidly acting than aqueous and are always preferred. Care is necessary to ensure the skin is dry particularly if diathermy is used.

Where there is a special hazard from clostridia, the application of a compress of 7.5% aqueous povidone-iodine for 30 minutes may be useful through killing many bacterial spores, but antibiotic prophylaxis is a more important measure. The skin should be washed with soap and water and dried before disinfection. Soap for shaving should be applied with a sterile gauze swab, not with a shaving brush. If it is considered necessary to shave the site of operation, this should be deferred until the day of operation because of the risk of causing small abrasions which may become heavily colonized with bacteria. Shaving should be avoided if possible; clipping or use of depilatory creams are preferable if removal of excess hair is considered essential.

For disinfection of mucous membranes, an aqueous solution of iodine (e.g. Lugol's or povidone-iodine) or aqueous chlorhexidine is generally recommended; alcoholic solutions appear to be less effective on the oral mucous membranes, probably because of dilution by saliva.

For disinfection of the urethra, 1 ml of 1% chlorhexidine obstetric cream should be instilled immediately before the patient is taken to the theatre for cystoscopy or before catheterization; the instillation of a diluted solution (1/5000) of chlorhexidine for disinfection of the bladder after gynaecological operations is also useful. A pad of plastic foam kept moist with chlorhexidine jelly may be attached to indwelling catheters at the urethral meatus in female patients to prevent movement of the catheter (see also Chapter 7).

11.4.4   PRE-OPERATIVE BATHS AND SHOWERS

It is customary for patients to have a bath or shower before elective operations. This cannot be expected to reduce the chances of postoperative infection unless an antiseptic detergent used at the time causes a significant reduction in the skin flora. Davies and others (1977) found that a chlorhexidine detergent preparation used in the bath or shower caused some reduction in the density of the skin flora; this effect, as would be expected, was much smaller than that of using the same preparation for disinfection of limited areas – the hands or the operation site. Assessments of the effect of whole-body antiseptic ablutions on the incidence of postoperative sepsis have been varied. Cruse and Foord (1973) and Hayek *et al.* (1987) have reported a reduction in postoperative sepsis associated with pre-operative antiseptic baths and showers, but other studies, including some recent large-scale controlled trials, showed no such effect of one or two whole-body antiseptic baths or showers (Ayliffe *et al.* 1983; Leigh *et al.* 1983; Rotter *et al.* 1988). The effect, if any, is marginal and sporadic.

11.4.5   TRANSPORT OF THE PATIENT TO THE OPERATING SUITE

The patient should be provided with freshly laundered theatre clothes and disinfected blankets immediately before he is taken to the operating suite. The porters should hand over the patient on his trolley to theatre staff in the inter-change area. There is no evidence that transfer of the patient to a clean trolley reduces the chances of contamination of the theatre, so this procedure (and the availability of a trolley transfer area in the theatre suite) can be omitted (Ayliffe *et al.* 1969; Lewis *et al.* 1990). The patient can be transferred in a bed from the ward to the anaesthetic room or to the operating room without additional risk of infection provided ward bedding and clothing is removed before admission to the operating room. Parents of small children may accompany the patient to the anaesthetic room.

11.4.6   TOWELLING TECHNIQUES

Sterile drapes provide sterile cover for areas away from the immediate site of the operation and for instrument trays and other equipment. To prevent the loss of protectiveness on wetting, a layer of sterilized waterproof material under the drape or the use of waterproof towels is advantageous. There is evidence that adhesive plastic drapes do not protect the wound against contamination from the adjacent skin or reduce the incidence of sepsis. Their use for the prevention of infection of the operation wound can therefore not be recommended.

11.4.7 OPERATIONS ON CONTAMINATED ORGANS

The incidence and mortality from sepsis is higher after operations on the bowel than after operations on other sites. It is therefore rational to remove colonic bacteria when this can be done without risk. Colonic washouts have been widely used, but are unlikely to reduce the density of colonic bacteria or the incidence of sepsis. Non-absorbed aminoglycoside antibiotics (neomycin, framycetin) given by mouth can greatly reduce the aerobic flora, but they are ineffective against anaerobes; metronidazole has been shown to reduce the incidence of anaerobic postoperative sepsis, and a short course in combination with an aminoglycoside is an effective prophylactic (see Chapter 13).

In operations involving section of the alimentary tract or other heavily colonized viscera, gross soiling of tissue should be avoided by careful technique and by the use of packs (perhaps containing a layer of impervious material) and swabs. Instruments used on the opened viscus must be regarded as contaminated and should be kept separate from the rest of the instruments in the tray; they should be discarded after completion of anastomosis or excision.

11.4.8 TISSUE HANDLING TECHNIQUES

Good surgical technique is a major factor in reducing infection risk. Tissues must be handled gently, and no more foreign material must be left in a wound than is essential for the success of the operation. Careful haemostasis is important; dead tissue and haematoma must be removed, and their formation must be prevented.

The practice of picking up with artery forceps only the bleeding vessel with little or no surrounding tissue, and the use of diathermy to coagulate the smaller bleeding points reduces the amount of dead or foreign material in the wound. The thinnest ligature which has the required strength should be chosen.

Whenever primary suture is intended, care must be taken to avoid contamination from the skin. Techniques to avoid sharps injuries are being increasingly developed to reduce risk of acquisition of HIV infection (Sim and Jeffries 1990).

11.4.9 WOUND DRAINAGE

A wound that is drained is more likely to become infected than a closed wound; drainage should therefore be used only when there is a definite indication for it (e.g. to prevent accumulation of fluid such as when a serous cavity has been opened, when infection is present, when there is a fistula, or when there is much oozing of blood, lymph or serum into the wound).

The risk of infection may be reduced by the use of a closed system of drainage. The drain should be removed as soon as possible; for example, oozing of blood will stop after a few hours, and a drain inserted to meet this hazard can normally be removed after 24 hours or less. For deeper wounds, the drain should be long, extending to a bottle below the level of the bed; an underwater seal should be used for chest drains. Suction drainage provides a closed system which should help to prevent ascending infection.

11.4.10   DISPOSAL OF USED MATERIAL

Contaminated swabs and other articles should be placed in impermeable bags, which are sealed to prevent liberation of bacteria during handling and removal for cleaning and sterilization.

11.5   Chemoprophylaxis (see also Chapter 13)

When the antibiotics were new they were often used uncritically and needlessly for prophylaxis in surgery. This indiscriminate use encouraged the emergence of a predominantly resistant hospital flora. There was evidence, too, that patients were obtaining no clinical benefit from such prophylaxis, and when sepsis appeared it was likely to be caused by organisms resistant to the available antibiotics. The outcome was a general and somewhat uncritical condemnation of chemoprophylaxis in surgery.

A number of controlled trials and microbiological studies in recent years has led to a reappraisal of the situation. While routine systemic chemoprophylaxis is still seen as likely to do more harm than good, the use in selected patients of antibiotics which are likely to cover the range of probable invaders can undoubtedly give valuable protection. Selective prophylaxis against known organisms of usually predictable sensitivity, used as an adjunct of careful asepsis, is appropriate when the consequence of infection would probably be serious.

The drug should be given in standard or large doses, covering the peri-operative period; a single dose should be adequate for most operations. Such a short period of treatment is unlikely to encourage the emergence of resistant variants, but it protects the patient during his/her most vulnerable period of exposure. There have been many publications which show the great importance of non-sporing anaerobic bacilli as a cause of postoperative sepsis after operations on the gastrointestinal tract. Such organisms greatly outnumber the aerobic organisms, including *E. coli*, in the faeces, and they are resistant to the aminoglycoside antibiotics, such as neomycin, which have been in common use for pre-operative disinfection of the gut. Prophylactic metronidazole may be expected considerably to reduce anaerobic sepsis after operations in which the anaerobic sepsis rates are usually high; similar prophylactic results have been obtained in patients having appendicectomies and hysterectomies.

Chemoprophylaxis is indicated in patients having colorectal oper-ations because they are exposed to massive contamination. Detailed recommendations for chemoprophylaxis in abdominal surgery are pre-sented in Chapter 13. In operations on ischaemic lower limbs (e.g. amputation for diabetic gangrene) a short course (five days) of prophy-laxis with a narrow-range antibiotic active against *Cl. perfringens* and other gas gangrene clostridia (usually a penicillin) is indicated because of the known risks of gas gangrene through contamination of ischaemic muscle with *Cl. perfringens* (faecal contaminants) on the skin of the buttocks and thighs.

After total hip or knee replacement operations, deep joint infection may develop several years later. Short courses of systemic chemopro-phylaxis by a semi-synthetic penicillin (e.g. flucloxacillin) or by an anti-biotic (or combination of antibiotics) active against both Gram-positive and Gram-negative organisms (e.g. cephazolin) have been found to reduce this hazard (Hill *et al.* 1981; Lidwell *et al.* 1982). Another method which has been associated with exceptionally low sepsis rates is the use of acrylic cement containing gentamicin, which is released very slowly and does not lead to any detectable concentration of the anti-biotic in the blood after the first few days (Buchholz *et al.* 1984).

After heart transplant operations the hazard of infection, especially by such 'commensal' organisms as toxoplasma and cytomegalovirus, can be reduced by less drastic immunosuppressive therapy. Risk of postoperative pneumonia (e.g. through inhalation of aspergilli) can be reduced by protective isolation of the patient after operation in a room ventilated with HEPA filtered air (Newsom 1984).

Other operations in which chemoprophylaxis is recommended include dental operations in patients with endocardial disease to pre-vent infective endocarditis (penicillin or, in penicillin-sensitive patients, erythromycin or a cephalosporin, are appropriate agents). Patients with infected urine should have prophylaxis with an antibiotic selected on the basis of sensitivity tests before operation. In patients undergoing operations for insertion of heart valve prosthesis, prophylactic treat-ment is indicated with, for example, a penicillinase-tolerant penicillin (British Society of Antimicrobial Chemotherapy 1990).

The use of volatile sprays containing neomycin, bacitracin and poly-myxin has been found to reduce the incidence of sepsis in general surgery and in neurosurgery. It has also led to the emergence, through selection, of staphylococci resistant to neomycin and bacitracin. This method should therefore be used only in 'high-risk' patients. Its use should be controlled by the microbiologist and the antibiotics chosen should be active against all the staphylococci and most of the Gram-negative bacilli isolated in the hospital. The use of a povidone-iodine spray is an alternative to topical antibiotics. Instillation into the wound before closure of 1 g cephaloridine in 2 ml water has been reported to reduce the incidence of sepsis. Resistant bacteria are likely to emerge if this method is used, so it should be reserved for patients in whom there is a high risk of infection (see Chapter 13). Oral pre-medication with antibiotics before colonic operations is discussed above (operations on contaminated organs); super-infection with resistant organisms not only reduces the value of this method, but may be a dangerous complication. Nasal chemoprophylaxis with neomycin-containing creams has been found effective when combined with other methods, but should be reserved for 'high-risk' or epidemic situations; a mupirocin-containing cream is a preferable alternative today. Disinfection of the urethra before instrumentation may prevent postoperative infection of the urinary tract and bacteraemia.

References and further reading

Altemeier, W.A. (1963) Prevention of postoperative infections: operating theatre practice. In *Infection in Hospitals* (eds. R.E.O. Williams and R.A. Shooter) p. 207, Blackwell Scientific Publications, Oxford.

Altemeier, W.A., Burke, J.F., Pruitt, B.A. *et al.* (1984) *Manual on Control of Infection in Surgical Patients*. Lipincott, Philadelphia.

Ayliffe, G.A.J., Babb, J.R., Collins, B.J. and Lowbury, E.J.L. (1969) Transfer areas and clean zones in operating suites. *Journal of Hygiene (Camb)*, **67**, 417.

Ayliffe, G.A.J., Brightwell, K.M., Collins, B.J., Lowbury, E.J.L., Goonatilake, P.C.L. and Etheridge, R.A. (1977) Surveys of hospital infection in the Birmingham Region: effect of age, sex, length of stay and antibiotic use on normal carriage of tetracycline-resistant *Staphylococcus aureus* and on postoperative wound infection. *Journal of Hygiene (Camb)* **79**, 299.

Ayliffe, G.A.J., Noy, M.T., Babb, J.R., Davies, J.G. and Jackson, J. (1983) Preoperative bathing and infection. *Journal of Hospital Infection*, **4**, 237–44.

British Society of Antimicrobial Chemotherapy. (1990) Report: Antibiotic Prophylaxis of Infective Endocarditis. Recommendations from the Endocarditis Working Party. *Lancet*, **1**, 88.

British Standards Institution (1967) Electrically operated surgical suction apparatus of high vacuum and high air displacement type BS 4199; Part 1. BSI, London.

Buchholz, H.W., Elson, R.A. and Heinert, K. (1984) Antibiotic-loaded acrylic cement: current concepts. *Clinic Orthopaedics*, **190**, 96.

Casewell, M.W., Slater, N.P.G. and Cooper, J.E. (1981) Operating theatre water-baths as a cause of pseudomonas septicaemia. *Journal of Hospital Infection*, **2**, 237.

Charnley, J. (1979) *Low Friction Arthroplasty of the Hip*. Springer Verlag, Berlin, Heidelberg, New York.

Cruse, P.J.E. and Foord, R. (1973) A five year prospective study of 23,649 surgical wounds. *Archives of Surgery*, **107**, 206–10.

Davies J.G., Babb, J.R., Ayliffe, G.A.J. and Ellis, S.H. (1977) Effects on the skin flora of bathing with antiseptic solutions. *Journal of Antimicrobial Chemotherapy*, **3**, 473–81.

Fitzgerald, R.H., Nolan, D.R., Ilstrup, D.M. and Van Scoy, R.E. (1977) Deep wound sepsis following total hip arthroplasty. *Journal of Bone and Joint Surgery*, **59a**, 847.

George, R.H., Symonds, J.M., Dimock, F., Brown, J.D., Arabi, Y., Shinagawa, N., Keighley, M.R.B., Alexander-Williams, J. and Burdon, D.W. (1978) Identification of *Clostridium difficile* as a cause of pseudomembranous colitis. *British Medical Journal*, **i**, 695.

Hambraeus, A. and Laurell, G. (1980) Protection of the patient in the operating suite. *Journal of Hospital Infection*, **1**, 15.

Hayek, L.J., Emerson, J.M. and Gardner, A.M.N. (1987) Pre-operative chlorhexidine bath. *Journal of Hospital Infection*, **10**, 165–72.

Hill, C., Flamant, R., Mazas, F. and Evrard, J. (1981) Prophylactic cephazolin versus placebo in total hip replacement. *Lancet*, **1**, 795.

Johnston, I.D.A. and Hunter, A.R. (1984) *The Design and Utilization of Operating Theatres*. Edward Arnold, London (for the Royal College of Surgeons).

Keighley, M.R.B. and Burdon, D.W. (1979) *Antimicrobial Prophylaxis in Surgery*. Pitman Medical, London.

Leigh, D.A., Stronge, J.L., Marriner, J. and Sedgwick, J. (1983) Use of 'Hibiscrub' with surgical patients. *Journal of Hospital Infection*, **4**, 229–35.

Lewis, D.A., Weymont, G., Nokes, C.M. *et al.* (1990) A bacteriological study of the effect on the environment of using a one or two trolley system in theatre. *Journal of Hospital Infection*, **15**, 35.

Lidwell, O.M. (1984) The cost implication of clean air systems and antibiotic prophylaxis in operations for total joint replacement. *Infection Control*, **5**, 36.

Lidwell, O.M., Lowbury, E.J.L., Whyte, W., Blowers, R., Stanley, S. and Lowe, D. (1982) Effect of ultraclean air in operating rooms on deep sepsis in the joint after operation for total hip or knee replacement: a randomised study. *British Medical Journal*, **285**, 10.

Lidwell, O.M., Elson, R.A., Lowbury, E.J.L., Whyte, W., Blowers, R., Stanley, S.J. and Lowe, D. (1987) Ultraclean air and antibiotics for prevention of post-operative infection. *Acta Orthopaedica Scandinavica*, **58**, 4.

Marshall, R.J., Ricketts, V.E., Russell, A.J. and Reeves, D.S. (1991) Theatre overshoes do not reduce operating theatre floor bacterial counts. *Journal of Hospital Infection*, **17**, 125.

Medical Research Council (1962) Design and ventilation of operating suites. *Lancet*, **ii**, 943.

Medical Research Council (1968) Aseptic methods in the operating suite. *Lancet*, **i**, 705, 763, 831.

Newsom, S.W.B. (1984) Infection control for heart transplant operations. *Journal of Hospital Infection*, **5**, 118–20.

Orr, N. (1981) Is a mask necessary in the operating theatre? *Annals of the Royal College of Surgeons of England*, **63**, 390.

Rotter, M.L., Larsen, S.O., Cooke, E.M. *et al.* (1988) The European Working

Party on Control of Hospital Infection. Pre-operative whole body bath. *Journal of Hospital Infection*, **11**, 310–20.

Salvati, E.A., Robinson, R.P., Zeno, S.M. (1982) Infection rates after 3175 total hip and total knee replacements performed with and without a horizontal undirectional filtered airflow system. *Journal of Bone and Joint Surgery*, **64-A**, 525.

Sim, J.W. and Jeffries, D.J. (1990) *AIDS and Surgery*. Blackwell Scientific Publications, Oxford.

Wheeler, M.H. (1979) Abdominal wound protection by means of plastic drapes. In *Surgical Sepsis* (eds. C.J.L. Strachan and R. Wise) Academic Press, New York.

Whyte, W. (1988) The role of clothing and drapes in the operating room. *Journal of Hospital Infection*, (Supplement C: Infection Control in Orthopaedic Surgery), 2–17.

Willis, A.T. (1979) Infections with obligate anaerobes. In *Recent Advances in Infection 1* (eds. D. Reeves and A. Geddes) Churchill Livingstone, Edinburgh, London, New York.

12 *Laundry, kitchen hygiene and refuse disposal*

12.1 Laundry hygiene and handling of contaminated linen

Clothing or bed linen used by hospital patients is a possible infection risk to staff handling it on the ward, during transport to, or during processing in the laundry. Inadequately disinfected or recontaminated clean laundry may also be a risk to subsequent users.

Used linen may be heavily contaminated with bacteria, but these are mainly Gram-negative bacilli from the intestinal tract or coagulase-negative staphylococci from the skin. These organisms are common environmental contaminants and unlikely to cause infection in staff handling linen. *Staph. aureus* may be present, usually in small numbers (less than 1% of total) and presents little hazard if normal precautions are taken.

Used linen that has been in contact with patients infected with specific pathogens (e.g. *Salmonella* spp., *Shigella* spp. and Mycobacterium tuberculosis) is a potential infection hazard, if excretions or secretions are present. Linen from patients infected with, or carriers of HBV, or HIV is unlikely to be hazardous unless bloodstained.

The Department of Health and Social Security (1971) recommended that all laundry should be categorized either as (1) **foul or infected**, or (2) **soiled**, and that both groups should be heat disinfected during the wash process. **Foul or infected** linen requires special facilities for storage and processing, and it was recommended that items in this category should not be sorted by hand. This recommendation was often found to be impractical, since bags labelled **foul or infected** still required sorting to ensure that different fabrics received appropriate treatment and hazardous extraneous items, e.g. scissors, etc, were removed from the load.

Visibly fouled linen is usually contaminated with the same range of organisms as other used linen, although the numbers are usually higher. Fouled linen, if handled with reasonable care, is unlikely to infect laundry workers. Many laundry workers did not follow the 1971 recommendations and continued to hand-sort linen in the foul or infected group and therefore inadvertently handled linen from patients with a known specific infection in the higher risk group because it was not specifically identified.

To overcome these problems, the DHSS (1971) report has been reviewed and laundry now categorized as: (1) **used**, (2) **infected**, or (3) **heat-labile** (DHSS 1987a). Linen categorized as *infected* will be from patients with specified infections with a potential to infect healthy staff (see Chapter 9). Such infections will include enteric diseases, dysentery, and open tuberculosis. Although the risk from handling linen from these patients is small, it was felt that handling by laundry workers should be avoided. Linen from most notifiable diseases (e.g. measles, chickenpox etc.) is not hazardous and can be treated as used linen.

Linen from infected patients, including bloodstained linen from patients with HBV or HIV infection, should be sealed in an alginate stitched, or hot water-soluble bag, as soon as it is removed from the patient. This bag should then be placed in a clearly identifiable impermeable outer bag for storage or transport. On arrival in the laundry, the alginate or water soluble bag should be removed from its outer bag, or bags, and placed unopened in a washing machine with a suitable heat-disinfection cycle. Alginate or water soluble bags are designed to dissolve, or partly dissolve, releasing their contents into the washing machine at an early stage in the cycle. Infested linen (e.g. with lice or fleas) should be dealt with in the same way. The outer bag should be washed at the same time as the contents.

Linen or clothing from patients with particularly hazardous infections (e.g. Lassa fever or anthrax) may require autoclaving before laundering, but if there is any uncertainty the infection control department should be consulted (see Chapter 9). The sorting of fouled linen is undesirable; it can be separated from other used linen if preferred by the laundry manager.

It is recommended that all hospital linen should be heat-disinfected during the wash process by raising the temperature to either 65°C (150°F) for ten minutes or 71°C (160°F) for three minutes. This has been found to be effective, but in practice higher temperatures or longer times are usually used. Mixing times of 4–8 minutes should be included in the cycle depending on the machine. Although 93°C for ten minutes was recommended for linen during outbreaks of hepatitis, this temperature was difficult to achieve in most washing machines and rarely used. The dilution of virus particles on washing associated with the temperatures suggested (e.g. 71°C for three minutes) should render linen from these patients safe to handle. Non-sporing bacteria, HIV and most other viruses, are readily inactivated or killed at this temperature.

The time/temperature relationships recommended in the DHSS report (1987a) are rather restrictive and not necessarily the most effective; 65°C is close to the minimum temperature required to kill the more resistant vegetative organisms in a realistic time. Recent tests have shown that if contaminated surfaces are raised to any of a defined range of temperatures, for example 70°C for two minutes, 80°C for one minute (Central Sterilizing Club 1986), all vegetative organisms and enteroviruses are likely to be killed, but measuring the temperature at the interface between linen and water is difficult. All washing machines should be fitted with recording thermometers to indicate the temperature reached during the disinfection cycle. The relationship between the indicated temperature and the coolest part of the largest load used should be established. Experimental evidence suggests that differences as great as 20°C can occur. However, most organisms surviving the disinfection cycle are killed during subsequent heat-drying and finishing.

The requirement to heat-disinfect all linen is becoming more difficult to achieve because of the increasing use of fabrics likely to be damaged at disinfecting temperatures. However, heat-disinfection is still advised wherever practical. A new category of 'heat-labile' has therefore been introduced. Thorough washing and rinsing at low temperatures (e.g. 40–50°C), will remove most organisms and should be satisfactory in most instances, particularly in domestic-type washers. For infected linen, a chemical disinfectant, such as hypochlorite (250 parts per million [ppm] av Cl_2), can be introduced into the second rinse. Other disinfectants, e.g. hydrogen peroxide, may be appropriate, but have not been adequately tested in the UK.

The efficiency of the disinfection cycle should be checked when commissioning new machines, at regular intervals, during major outbreaks, and in disputes with private laundries. Because of the difficulties in accurately measuring load temperatures, microbiological methods may be required in some of these situations, e.g. in disputes with private laundries (Collins *et al.* 1987).

Tests for survival of relatively heat-resistant vegetative organisms, for example, *Streptococcus faecalis* cultures applied to patches of material or sealed in narrow-bore plastic tubing and attached to an item of linen in the load are commonly used (Collins *et al.* 1987). Although microbiological testing of linen after processing is rarely required, it may also occasionally be useful if there is evidence or suspicion that infection has been transmitted by this route. Contact plates taken from processed linen awaiting distribution should not normally show more than 1 colony forming units (cfu) per sq cm and should not average more than 2. The organisms isolated should be predominantly Gram-positive cocci and aerobic spore-bearing bacilli. Gram-negative bacilli should not be present. Since some of the bacteria on linen are destroyed during the heat-drying and finishing process, counts taken from the load after washing, but before drying, are likely to be higher. The presence of substantial numbers of Gram-negative bacilli in these samples taken after washing but before drying may be evidence of recontamination from the surrounding environment or from contaminated water used to rinse after heat-disinfection. Tests on a number of machines, including batch, tunnel, and continuous washers, if properly adjusted, have shown that all would adequately disinfect the load (Collins *et al.* 1987).

Since all used linen is likely to be contaminated and may contain sufficient moisture to allow microbes present to continue to multiply, it should be enclosed as soon as possible in bags which are impermeable to microbes. All used linen should be handled with minimum disturbance to avoid dispersal of organisms. Once enclosed in a suitable bag, it can be safely transported through wards and corridors. The bag, if not disposable, should be processed through a suitable heat-disinfection cycle before re-use. Used linen is usually enclosed in white bags, and the water-soluble bags containing infected linen are placed in red bags, or in white bags with a red line. If temporary storage of used linen is necessary, it should be stored in a properly designated area where it is secure from pilfering and protected from pests. Facilities for keeping the area clean must be available, for example by installing hose points for water/steam. There is probably no reason for providing separate storage facilities for infected linen where it is enclosed in water-soluble bags contained in a secure identifiable outer bag. The use of large continuous operating machines may also make the separate provision of machines for processing 'infected' linen uneconomical. Provided that the disinfection cycle is tested and monitored regularly, special machines should be unnecessary. Organisms can grow overnight in continuous or batch washers and it is suggested that the machine is run until empty. If not, the linen should be heat disinfected before restarting on the following day.

When handling used linen, laundry staff should wear aprons, gloves and overalls and should be provided with adequate facilities for washing and changing when starting and finishing each period of work. Staff handling used linen should be given training to ensure that they understand the measures required to protect themselves and others. Staff should be offered immunization against poliomyelitis and tetanus and BCG vaccination if they are tuberculin-negative. Staff with unhealed lesions, rashes, or any exfoliative skin condition, should not handle clean laundry.

Linen returned after processing should not normally be carried in the same vehicle as used linen of any category. Exceptions could be made where the vehicle is divided into two compartments with separate loading doors and the partition is impervious and complete. In small units where the use of two vehicles is uneconomical, a single vehicle may be used if it is adequately cleaned between transport of clean and used linen.

Domestic-type washers used in some small units for personal clothing may be acceptable where the patients are physically healthy, but arrangements must be made for the adequate disinfection of items that would normally be classified as infected. Further work on the requirement and provision of disinfection cycles in this type of machine is required, but microbiological standards lower than those obtainable in the commercial machines used in hospitals should not be accepted without careful consideration of the infection risk in the proposed area of use. Education of ward staff should make it less common for laundry bags of used linen to contain objects that should not have been placed in them. The presence of sharp objects, particularly needles, represent a major hazard to laundry sorting staff. Labelling bags with ward of origin may help to reduce these hazardous practices.

If an outside contractor is responsible for hospital laundering, a similar policy to that used in hospital should be used, including immunisation and training of staff in hygienic methods.

12.2   Kitchen hygiene (DHSS 1987b)

All patients commonly receive food from a single kitchen, and poor hygiene in food preparation may be followed by an outbreak of infection involving the whole hospital. The cook-chill method of preparation is likely to include staff meals in possibly more than one hospital and could further increase the risk, although if controls are adequate the risks may be less than with conventional catering. Infection from contaminated food is particularly hazardous in debilitated or elderly people and can cause severe illness or even death. It is also important to prevent foodborne infection among the staff, since subsequent transfer to patients would have similar unfortunate results.

Outbreaks of bacterial food poisoning are usually caused by *Salmonella* spp., or the toxins of certain strains of *Staph. aureus*, *Clostridium perfringens* and *Bacillus cereus*. *Campylobacter* spp. is now the most common cause of foodborne infection although outbreaks in hospitals are infrequent. These organisms, especially *Salmonella* spp., may be transferred to the patient directly from contaminated raw foods (e.g. meat and poultry if inadequately cooked), or indirectly from initially uncontaminated food via the hands of staff, or from inadequately cleaned surfaces or equipment. Staphylococcal and salmonella carriers on the staff may also contaminate food if their personal hygiene is poor, but are infrequently responsible for outbreaks. Inadequately cooked food which is left without refrigeration for several hours, and particularly if subsequently warmed, is an important source of infection; any food capable of supporting bacterial growth should be stored either below 5°C or above 63°C) and should not normally be allowed to remain between these temperatures for more than two hours and sufficient time must be allowed for complete thawing before cooking. Food hygiene regulations in the UK state that 8°C is satisfactory for cold storage, but 5°C is preferred if possible. Some bacterial species (e.g. listeria) can grow slowly at low temperatures and chilled food should be kept at a temperature of 0–3°C (see p. 243)

Good personal hygiene of kitchen staff and effective methods of cleaning food preparation areas and equipment is of major importance in preventing the spread of infection. The general kitchen structure, e.g. walls, floors and ceilings, though of little direct relevance in the spread of infection, should be kept clean and in good condition.

12.2.1   MEDICAL EXAMINATION OF STAFF

The prospective employee should be questioned for a past history of typhoid or paratyphoid fever, dysentery, persistent diarrhoea, or attacks of diarrhoea and vomiting lasting for more than two days within the past two years, tuberculosis, boils, skin rashes, discharges from eye, ear, nose or other site, also the place and date of visits abroad. A questionnaire on the above illnesses and other relevant information is filled in by the catering manager or a member of the occupational health department and signed by the proposed employee (see Appendix 12.2). The catering manager may provisionally accept the applicant pending a satisfactory assessment by a medical officer, who may require a more detailed medical examination. A tuberculin skin test is advisable and, if negative, BCG should be offered. Examination of blood, faeces, other laboratory tests, or a chest x-ray, need not be carried out unless indicated by past history. The microbiologist or infection control doctor should be consulted if laboratory tests are considered necessary. If an examination of faeces is required, at least three samples on successive days should be examined.

12.2.2   SICKNESS

A system for recording all incidents of diarrhoea and vomiting in both patients and staff is required; it is of particular importance for catering staff. An example of a reporting scheme for staff is shown in Appendix 12.3. General practitioners may regard hospital staff as fit to return to work when they are still excreting salmonella or shigella; an assessment of fitness to return to food-handling duties may therefore have to be made in the hospital. In addition, all catering staff exposed to enteric infection require counselling on handwashing technique and on other measures required to prevent possible spread.

Food-handlers suffering from diarrhoea and/or vomiting while at work should be immediately referred to an appropriate authority for assessment; this could be the occupational health or the infection control department, or the staff medical officer, depending on the system used. They should, where possible, be referred before leaving for home to ensure that specimens are obtained where appropriate and that the incident is properly documented. If it is then decided that they are unfit for further duty, they should be reminded that they must report back before returning to normal duties. Skin rashes, boils, and other lesions or rashes should be reported in a similar manner.

All food handlers should report to the occupational health department, staff medical officer, or infection control nurse if:

1. they have been off sick with one of the above conditions;
2. they have suffered from diarrhoea or vomiting lasting more than two days while on leave;
3. other members of the household are suffering from diarrhoea or vomiting.

If, on reporting, they are considered fit for return to work, they should be counselled on the importance of a good handwashing technique and general hygiene, and given a note for their manager specifying whether they can or cannot return to food preparation duties. To encourage prompt reporting of such conditions, staff should be made aware that being sent off duty will not lead to loss of salary.

12.2.3 TRAINING

All food handlers should be given training in personal and kitchen hygiene on employment and at intervals afterwards. A booklet containing rules of hygiene should be provided for each member. Posters demonstrating different aspects of hygiene should be prominently displayed in catering food storage areas and changed at frequent intervals (see Appendix 12.4).

12.2.4 PERSONAL HYGIENE

The main route of transfer of infection to food is on the hands of staff. Hands should be washed frequently, especially after using the toilet and before handling food. In addition to the hands and fingernails, the face and other parts of the body should be kept clean, including hair and scalp, and the forearms when short sleeves are worn. The nose, lips and hair should not be touched while handling food. Nails should be kept short. Hands cannot be assumed to be free from pathogenic organisms after washing, and food should be handled as little as possible. Hands should be washed in hot water using the recommended soap or detergent and must then be well rinsed and thoroughly dried on a fresh paper towel. Since they may damage the skin, nail brushes should be used only if they are required to remove heavy soiling which cannot be removed without their use. Nail brushes lying in soap dishes are likely to be heavily contaminated with Gram-negative bacilli; their use may then both damage the skin and inoculate it with bacteria. A small number of sterile or adequately decontaminated nail brushes should be available on request; arrangements should be made for these to be reprocessed after use. Wash-basins must be provided in each food preparation area and plain bar or liquid soap or detergent provided. Bar soap should be kept in a dry state between uses. If liquid soap dispensers are used, they must be thoroughly cleaned at regular intervals and must not be refilled without prior cleaning and disinfection. The liquid soap should contain a preservative. Antibacterial soaps and detergents (e.g. chlorhexidine-detergent preparations, iodophors, triclosan) may be required during an outbreak of staphylococcal infection, but should be used only on advice from the infection control staff. The catering staff should be provided with good changing and sanitary accommodation. Food handlers should keep their personal clothing and overalls clean and should change their protective clothing daily or more frequently if necessary. Protective clothing should only be worn for catering duties and should not be worn in other departments. Laundering should be arranged by the hospital authorities. Uniforms and other protective clothing should not be taken home for laundering or any other purpose. Staff should not smoke while handling food or while in a room where food is exposed. All cuts and grazes must be completely covered with a waterproof dressing.

12.2.5   CLEANING AND MAINTENANCE

Detailed schedules should be produced defining methods and responsibility. Floors should be constructed to facilitate cleaning and should be well maintained. Walls and ceilings should have smooth impermeable surfaces and cooking equipment should be so sited that areas below and around can be easily cleaned. All cleaning should be carried out with a freshly prepared and accurately diluted detergent solution. Cleaning equipment, such as scrubbing machines and mops, should remain in the kitchen but not in the food preparation area (for methods of disinfection see Chapter 6) and should be examined at defined intervals. If worn or damaged, equipment should be repaired or replaced. Special attention should be paid to the cleaning of food preparation surfaces and meat slicers. Preparation surfaces should be impervious to water and should be maintained in a good condition. Stainless steel surfaces are advised, although composition chopping boards and blocks are suitable. Wherever possible, preparation surfaces should be used for one purpose only. Food requiring no further cooking (e.g. sandwiches, cooked meat, etc.) must not be prepared on surfaces which have previously been used for preparation of raw meat, fish, poultry or vegetables. In small units with limited working areas, it may be necessary to use surfaces for more than one purpose; thorough cleaning and drying between different uses is required in such cases. Preparation surfaces should always be cleaned with a recently prepared hot cleaning solution and a fresh disposable or freshly laundered cloth. There is little point in providing separate surfaces for different types of food if all surfaces are cleaned with the same cleaning solution and cloths; contamination will be transferred from one surface to another. Each individual surface should be dried with a disposable or freshly laundered dry cloth; most Gram-negative bacilli die on drying, if the surface is initially clean.

Disinfectants are usually unnecessary, but may be recommended by the infection control doctor or microbiologist during outbreaks of infection (hypochlorite solutions containing at least 250 ppm av Cl_2 are often used).

Transfer of contamination from one product to another is particularly likely with meat mincers and slicers. Cooked and uncooked meats must never be processed with the same machine without thorough cleaning between operations.

12.2.6 CROCKERY AND CUTLERY: POTS AND PANS

Crockery and cutlery should be machine-washed at a minimum temperature of 60°C and a final rinse of at least 80°C or another appropriate temperature and time (see Chapter 4; Central Sterilizing Club 1986). A central washing-up machine is preferred and washing-up by hand on the ward should be avoided whenever possible. A washing-up machine on the ward is, however, a satisfactory alternative. When machine washing is not available and crockery and cutlery have to be washed by hand, twin sinks should preferably be used to ensure efficient rinsing. Detergent solutions and rinsing water should be changed frequently and should be as hot as possible. Re-usable washing-up cloths should not be used; they should be replaced by disposable cloths. Nylon brushes, washed and thoroughly dried after each use, are preferable to cloths, but should not be used in preference to disposable materials.

It is important that all crockery, cutlery, pots and pans and kitchen equipment should be thoroughly dried after cleaning. The use of linen drying cloths (tea towels) should be discontinued whenever possible and replaced by a system of heat-drying or air-drying in racks. When drying by hand is necessary, a disposable towel is preferred.

Crockery, cutlery, pots and pans should be examined regularly.

Worn, chipped, stained or broken items should be replaced. When not in use, they should be stored clean and under conditions in which recontamination is reduced to the minimum.

12.2.7 STORAGE AND TRANSPORTATION OF FOOD

Certain food, such as raw meat, fish and poultry, may carry harmful bacterial contaminants and should be prepared and cooked in such a way that these organisms are destroyed before serving; periodic checking of temperatures with a probe thermometer in the coldest part of the food is recommended. Poultry may be contaminated with *Salmonella* spp. and inadequate thawing of frozen poultry before cooking may enable these organisms to survive the cooking process. The multiplication of bacteria should be prevented by careful storage of food at the correct temperature before and after cooking; for example, *Cl. perfringens* is a common cause of food-poisoning and its spores may survive the cooking process. These bacteria may multiply if cooked food is left without refrigeration for longer than two hours. Subsequent reheating may further increase the numbers of bacteria, and when large numbers are eaten, toxins may be released into the intestine and cause food-poisoning.

Food must be stored so that raw meat, fish and uncooked vegetables (whether prepared or unprepared) do not come in contact with food which is to be served without further heat-treatment. These foods must be separated by storing in separate refrigerators or in closed compartments within the same refrigerator or cold room. Food must not be stored on the floor of cold rooms or below foods which may leak or be spilt.

Food requiring cooling must not be left in the kitchen area but should be transferred to a cooling area and cooled rapidly to at least 8°C (see also cook-chill). Stored food should be protected from recontamination. Food which is transported within the hospital, for example from stores to kitchen, or from kitchen to ward, should be transported under clean conditions and properly covered to prevent contamination. It should be carried in a clean closed container, especially if the vehicle is used for other purposes. Vehicles used for this purpose should be appropriately designed, kept clean and in good repair. Contaminated materials, such as refuse or soiled linen, must not be carried in these vehicles.

Refuse and food waste (swill) must not be allowed to accumulate in the kitchen, and should be removed at frequent intervals (see section 12.4).

The amount of time during which food is allowed to stand on hot plates and trolleys must be kept to a minimum. Trolleys, hot cupboards and containers must be maintained at the correct temperature and checked at regular intervals (e.g. monthly).

Food should be served by staff trained in food hygiene. Clean overalls should be worn and adequate serving equipment provided to prevent unnecessary handling. Patients should not take part in food preparation or washing-up procedures unless agreed by the ward sister; this applies particularly to psychiatric hospitals where it is difficult to instruct patients in good food hygiene. Left-over food in ward refrigerators should be discarded daily; swill must not be retained or stored on the ward.

12.2.8 GOOD CATERING PRACTICE

Where possible, standardized recipes should be used so that internal temperatures can be measured and reproduced to ensure adequate cooking. Policy decisions should be made for each type of food concerning the minimum internal temperature required, maximum time allowed at room temperature after cooking, and how long it can be kept refrigerated before use or disposal. Whenever possible meat should be cooked on the day it is served. There should also be a strict policy on the maximum time sandwiches, salads, etc. are kept at room temperature, or in chilled storage, before they are discarded.

12.2.9 RETAINING FOOD FOR TESTING

Food poisoning organisms, when present, are not uniformly distributed throughout contaminated food and, whatever the conditions of storage, the numbers of bacteria/gm of food will vary from sample to sample examined over the storage period. The absence of food poisoning organisms in a sample does not indicate that the item contained no such organisms, and the numbers present at the time of testing does not necessarily reflect the numbers present when the food was eaten. The results obtained from stored samples can be misleading. Sampling needs careful planning, proper supervision and extensive documentation. The amount and type of food stored and the particulars of the storage container should be defined. The full cooperation of the microbiologist is necessary. Even where only representative samples of those items likely to be associated with food poisoning are saved, the value of sampling for intestinal pathogens is unlikely to justify the substantial resources required and cannot be recommended as a routine procedure. Although outbreaks of food poisoning in an individual hospital are very rare, some monitoring may be required, particularly during the setting up of a cook-chill service. Control of processes by good techniques is much more important than microbiological sampling.

12.2.10   COOK-CHILL MEAL SERVICES (DHSS 1989)

Good catering practices should be followed as with conventional catering. A flow chart should be prepared at each stage and examined for potential infection risk. Monitoring systems should be set up to ensure agreed standards are met and all stages should be documented. A system of monitoring based on hazard analysis critical control points (HACCP) is now commonly used. This involves defining and controlling microbiological or other hazards at certain critical points during the processing of food (Wilkinson *et al*. 1991). The responsibility for maintaining standards should be clearly defined. The present DHSS guidelines should generally be followed and not modified unless the microbiologist or environmental health officer agree that a modification is acceptable.

The following should be observed.

1. Raw foods of good microbiological quality should be chosen and correctly stored.
2. Areas for handling raw and cooked foods should be separate.
3. During cooking, food should reach a temperature of 70°C (and preferably be retained at this temperature for two minutes to destroy listeria).
4. The food should be chilled to a temperature of 0–3°C within 90 minutes. Special arrangements may be required for joints and poultry. Either slice hot and transfer to rapid chiller within 30 minutes, or reduce temperature of joints to 10°C or less in two and a half hours. When the temperature has reached this level the joints should be sliced in a temperature controlled room and transferred to the rapid chiller without delay.
5. Food should be stored at 0–3°C for no longer than five days. If the temperature exceeds 5°C but remains less than 10°C, the food should be eaten within 12 hours. If the temperature exceeds 10°C, destruction of the stored food should be considered. Advice should be obtained from the microbiologist.
6. Food should be transported in a refrigerated or insulated trolley and the temperature should not exceed 10°C before reheating to 70°C. If refrigeration is not available maximum transport times should be agreed.
7. Food containers should either be disposable or cleaned, disinfected by heat and dried after use. Times and temperatures should be regularly checked and recorded to ensure that no bacterial growth can occur during the process. A probe thermometer should be used to confirm that the necessary temperatures are reached in each of the processes. Most pathogenic organisms fail to grow at tempera-

tures below 5°C and significant growth is unlikely to occur in less than two hours at room temperature.

Although routine microbiological testing should be unnecessary if process control is reliable, tests are usually carried out with a recently set-up service or if changes are made; a suggested standard is as follows:

A sample of 100 g of each item of food from each batch to be tested should be taken immediately before re-heating.

The following criteria are suggested (Sandys and Wilkinson 1988):

1. total aerobic count – less than 100 000 per g (agar plates incubated at 37°C for 48 hours);
2. *Salmonella* spp and *Listeria monocytogenes* should not be detected in 25 g;
3. *E. coli* – less than 10 per g;
4. *Staph. aureus* and *Cl. perfringens* – less than 100 per g;
   Listeria monocytogenes has recently emerged as a potential hazard as it will grow at lower temperatures than most other pathogens. It is commonly found in the environment and as a contaminant of raw foods, but the number of food-borne infections remains low. Although the number of clinical infections reported has increased in recent years, the overall number is still relatively small. Nevertheless, susceptible groups (e.g. pregnant women or immunocompromised patients) should not eat food likely to contain listeria.

12.2.11 RESPONSIBILITY

The catering manager is responsible for hygiene and cleaning in his/her department. The responsibility for maintenance of structure and equipment should be clearly defined. At least one annual inspection should be made by the catering manager, infection control doctor, or a member of the infection control team, and a member of the engineering or building staff to examine aspects of hygiene in the catering area. A check list for kitchen inspections is shown in Appendix 12.1. Occasional inspections should also be made by an environmental health officer (EHO). The infection control doctor and committee are responsible for advising the District manager or administrator on all hygienic matters, including catering, and reports should be referred to them before action is taken.

12.3 Pests: eradication and control

The infestation of hospital premises (kitchens, staff restaurants, laundries, nurses' homes, etc.) with pests, particularly cockroaches,

Pharaoh's ants and mice, is a common but undesirable occurrence. Although it may be difficult to keep some old premises free of pests, every effort should be made to achieve a reasonable level of control or eradication, whichever is practicable. This will depend on the type of pest, extent of infestation, complexity of the buildings and other local factors (Baker 1981).

The role of pests in the transmission of hospital-acquired infection is uncertain, but reports indicate that carriage of specific pathogens, including *Salmonella* spp., may occur. Apart from the possibility of disease transmission, food may be tainted and spoiled, and fabrics and building structure damaged. Pharaoh's ants have been responsible for the penetration of sterile packs and the invasion of patients' dressings, including those in use on a wound.

Treatment with insecticides and rodenticides alone is seldom sufficient; attention must also be paid to good hygiene and structural maintenance. Pests require food, warmth, moisture, harbourage, and a means of entry; hospital staff should be encouraged to keep food covered, to remove spillage and waste, and to avoid accumulations of static water. Buildings should be of sound structure and well maintained, drains should be covered, leaking pipework repaired, and damaged surfaces made good. Cracks in plaster and woodwork, unsealed areas around pipework, damaged tiles, badly fitting equipment and kitchen units, are all likely to provide excellent harbourage. Close-fitting windows and doors, the provision of fly screens and bird netting, all help to exclude pests from hospital buildings.

Many pests are nocturnal, for example cockroaches and mice, and infestation surveys are best carried out at night and when the rooms are unoccupied. In addition to seeing the pests themselves, droppings, nests, runs, rodent smears, insect fragments, structural and fabric damage are all signs of infestation. Also, sticky detectors or traps are now available for monitoring the control of cockroaches and other crawling pests. Pyrethrum aerosols are useful for flushing cockroaches and other insects from their harbourage, and liver baiting is useful for assessing infestation with Pharaoh's ants.

In most hospitals, the task of pest control is given to a commercial company specializing in this work. Nevertheless, the hospital should appoint an officer to co-ordinate local pest control activities, initiate a reporting system, carry out preliminary and routine assessments of control measures, and negotiate with and follow up the recommendations of the servicing company (NHS, 1991).

Standard NHS Pest Control Contracts require that premises be 'rid' of certain pests within a finite period of time. Thereafter there is a contractual obligation upon the servicing company to ensure the premises remain free of those pests. Integrated into this type of strategy are inspection and reporting procedures.

The pesticides used will have been approved under the Pesticides Regulations and furthermore will have been considered by the Health Authority suitable for use within its premises.

Advice on all aspects of pest control is available from the Environmental Health and Food Safety Division (EHF4A) of the Department of Health.

12.4 Disposal of refuse and food-waste

There is no evidence that waste from hospitals is a greater infection risk than that from domestic and commercial premises, or that hospital waste has been the cause of outbreaks of infection in the community. Some waste however, is more likely to be a source of infection, and to be found in hospitals than elsewhere. If the risk is sufficiently high, additional measures may be justified. Infection risk is related to the number and type of microbes present, their ability to survive in the environment and the probability that those organisms will reach a susceptible site. These factors are not usually known and the decision to adopt additional measures is often based on other reasons. Although aesthetic reasons have some justification, the hazard of waste should be mainly assessed on scientific data (Hedrick 1988). Waste requiring additional measures should be clearly identified. Black plastic bags are used for domestic waste and yellow for waste requiring incineration (Health Services Advisory Committee 1982). Waste bags should not be over-filled and should be securely closed as soon as they are full. Intact sealed bags are not an infection risk to handlers.

12.4.1 CATEGORIES OF HOSPITAL WASTE

Categories of hospital waste requiring additional measures for disposal are as follows.

1. Used sharp instruments for disposal (e.g. syringes, needles and scalpel blades). These must be disposed of in containers to an approved standard (DHSS 1982; Health Service Advisory Committee 1982). Containers should be stored under secure conditions to prevent any unauthorized access (syringes and needles are an attraction to children and drug addicts). Final disposal must be by incineration.
2. Recognizable animal or human tissue (e.g. amputated limbs). Place in a yellow bag and arrange for supervised transport to an operating incinerator for immediate disposal. If transport outside the hospital

is necessary, the bag should be placed in a rigid locked container labelled with instructions as to who should be contacted in the case of breakdown or accident.

3. Potentially offensive material which is not necessarily an infection risk (e.g. soiled dressings, incontinence pads, and wipes used for cleaning patients). This material is unlikely to be an infection risk to handlers since the organisms present, even in large numbers, are likely to be common environmental contaminants present in almost any moist waste. Material of this type may be a substantial proportion of hospital waste and if disposed of by landfill and not immediately covered, may be noticed by the public and cause offence; incineration is the preferred method of disposal. It may, however, be possible to make other acceptable arrangements (e.g. deep land fill) with the waste disposal authority. Large quantities of similar material is disposed of in waste from private dwellings without apparent harm. This category is recommended as requiring inclusion, as 'clinical waste' in present guidelines (Health Service Advisory Committee 1982), but this is unnecessarily expensive and creates major problems in the community. It is suggested that 'clinical waste' is subdivided and a separate category included for 'infected' waste as with laundry.

4. Infected (or potentially hazardous) clinical waste is waste material likely to be contaminated by contact with patients with specific infections which could be transferred to anyone handling it (e.g. HBV or HIV infection, pulmonary tuberculosis, salmonella and shigella infections). This material must be sealed in yellow plastic bags at the point of generation. Secure storage, which protects the material from pests which could spread the infecting organisms, is important. Final disposal must be by incineration.

5. Laboratory waste (e.g. bacterial cultures and clinical specimens). Laboratory waste is usually autoclaved in the laboratory before disposal. This will render it safe for subsequent disposal, but secure storage to prevent spread of infection by pests prior to autoclaving should be considered. Incineration without autoclaving could be acceptable provided adequate precautions are taken during transport. Special arrangements are also required for:
   (a) certain exotic diseases, such as Lassa fever;
   (b) radioactive material;
   (c) cytotoxic drugs.

Those involved with the use of these materials should be aware that there is legislation governing safe disposal. There may also be a requirement to separate broken glass which should be stored in puncture-proof containers and used aerosol canisters which can explode if incinerated.

12.4.2 DOMESTIC WASTE

All other materials can be regarded as domestic waste and can be placed in black plastic bags for disposal. In situations where all hospital waste can be incinerated at acceptable cost, this should be done and would make it unnecessary to have separate categories of waste requiring different methods of disposal.

12.4.3 WASTE STORAGE AREAS

Any area used for the storage of waste should be easy to clean, roofed, properly drained and bird and rat-proof. A water supply for hosing down is essential.

12.4.4 FOOD WASTE

Food waste from wards should be enclosed in a suitable container and returned to the central area for disposal, so that some check can be kept on the amount of food not being eaten. Prompt disposal by a disposal unit is preferred to selling to contractors. Proper storage of food waste before collection by contractors is difficult to control. Containers should be of good quality with well-fitting lids which are kept closed, and should be cleaned at regular intervals. Storage areas should be properly designed and kept clean. This is rarely achieved. However, if sold, waste should only be disposed of to contractors licensed in accordance with the requirements of the Disease of Animals (Waste Food) Order (1973), and every effort should be made to ensure that storage areas and containers are maintained to a reasonable standard.

Appendix 12.1   Inspection of kitchens

A check list should be produced from the following guidelines.

DELIVERY

Food should be properly transported, delivered in good condition and at the right temperature.
   Check that:

1. transport is clean, not used for any other purpose, and refrigerated if specified;
2. food is properly contained and at the right temperature (deep frozen should be at −18°C or below; chilled should be between 0°C and +3°C);

3. a probe thermometer should be used to check the temperature, which should be recorded. Is the food properly wrapped and handled? Does packaging give any information on origin? Is it dated? Is the person unloading the van wearing clean clothing etc?

HANDLING ON ARRIVAL

Food should be transferred to the correctly designated storage area at the appropriate temperature as soon as possible. It should be transferred with minimal handling and without coming into contact with other foods.

Check wet stains on the bottom of boxes of frozen food, suggesting it has been defrosted and refrozen. If boxes are stacked, check contents to ensure thawing meat is not dripping into butter, cheese etc.

STORAGE TEMPERATURE

Any food capable of supporting microbial growth should either be stored below 5°C or above 63°C (cook-chilled food should be stored below 3°C).

Check temperature at which food items should be stored. Question staff if food is at room temperature; ask two different people, not present at the same time, how long it has been there. Use probe to check temperature of food being served or plated.

FOOD STORES

Food stores should be generally clean, uncluttered and with good access for cleaning. Food in boxes or sacks should not be stored directly on the floor. Shelving should be easy to clean and if not movable, easy to clean under, around and behind.

Check evidence of infestation, lids left off bins, packets left open. Determine that there is a proper stock rotation system and products are clearly identified. There should be no staff clothing, handbags etc. in the storage area. Any opening skylights or windows should be bird proofed, door bottoms should be rat proofed and all pipes etc. sealed into the wall.

FOOD SEPARATION

Any food likely to be naturally contaminated with organisms capable of causing food poisoning (e.g. raw poultry, meat and fish) should be prevented from coming into direct or indirect contact with any food that will be eaten without further cooking.

Check – question staff on requirements for food separation.

Look for the following – the use of the same surface for preparation of different foods, use of common cloths or knives; staff not washing hands.

Note – good practice includes separate bays for each task, colour coded cloths, satisfactory cleaning of knives, preparation surfaces and chopping blocks.

ADEQUATE COOKING

The use of approved detailed recipes should include minimum internal temperatures before starting cooking and at the end. The type of container used should also be specified. For each type of food there should be clear guidelines on whether unserved portions can be used as a basis for other dishes and whether all processes for the particular meal are completed in the same day. Clear guidelines must also exist as to how long the food can be retained after it is cooked and before it is served, and at what temperature it should be stored. Is reheating allowed? Under what circumstances and to what temperature.

Check details of at least one commonly prepared dish and question staff in detail to ensure that guidelines are known, understood and followed.

STAFF HYGIENE

All staff handling food should be trained in personal and catering hygienic methods.

Check numbers of wash-hand basins and whether they are correctly sited, the presence of soap and paper towels and evidence of recent use. Is it the clearly defined responsibility of a named individual to ensure that soap and towels are always available? Are staff aware under what conditions they should report sick and to whom? Is counselling on the need for care in handwashing given after each absence for illness if diarrhoea or sickness is involved? What is the availability of clean uniforms and are they sufficient?

Question staff on training courses and their content and existing knowledge.

WARD KITCHENS ETC.

Ensure that all the food preparation and service areas (including ward kitchens) are included in inspections and that they are covered by an agreed policy.

CLEANING

Every area and item in the kitchen should have an agreed cleaning procedure. Methods, materials and frequency should be defined, including an order of priority during periods of staff shortage. These should be displayed and known by staff concerned. It should be known where the cleaning equipment is stored and who is responsible for cleaning and notifying any need for repair or replacement.

Appendix 12.2   Questionnaire for catering staff

	Yes	No	When (year)	How long off work	If yes Name of doctor or hospital
1. Have you ever had any of the following: Typhoid fever? Paratyphoid fever? Dysentery? Persistent diarrhoea? Tuberculosis?					
2. Have you suffered from any of the following within the past two years: Diarrhoea and/or vomiting for more than 2 days? Skin rash? Boils? Discharge from eye? ear? nose? Other infections?					

3. Have you ever been abroad? If yes:	Yes Where	No When	

I declare that all the foregoing statements are true and complete to the best of my knowledge and belief.

....

4. *Investigations:*
   Chest X-ray
   Faeces
   Blood
   Other

Comments

Appendix 12.3 Catering staff agreement to report infection

I agree to report to the Catering Officer or his deputy

1. If suffering from an illness involving:
   Vomiting
   Diarrhoea
   Skin rash
   Septic skin lesions (boils, infected cuts etc., however small)
   Discharge from ear, eye or nose
2. After returning and before commencing work following an illness involving vomiting and/or diarrhoea, or any of the above conditions.
3. After returning from a holiday during which an attack of vomiting and/or diarrhoea lasted for more than two days.
4. If another member of my household is suffering from diarrhoea and/or vomiting.
   I have read (or had explained to me) and understood the accompanying rules on personal hygiene.

Signed   Date

Appendix 12.4 Kitchen and food-handling staff: rules of personal hygiene

Patients in hospital may develop severe infection with germs which are not harmful to healthy people.

The following rules must be observed to prevent germs from entering food:

1. **WASH THE HANDS FREQUENTLY**, ESPECIALLY AFTER USING THE TOILET AND BEFORE HANDLING FOOD. THIS IS THE MOST IMPORTANT METHOD PREVENTING THE SPREAD OF INFECTION. In addition to hands and particularly nails, the face and other parts of the body likely to come into contact with food should be kept clean, e.g. the hair and scalp, and the forearms when short sleeves are worn. Avoid touching the nose, lips and hair while handling food.
2. Personal clothing and overalls must be kept clean. Protective clothing provided by the Hospital must be worn.
3. All open cuts and grazes must be completely covered with a waterproof dressing.
4. You must not smoke while handling 'open' food or while in a room where there is such food.
5. Other hygienic rules as indicated by the Catering Manager.

References and further reading

Baker, L.F. (1981) Pests in hospitals. *Journal of Hospital Infection*, **2**, 5.
Central Sterilizing Club (1986) Working Party Report No. 1. *Washer/disinfection machines*. Obtainable from Hospital Infection Research Laboratory.

Collins, B.J., Cripps, N. and Spooner, A. (1987) Controlling microbiological decontamination levels. *Laundry and Cleaning News*, 30.

Department of Health and Social Security (1971) *Report on Hospital Laundry Arrangements*. HM(71)49. HMSO, London.

Department of Health and Social Security (1981) *Domestic Services Management Advice Note 6. Pest Control: Contract Management*. DHSS, London.

Department of Health and Social Security (1982) *Specifications for Containers for Disposal of Needles (TSS/S/330.075)*. HMSO, London.

Department of Health and Social Security (1984) *Domestic Services Management Advice Note 5. An Introduction to Pest Control in Hospitals*, 2nd edn. DHSS, London.

Department of Health and Social Security (1987a) *Hospital Laundry Arrangements for Used and Infected Linen HC(37)30*. HMSO, London.

Department of Health and Social Security (1987b) Health Service Catering Hygiene.

Department of Health and Social Security (1989) *Health Service Guidelines on Pre-cooked Chilled Food*. HMSO, London.

Health Service Advisory Committee (1982) *HN(82)22. The Safe Disposal of Clinical Waste*. HMSO, London.

Hedrick, E.R. (1988) Infectious waste management – will science prevail? *Infection Control and Hospital Epidemiology*, **9**, 488.

Hobbs, B.C. and Roberts, D. (1987) *Food poisoning and Hygiene*, 5th edn. Edward Arnold, London.

National Health Service (1991) Conditions of contract for pest control. NHS Management Executive Procurement Directorate.

Sandys, G.H. and Wilkinson, P. (1988) Microbiological evaluation of a hospital delivered meals service using pre-cooked chilled foods. *Journal of Hospital Infection*, **9**, 209.

Wilkinson, P.J., Dart, S.P. and Hadlington, C. J. (1991) Cook-chill, cook-freeze, sous vide: risks for hospital patients. *Journal of Hospital Infection*, **18** (Supplement A), 222.

13 Use of antibiotics and chemotherapeutic agents

In this chapter the word **antibiotic** refers to both synthetic compounds (antimicrobial chemotherapeutic agents) and naturally produced agents (antibiotics). Some of these substances (e.g. the penicillins) are almost without toxicity to man (except for those persons who are hypersensitive to them) but will kill many pathogenic bacteria. Certain antibiotics (e.g. bacitracin) are so toxic to man that they cannot safely be given parenterally and are reserved for topical treatment of superficial infections, or are given orally to disinfect the gut, if non-absorbed.

If a patient is known or suspected to be suffering from an infection the clinician must decide which organism is known or likely to be responsible and to which antibiotic it will or will probably be sensitive. Other factors which need to be considered include the expected value of treatment and the possible side-effects of the antibiotic.

The aim of chemotherapy is principally to aid the natural defences of the body to eliminate the microbes from tissues by preventing their multiplication. To have this effect the blood and infected tissues must contain a concentration of the antibiotic higher than the **minimal inhibitory** (i.e. bacteriostatic) **concentration** (MIC) of the antibiotic for the infecting organism. In very severe infections, especially septicaemia, endocarditis, osteomyelitis, pyelonephritis, and infections in patients with poor natural defences or in those receiving immunosuppressive drugs or steroids, chemotherapy must aim to kill the infecting organisms; i.e. tissue fluids must contain more than the **minimal bactericidal** (i.e. killing) **concentration** (MBC) of the antibiotic. To achieve this the drug must be given by the proper route – for example, drugs not absorbed from the intestine must not be given by mouth unless local action in the bowel is required. If the drug does not reach the tissues in sufficiently high concentration, local administration may occasionally be required in addition to systemic therapy. If high blood levels are important, as in severe infections, injection rather than oral administration is preferable, and for the initial treatment of life-threatening infections the route may need to be intravenous. It should be borne in mind that intravenous lines for infusion are a significant source of infection in hospital. Intravenous lines for administration of antibiotics carry similar risks. Several new antibiotics are well absorbed when given by mouth, and the oral route is preferable to the parenteral wherever possible. New quinolones, β-lactam inhibitors and recently described macrolides and oral cephalosporins are examples of the types of antibiotics which should be considered in this regard.

Antibiotic-resistant strains of certain organisms are common in hospital. *Staphylococcus aureus* and certain Gram-negative bacilli causing hospital infection have become increasingly resistant to the commonly used antibiotics. These resistant organisms may have appeared either as the result of the selection of intrinsically resistant strains by extensive and often indiscriminate use of antibiotics, or by mutation of previously sensitive bacteria, and selection following exposure to the antibiotics. Some resistant organisms, especially Gram-negative bacilli, can transfer antibiotic resistance to other bacteria.

Whereas the majority of hospital staphylococci and also most strains in the community are now resistant to penicillin, all haemolytic streptococci of *group A* (*Streptococcus pyogenes*), clostridia and the treponema of syphilis remain sensitive to this antibiotic – an example of the extreme variability of bacterial resistance.

In view of the large number of available antibiotics, there is need for guidance on their use. This chapter provides concise information about antibiotics and recommendations for their safe and effective administration in treatment and (where indicated) in prophylaxis. Methods of delaying the emergence of resistance (especially by avoidance of unnecessary or inefficient use) are stressed. (For detailed information on antibiotics see Garrod *et al.* 1981; Kucers and Bennett 1987).

13.1   Classification of antibiotics

Antibiotics have been classified in many different ways. The most useful way for clinical use is to classify them as to which micro-organism they are likely to affect. In practice, the acquisition of resistance may render antibiotics less useful, and knowledge of the local epidemiology of resistant bacteria is necessary in selection of the most appropriate agent. Table 13.1 is condensed from the classification used in Parker and Collier (1990) and indicates which groups of bacteria are sensitive to the different classes of antibiotics.

Antibiotics can also be classified as bactericidal (killing bacteria) or as **predominantly bacteriostatic** (preventing their growth). The latter are satisfactory for most purposes, but the former are required for the successful treatment of severe infections or in patients with poor natural resistance. Some bactericidal agents (penicillins) may be antagonized by bacteriostatic agents and are best not used in combination with them.

Table 13.1 Classification of antimicrobial agents according to activity

Activity against Gram-positive bacteria and Gram-negative cocci	Main activity against Gram-negative bacteria	Broad-spectrum antibiotics	Specific antibacterial agents	Antifungals and antivirals
Benzylpenicillin	Ampicillin[a]	Sulphonamides	*Anaerobes*	*Antifungals*
Phenoxymethyl- penicillin	Mezlocillin[a]	Co-trimoxazole	Clindamycin	Nystatin
	Piperacillin	Cephalosporins	Metronidazole	Amphotericin B
Flucloxacillin	Ciprofloxacin	Imipenem	*Tuberculosis*	5-Fluorocytosine
Erythromycin	Ofloxacin	Tetracyclines	Isoniazid	Imidazoles
Clindamycin	Temocillin	Chloramphenicol	Rifampicin	Griseofulvin
Rifampicin	Aztreonam		Ethionamide	*Antivirals*
Vancomycin	Gentamicin		Pyrazinamide, etc.	Idoxuridine
Teicoplanin	Amikacin		*Chlamydia*[c]	Amantadine
	Nitrofurantoin[b]		Erythromycin	Ganciclovir
	Nalidixic acid[b]		Rifampicin	Azidothymidine
			Tetracycline	
			Chloramphenicol	
			Campylobacter spp.	
			Erythromycin	
			Ciprofloxacin	
			Legionella spp.	
			Erythromycin	
			Rifampicin	

(a) Some activity vs. Gram-positive cocci
(b) Urinary tract infection only
(c) Also Mycoplasma, Legionella, Rickettsia

Broad spectrum antibiotics should not be used for treating specific pathogens sensitive to narrow range agents (e.g. *Strep. pyogenes*).

13.2 Use of individual antibiotics

For guidance on complex treatment and its control, the clinician should consult a clinical microbiologist or a physician experienced in chemotherapy. The *British National Formulary*, which should be available in all wards and departments, contains up-to-date information on all available antibiotics.

13.3 Application of antibiotics to tissues

Most infections with sensitive organisms respond to systemic antibiotic therapy. However, there are times when local application of chemotherapeutic agents may be indicated. Chloramphenicol is used for the treatment of purulent conjunctivitis. Suppurative external ear conditions are treated with antibiotic ear drops. 0.5% silver nitrate solution is an effective chemoprophylactic agent for severe burns: silver sulphadiazine cream is a more convenient and very effective application for this purpose, though sulphonamide-resistant bacteria may be selected through its use in a burns unit. Gentamicin should not be used topically for routine prophylaxis because of the risk of promoting resistance. Streptococcal infections of burns should be treated with a systemic antibiotic (flucloxacillin or erythromycin; see Chapter 16, p. 301) and not topical therapy; in general it is best to avoid applications of penicillins or neomycin to the skin as sensitization may result. Furthermore, neomycin should not be applied to severe burns as it may lead to absorption and subsequent deafness through damage to the auditory nerve. Intrathecal administration of antibiotics is potentially hazardous and should be avoided. Antibiotics may be instilled into the pleural and peritoneal cavity in addition to parenteral therapy in the treatment of purulent effusions or peritonitis.

13.4 Antibiotic combinations

Most infections respond satisfactorily to treatment with a single antibiotic. In the following circumstances, however, combined therapy may be valuable:

13.4.1 PREVENTION OF DEVELOPMENT OF BACTERIAL RESISTANCE

Tuberculosis is the outstanding indication for obligatory combined chemotherapy for this purpose.

13.4.2 INFECTIONS CAUSED BY MORE THAN ONE ORGANISM (MIXED INFECTIONS)

Intra-abdominal sepsis is usually caused by both aerobic and anaerobic bacteria, and for this reason a combination of gentamicin or a cephalosporin with metronidazole is commonly used.

13.4.3 SEPTICAEMIA AND ENDOCARDITIS

Combinations of antibiotics are sometimes required for treatment of septicaemia and certain forms of endocarditis. A combination of penicillin and gentamicin may be used to treat endocarditis caused by viridans streptococci if the organism shows reduced susceptibility to benzyl penicillin, and penicillin or ampicillin plus gentamicin is suitable for *Ent. faecalis* endocarditis. Ticarcillin or another appropriate penicillin or cephalosporin may be used in combination plus gentamicin (they must be injected separately) for the treatment of pseudomonas septicaemia, and combined therapy (e.g. flucloxacillin and fusidic acid) can be employed for staphylococcal septicaemia. However, most infections mentioned under this heading can be treated successfully with a single antibiotic.

13.4.4 WHEN A COMBINATION IS SUPERIOR TO A SINGLE AGENT (SYNERGY)

Ampicillin and clavulanic acid is such a combination. Laboratory methods are available for synergy testing of chemotherapeutic agents.

13.5 Selection of an antibiotic

The selection of an antibiotic should never be a haphazard choice but must be based on careful consideration of the following factors.

13.5.1 THE SENSITIVITY (OR PROBABLE SENSITIVITY) OF THE INFECTING ORGANISM

Before the infecting organism and its sensitivity are known, it is useful to make a presumptive diagnosis of its possible identity and antibiotic sensitivity of the organism by consideration of the clinical picture, so that treatment with a potentially appropriate antibiotic can be started; e.g. in infective endocarditis, where the commonest infecting organism is a viridans streptococci or in purulent meningitis, in which the organisms are usually meningococci, pneumococci or *Haemophilus influenzae*. Severe infections such as endocarditis and meningitis require detailed sensitivity testing, including the determination of the MIC and MBC of the organism.

13.5.2 THE CLINICAL PHARMACOLOGY OF THE VARIOUS ANTIBIOTICS

Particularly important factors are their absorption, excretion and distribution. Certain antibiotics (e.g. ampicillin) are excreted in bile and urine while some (e.g. chloramphenicol and the penicillins) penetrate the inflamed 'blood-brain barrier' and pass on to the cerebrospinal fluid (CSF).

13.5.3   ROUTE OF ADMINISTRATION

Oral therapy is satisfactory for the treatment of many infections. Severe infections, however, may require intravenous injections. To achieve adequate blood levels antibiotics given intravenously should normally be administered by 'bolus' and not added to the drip bottle unless slow IV infusion is the recommended method of administration. Topical application of antibiotics may be sufficient for certain eye, superficial skin and external ear infections.

13.5.4   TOXICITY OF ANTIBIOTICS

All antibiotics have side-effects and toxic drugs should not be used when safer agents are available. Chloramphenicol, for example, can cause fatal aplastic anaemia and should normally be reserved for the treatment of *H. influenzae* meningitis, or typhoid fever where the organism is not susceptible to other relevant antibiotics. Aminoglycoside antibiotics cause eighth nerve damage if blood levels are allowed to exceed accepted safe levels; in the presence of renal failure longer intervals between doses are required to prevent toxic blood levels.

13.5.5   PROPHYLAXIS

There are several well-defined indications for prophylactic antibiotics (p. 264).

Antibiotic prophylaxis should not be given as a routine to unconscious patients or usually before 'clean' surgical operations, or to patients with bladder catheters.

13.5.6   COST OF ANTIBIOTICS

When other factors are equal, the least expensive drug should be selected.

13.6   Treatment of specific infections

13.6.1   URINARY TRACT INFECTIONS

In domiciliary practice most urinary tract infections are caused by *Esch. coli*, one third of which will be resistant to ampicillin. Trimethoprim is usually effective against ampicillin-resistant strains. Patients with chronic or recurrent infections and those with hospital-acquired infections often have organisms in their urine resistant to many antibacterial agents and the choice of antibiotic must then be made when the results of sensitivity testing are available. Acute pyelonephritis must be treated as soon as the diagnosis is suspected with a parenteral drug active against a wide range of Gram-negative bacilli, such as a cephalosporin or augmentin.

13.6.2   ALIMENTARY TRACT INFECTIONS

Antibiotics are not indicated for the treatment of most gastrointestinal infections. Exceptions to this rule are:

1. invasive salmonella infections and those which are clinically severe; typhoid fever is treated with chloramphenicol or ciprofloxacin; co-trimoxazole and ciprofloxacin are effective in invasive and non-invasive severe infections caused by salmonella organisms other than *Salmonella typhi* and *Salmonella paratyphi B*;
2. staphylococcal enterocolitis is treated with flucloxacillin;
3. co-trimoxazole or ciprofloxacin are indicated for severe bacillary dysentery;
4. perforation of the bowel (including the appendix) leads to peritonitis, often with a mixed flora, the principal organisms being Gram-negative bacilli and anaerobic bacteria, especially *Bacteroides* spp.; the treatment of choice is gentamicin or cefuroxime plus metronidazole (or clindamycin), or cefoxitin; augmentin is an alternative;
5. acute cholecystitis and cholangitis should be treated with gentamicin or a cephalosporin;
6. campylobacter enteritis, if severe, is treated with erythromycin or ciprofloxacin.

13.6.3   TUBERCULOSIS

Material such as pus, sputum, or CSF, from which tubercle bacilli may be cultured, should be sent to the laboratory before chemotherapy is commenced. Tubercle bacilli readily acquire resistance when exposed individually to one of the three principal drugs (isoniazid, rifampicin and streptomycin) and also to the drugs of second choice (e.g. ethambutol) which are used when the infecting strain is resistant to the standard drugs. For this reason two or three drugs must always be used in combination. Treatment should be supervised by a physician with experience in the management of tuberculosis.

13.6.4   RESPIRATORY TRACT INFECTIONS (OTHER THAN TUBERCULOSIS)

Upper respiratory tract infections are frequently viral, and antibiotic therapy is only indicated when a bacterial aetiology is known or suspected. The commonest bacterial cause of acute sore throat is the haemolytic streptococcus of group A for which benzylpenicillin or phenoxymethylpenicillin are the drugs of choice (except in mixed infections with β. lactamase producing *Staph. aureus* (e.g. in burns) when flucloxacillin or erythromycin are indicated. Acute sinusitis and otitis media usually respond satisfactorily to erythromycin or ampicillin. For oral candidiasis (thrush), local applications of nystatin are effective.

Acute infections of the lower respiratory tract acquired outside hospital are usually due to *Strep. pneumoniae* or *H. influenzae*. Both organisms are usually sensitive to ampicillin and co-trimoxazole. Benzylpenicillin is the drug of choice for pneumococcal infections. Some strains of pneumococci, *H. influenzae* and haemolytic streptococci of group A are resistant to tetracycline, erythromycin, ampicillin or trimethoprim. In debilitated patients or those suffering from viral infections such as influenza, *Staph. aureus* may cause a fulminating pneumonia which should be treated with high doses of flucloxacillin and fusidic acid. Acute epiglottitis is a very serious and sometimes fatal condition which is usually caused by *H. influenzae* and should be treated with parenteral chloramphenicol. Acute bronchitis and exacerbations of chronic bronchitis are treated with ampicillin or trimethoprim. Specific pneumonias are treated, initially, as follows:

Staphylococcal	flucloxacillin, fusidic acid or augmentin
Pseudomonas	gentamicin, ticarcillin, azlocillin or ciprofloxacin
Mycoplasma	tetracycline or erythromycin
Chlamydia	tetracycline
Legionella	erythromycin (plus rifampicin if severe)

13.6.5   WOUND INFECTIONS

Wounds are frequently colonized by bacteria without being grossly infected, and these respond satisfactorily to local measures, such as removal of sutures, drainage, application of antiseptics and frequent saline bathing.

Severe wound infections with spreading cellulitis and/or systemic illness are treated with an antibiotic, depending on sensitivity testing. Infected abdominal wounds in patients who have had operations of the gastrointestinal tract (including appendix and gall-bladder) are likely to be due to the patient's bowel flora, including aerobic and anaerobic organisms and should be treated with combinations of metronidazole and gentamicin or cefuroxime. Infections of clean stitched wounds when the intestine has not been opened are usually staphylococcal and should be treated with flucloxacillin. A combination of gentamicin or cefuroxime plus metronidazole may be necessary for 'mixed' wound infections or those where the severity is such that treatment must be commenced before the results of sensitivity testing are available. Augmentin is an alternative.

Burns must be cultured regularly and treated according to the results obtained. The isolation of *Staph. aureus*, *Ps. aeruginosa* or other Gram-negative bacilli is not an indication for chemotherapy except when there is evidence of clinical sepsis (severe illness, septicaemia, cellulitis). Flucloxacillin, erythromycin or clindamycin should be used rather than penicillin G for *Strep. pyogenes* (haemolytic streptococci of Group A) burns infections, for which chemotherapy is obligatory on all full-thickness lesions because of destruction of skin grafts by this organism.

13.6.6 MENINGITIS

Bacterial meningitis caused by identified organisms should be treated as follows.

Meningococcal Benzylpencillin 2,000.00 i.u. every 4–6 hours by 'bolus' injection.

Pneumococcal As for meningococcal.

Haemophilus influenzae Because of the increasing prevalence of peni-cillinase (β-lactamase) producing strains of *H. influenzae*, chloramphenicol or cefotaxime have become the initial therapy for presumptive *H. influenzae* meningitis – chloramphenicol 50–100 mg/kg/day or cefotaxime. When the organism is known to be ampicillin-sensitive a dose of 400 mg/kg/day ampicillin should be used.

Other forms of meningitis are treated according to predicted or known sensitivity of the organism. If the organism is unknown, give chloramphenicol and ampicillin to children and benzylpenicillin and chloramphenicol to adults. Cefotaxime is an alternative choice in both adults and children.

13.6.7 INFECTIONS IN NEONATES

Most superficial infections such as septic spots, 'sticky' eyes and umbilical sepsis respond to local treatment. Systemic infections are frequently caused by Gram-negative bacilli, including *Pseudomonas* spp,, and also by penicillin-resistant staphylococci. A combination of the cloxacillin with gentamicin or a cephalosporin such as cefotaxime should be used to treat seriously ill neonates with an undiagnosed infection.

13.6.8   PUERPERAL SEPSIS (AND SEPTIC ABORTION)

Infection is usually due to streptococci or anaerobic organisms, but also sometimes caused by Gram-negative bacilli; should be treated initially with a combination of metronidazole and gentamicin or cefuroxime until results of cultures are available.

13.6.9   EYE INFECTION

Gonococcal ophthalmia is treated with a combination of topical and parenteral penicillin. Most other forms of purulent conjunctivitis respond to topical chloramphenicol.

13.6.10   EAR INFECTION

Acute bacterial otitis media is usually caused by *Strep. pyogenes* pneumococci and *H. influenzae*. The majority of cases respond to amoxycillin co-amoxyclav or to erythromycin; children under the age of five should be given amoxycillin as *H. influenzae* is a common pathogen of that age group.

13.6.11   SEPTICAEMIA

This is a serious and potentially fatal condition which should be treated with a parenteral bactericidal antibiotic as soon as the diagnosis is suspected on clinical grounds. It is often possible to infer from the clinical features of the illness what organism is probably causing the infection. For example, acute pyelonephritis or cholangitis may be complicated by Gram-negative septicaemia and segmental pneumonia may be associated with pneumococcal septicaemia. Acute osteomyelitis is frequently secondary to staphylococcal septicaemia which can also accompany wound infection and skin sepsis. *Enterococcus faecalis* may enter the patient's bloodstream during operations on the genito-urinary tract or catheterization; it may cause endocarditis in elderly males after cystoscopy of prostatectomy, and in young women following gynaecological procedures.

When an organism is cultured from the blood it is important to carry out detailed sensitivity testing, including MIC and MBC determinations in cases of bacterial endocarditis with appropriate antibiotics. When there is a lack of response to treatment, serum levels of the antibiotic selected should be determined during treatment of endocarditis or septi-caemia to ensure that adequate concentrations are obtained in the blood.

The blind initial therapy of septicaemia requires the selection of a broad-spectrum agent such as imipenem or a combination of a penicillin and an aminoglycoside (with metronidazole if abdominal sepsis is present).

13.6.12   ENDOCARDITIS (British Society of Antimicrobial Chemotherapy 1985, 1990)

Infective endocarditis can be caused by many different organisms. How-ever, the commonest are the viridans group of streptococci and *Staphylo-coccus aureus*.

13.6.13   *VIRIDANS STREPTOCOCCI*

If the organism is fully sensitive to penicillin, treatment is with 14 days of intravenous penicillin plus low-dose (60 or 80 mg a day) gentamicin. For streptococci of reduced sensitivity to penicillin, continue treatment for four weeks.

13.6.14   *STAPHYLOCOCCUS AUREUS*

Treat with two antibiotics, usually flucloxacillin plus gentamicin or fusi-dic acid for four weeks.

13.6.15   FUNGAL INFECTIONS AND ACTINOMYCOSIS

Most fungal infections seen in the UK involve skin, nails or mucous membranes; systemic fungal infections (or mycoses) are relatively rare although they occasionally occur in debilitated patients, in immuno-deficient patients or following gastrointestinal surgery.

The commonest superficial fungal infection is candidiasis or thrush caused by *Candida albicans* which responds satisfactorily to topical appli-cations of nystatin or miconazole. Systemic candida infection is treated with intravenous injections of amphotericin B, a relatively toxic anti-biotic which may cause drug fever, nausea, vomiting and an increase in blood urea. Fluconazole is also effective against serious candida infections. Flucytosine is an alternative or may be used in combination with amphotericin B. Actinomycosis is treated with benzylpenicillin. Griseofulvin has a specific action against dermatophytes and is used for the treatment of fungal infections of hair and nails.

13.7   Indications for prophylaxis with antibiotics

13.7.1   SYSTEMIC CHEMOPROPHYLAXIS

There is a limited range of clinical conditions, both medical and surgical, in which the prophylactic use of antibiotics is indicated because there are special hazards of infection in such cases and because of the probable or known benefits of chemoprophylaxis. When chemoprophylaxis is not indicated (e.g. in most clean surgical operations) it should, for obvious reasons, be avoided; routine prophylactic use of antibiotics leads to an increase in the proportion of resistant organisms and may cause the replacement of sensitive by resistant strains and species in the patient's flora, increasing the hazards of infection. When prophylaxis is indicated it is important that the most appropriate antibiotic or antibiotics should be given, and that the dosage, duration of course and route of administration should be optimal; in prophylaxis against post-operative infection this involves very short peri-operative administration, which is most unlikely to cause the selection of resistant strains. In the early years of antimicrobial chemotherapy antibiotics were often used for prophylaxis without such precautions; such courses proved ineffective, and the concept of antibiotic prophylaxis fell under a cloud, from which it was eventually rescued by studies that demonstrated the value of antibiotic prophylaxis used with rational care.

When chemoprophylaxis is used, attention must be given to a number of factors, including the clinical state of the patient at operation, the procedure to be carried out and the presence or absence of existing infection. In the choice of antibiotics, alternatives must be available for patients who are hypersensitive to the agents of first choice, and the choice between oral and parenteral administration should take into account side effects that may appear. It may be necessary to change the regimen in order to meet changes in the pathogens carried by patients, for example the emergence of MRSA and enterococci.

In open heart surgery there is a very low incidence of infection, but the risk of mortality is high if infection (e.g. with coagulase-negative staphylococci) occurs; on theoretical grounds it should be possible to prevent lodgement at key sites in the heart or sternum at the time of the operation, and antibiotic prophylaxis is almost always given for this purpose. Some clinical trials suggest that this is beneficial.

Medical indications for systemic prophylaxis
1. Prevention of endocarditis in patients with heart valve lesions, septal defect, patent ductus or prosthetic valve (see *British National Formulary*).

2. For non-immune diphtheria contacts, give erythromycin 500 mg four times a day for one week.
3. For contacts of meningococcal infection, give rifampicin 600 mg twice a day for two days (or sulphonamide if strain is known to be sensitive).
4. Following acute rheumatic fever for at least five years or until child leaves school, give phenoxymethyl penicillin (penicillin V) in a dose of 125 or 250 mg twice a day by mouth.
5. Following splenectomy, especially in children, give long-term oral penicillin (and/or immunization against pneumococcal infection).

Indications for systemic prophylaxis in clean surgery
1. Arterial grafts.
2. Cardiac surgery.
3. Neurosurgical operations involving foreign materials.
4. Joint prostheses.
5. Severe injuries and burns (e.g. *Clostridium tetani* and *perfringens*).
6. High amputation of ischaemic legs (versus *Cl. perfringens*).

Wide cover is required not only against recognized pathogens but also against organisms which are not normally pathogenic, for example coagulase-negative staphylococci. Combined therapy is therefore necessary.

13.7.2 PROPHYLAXIS AGAINST SURGICAL SEPSIS

Indications Prophylaxis against surgical sepsis is advisable whenever an internal organ, the contents of which contain high concentrations of bacteria, is opened. The type and extent of bacterial colonization within the gastrointestinal tract is related to the site and the nature of any underlying disease. Prophylaxis should be used for the following groups of operations.

1. Operations on the stomach or oesophagus in patients with carcinoma or bile reflux gastritis.
2. Cholecystectomy in selected patients who may have infected bile. Patients at risk for sepsis can be selected on the basis of a history of jaundice, rigors, recent acute cholecystitis, age over 70 years, or a previous biliary operation.
3. All intestinal operations in patients with inflammatory bowel disease.
4. All colorectal operations involving resection and/or anastomosis.
5. Patients with a perforated gangrenous appendix should be given a therapeutic course of antibiotic. The need for prophylaxis in non-perforated, non-gangrenous appendicitis is not yet established.

6. There are also other indications for prophylaxis for which there is often no general agreement:
   (a) recurrent cystitis in women of child-bearing age with a normal upper urinary tract;
   (b) infants of mothers with sputum-positive tuberculosis (if the child cannot be separated from the mother);
   (c) siblings of patients with whooping cough;
   (d) all instrumentations in the presence of bacteriuria;
   (e) trans-rectal prostatic biopsy;
   (f) urethral dilatation.

Timing and route of prophylaxis in surgery   Prophylaxis is effective only if high blood and tissue levels of an appropriate antibiotic are present at the time of bacterial contamination of the surgical wound. Prophylaxis should not continue after completion of the operation. Intramuscular drugs should be given one hour before the start of the surgery and IV drugs during the induction of anaesthesia.

Choice of chemotherapeutic agent   This should be based upon the nature of the organisms likely to contaminate the operative field. For patients in groups 1 and 2, the organisms most likely to cause sepsis are streptococci, *E. coli* and other aerobic Gram-negative bacilli. Operations in groups 3, 4 and 5 require antibiotics active against anaerobic bacteria, *E. coli* and other aerobic Gram-negative bacilli. Anaerobic and micro-aerophilic bacteria are mainly responsible for pelvic sepsis in group 6 patients.

Suitable prophylactic regimens for the above groups are as follows.

Group 1   A single pre-operative dose of gentamicin or a cephalosporin by IM or IV injection.
Group 2   A single pre-operative injection of gentamicin or cephalosporin IM or IV.
Groups 3 and 4   A single pre-operative injection of gentamicin IM or IV and metronidazole is recommended. Pre-operative oral bowel preparation with antibiotics is often effective but, with the possible exception of neomycin plus erythromycin, is not recommended because of the risk of emergence of resistant Gram-negative bacilli.
Group 5   Metronidazole given as a suppository or IV is the most rational prophylactic for appendicectomy.
Group 6   Metronidazole combined with cefuroxime is effective prophylaxis against pelvic sepsis.

Chemoprophylaxis with antibiotics will almost inevitably lead to the selection of bacteria resistant to the prophylactic agent. For this reason indiscriminate prophylaxis should be avoided; narrow-range rather than broad-spectrum antibiotics should be used whenever possible (e.g. in prophylaxis against a particular pathogen, such as *Strep. pyogenes or Cl. perfringens*); short-term or single-dose prophylaxis should be used to cover short periods of hazard, such as exposure to microbial contamination during an operation; and a careful watch must be kept for the appearance of resistant bacteria.

13.7.3   PERITONEAL DIALYSIS

The dialysis fluid is an excellent culture medium for bacteria and may become infected from the outside (faulty technique) or the inside (pre-existing peritoneal infection or transperitoneal spread). Prophylactic addition of antibiotics to dialysis fluid is not recommended but is a useful route of administration should peritonitis occur. Intraperitoneal therapy with vancomycin and a cephalosporin is often started on clinical evidence of infection and treatment modified when cultures are available (see Chapter 18).

13.7.4   TOPICAL CHEMOPROPHYLAXIS

Local treatment of severe burns with 0.5% silver nitrate compresses, one of the most effective means of preventing infection with *Ps. aeruginosa* and *Proteus* spp. is less often used today than in the late 1960s. Patients having this treatment need supplements of electrolytes by mouth and laboratory control of serum electrolyte levels. Silver sulphadiazine cream is less effective against *Ps. aeruginosa* and *Proteus* spp., but more effective against many other Gram-negative bacilli. It is a valuable alternative to silver nitrate compresses, easier to use and more appropriate for the treatment of infants, also for smaller burns. Mafenide acetate (11%) cream applied daily and left exposed is an alternative to 0.5% silver nitrate compresses which can be used if silver nitrate solution is not appropriate (e.g. if serum electrolytes cannot be kept at normal levels); it is painful on burns in which the nerve endings are not destroyed and may cause acidosis, and patients require daily baths to remove dried cream. A cream containing 0.5% silver nitrate and 0.2% chlorhexidine gluconate is also effective and involves no hazard of emergence of resistant bacteria (Lowbury 1976).

13.8   Formulation of antibiotic policy

There are several reasons for having in each hospital an agreed policy for prescribing antibiotics.

1. It is a way of ensuring that patients receive appropriate therapy.
2. The restrained use of antibiotics means that the appearance of resistant organisms is delayed and their incidence in hospital is kept low. Resistant staphylococci remain a problem, and strains resistant to gentamicin or methicillin are found increasingly. Gentamicin-resistant Gram-negative bacilli, especially *Klebsiella aerogenes* and *Ps. aeruginosa*, have caused cross-infection problems in urological, intensive care and burns units. Resistance is commonly transferred from one organism to another, even when the organisms are unrelated. Transferable resistance to one antibiotic is often linked with resistance to other antibiotics, so that excessive use of one antibiotic may be the cause of a high incidence of resistance to several others.
3. Up-to-date information should be provided for the prescriber and adverse reactions should be reduced by restricting the use of certain potentially toxic agents.
4. Prescribing costs are reduced by controlling the use of expensive agents.

The type of policy must be adapted to the needs of the staff, the type of patients treated and the prevalent organisms in the hospital or unit. It must therefore be flexible and where necessary adapted to the needs of individual units, for example burns and intensive care. The policy could have the components described in the following paragraphs.

13.8.1   PERSONAL ADVICE AND EXAMPLE

By this is meant the effect which daily discussion between senior and junior doctors has on prescribing habits. Effective use of antibiotics requires experience and this is not readily obtained. Most hospitals have doctors (usually a medical microbiologist or infectious diseases consultant) with a special interest in and knowledge of antibiotics which should be available to other members of staff.

13.8.2   GENERAL ADVICE AND EDUCATION

Education of antibiotic prescribers can also be helped if some aide memoir is available on the wards. The *British National Formulary* is one source of information. Some hospitals or even Regions have their own booklets. It is particularly important that advice is available on the use of topical agents, on prophylaxis and on expensive preparations. Postgraduate lectures on chemotherapy are also helpful, but less important than personal advice and discussion.

13.8.3 PROVISION OF SURVEY DATA

The antibiotic policy depends to a considerable extent on the sensitivity pattern of currently isolated strains of bacteria. The percentage of *Staph. aureus* and Gram-negative bacilli resistant to a number of antibiotics varies greatly from one hospital to another and between different units in the same hospital. Similar variations will occur from time to time in the same hospital. Regular reports can be prepared from information available in most laboratories where sensitivity tests are carried out, and knowledge of the current resistance patterns gives the clinician a valuable guide to the therapy most likely to be of use. This type of information is complementary to that provided by the individual report on a particular patient.

The same type of information can be made available to general practitioners. Of particular use is the resistance pattern of urinary tract organisms isolated from domiciliary urinary tract infections. Such information need only be made available once a year in general practice because of the small changes in resistance of bacteria among the general community as compared to that found in hospitals.

13.8.4 RESERVATION OF ANTIBIOTICS

Some hospitals may find it valuable to group antibiotics into different categories in order to hold some in reserve for particular organisms or specific types of patient. There is no doubt that such a policy of restricting the use of specific compounds can preserve the useful life of an antimicrobial agent; in large hospitals, where there is a resident population of organisms 'waiting to acquire resistance' and large amounts of antibiotics may be used, it is essential to keep some in reserve.

Examples of the way in which antibiotics can be classified for this purpose are shown in Tables 13.2 and 13.3, which summarize the policy adopted in a general hospital (Table 13.2) and one for a hospital with many specialized services and departments (Table 13.3).

13.8.5 PURCHASING POLICY

New agents should be carefully considered by a pharmacy committee and only purchased if superior in one or more respects to existing

Table 13.2   Example of antibiotic policy used in a general hospital

---

Unrestricted use
  Penicillin
  Ampicillin and derivatives
  Flucloxacillin
  Tetracyclines
  Erythromycin
  Metronidazole
  Gentamicin
  Cefuroxime
  Co-trimoxazole (or trimethoprim)

Restricted use (on advice of infectious disease physician or microbiologist)
  Azlocillin
  Ceftazidime
  Netilmicin
  Clindamycin
  Vancomycin
  Chloramphenicol
  Ciprofloxacin

Not recommended (and not in stock in the hospital)*
  All other cephalosporins
  Amikacin
  Tobramycin
  Ureidopenicillins

---

* Some of these agents e.g. amikacin may be on the restricted list in some hospitals

drugs. In particular, by this means the clinician can be guided in the use of the numerous antibiotic preparations now available.

13.9   Changes in antibiotic policies

13.9.1   ACTION WHEN RESISTANCE TO AN IMPORTANT ANTIBIOTIC BECOMES COMMON

Sometimes stopping the use of the antibiotic in question will lead to a large reduction or even elimination of the resistant organisms. This happened more often in the early years of the antibiotic era, before multiple and genetically linked resistance became common in hospital bacteria. When multiple resistance is present, all of the antibiotics involved in the resistance pattern may need to be withdrawn and not used again until these strains are eliminated. In some outbreaks withdrawal of antibiotics has not been effective; transfer of all patients carrying or infected with strains showing the resistance pattern to one ward, which is kept closed to new admissions until all carriers of the

Table 13.3 Antibiotic policy employed by a complex teaching district with many specialist units

The antibiotics are divided into five categories with different degrees of accessibility. (A) Oral and parenteral compounds which are available for prescription by all doctors. (B) Compounds which are restricted to certain units or indications. (C) Compounds which can only be started by senior doctors, usually consultants. (D) Drugs which are undergoing trial in the hospital and only available to trialists. (E) All other antibiotics available in the UK. These are not in stock and can only be ordered via consultants.

Category A
Amoxycillin (O+P)
Phenoxymethyl penicillin
Cephalexin
Erythromycin stearate
Flucloxacillin (O+P)
Fusidic acid
Metronidazole (O+P)
Nalidixic acid
Nitrofurantoin
Ciprofloxacin
Co-trimoxazole
Trimethoprim
Chloramphenicol
Cefixime
Co-amoxiclav
Benzylpenicillin
Cefuroxime
Erythromycin lactobionate
Gentamicin
Piperacillin
Teichoplanin
Nystatin

Category B
Ampicillin/sulbactam (surgical prophylaxis)
Cefotaxime (STD; paediatrics)
Ceftazidime (ITU)
Dapsone (dermatology)
Doxycycline (STD; dermatology)
Minocycline (dermatology)
Netilmicin (renal unit)
Vancomycin (haematology, renal unit)
Piperacillin (haematology)
Anti-TB drugs (chest unit)

Category C
(a) Amikacin
    Aztreonam
    Ciprofloxacin (inj)
    Clindamycin
    Imipenem
    Rifampicin (inj)
(b) Category B compounds used
    for non-listed indications
(c) Antivirals:
    Acyclovir
    Ganciclovir
    Ribavirin
    Zidovudine
(d) Antifungals
    Fluconazole
    Amphotericin

Category D
Variable list

Category E
Variable list

(O+P) Oral and parenteral prescriptions of these compounds are available to all doctors resistant strain have been discharged, may be effective in such a situation.

The antibiotic resistance pattern is constantly changing in hospital and it is necessary to change a policy in response to alterations in resistance. Often one unit in the hospital may require a policy different from that used by other units. For example, methicillin-resistant *Staph. aureus* or cephalosporin resistant enterobacteria may appear in one unit but not in others. A change could then be made to a reserve antibiotic in the ward with the newly acquired resistant strains.

13.10   Antibiotics and the laboratory

The hospital clinician can use antibiotics rationally only if adequate laboratory services are available. There are several ways in which the laboratory can give such assistance: most important is the provision of accurate sensitivity tests on the relevant isolates from individual patients to the most appropriate antibiotics. The choice of agents and the susceptibility guidelines employed should be kept under regular review. In addition the laboratory should provide regular summary data on the prevalence of resistant bacteria and facilities for monitoring of some antibiotic levels (particularly aminoglycosides) should be available. Laboratories should report a limited number of sensitivities to appropriate antimicrobials to the clinicians to restrict the range of antibiotics used, e.g. sensitivity of *Staph. aureus* could be reported to flucloxacillin and erythromycin only.

References and further reading

British National Formulary. British Medical Association and the Royal Pharmaceutical Society of Great Britain. (Revised twice yearly).

British Society of Antimicrobial Chemotherapy (1985) Working Party Report. Antibiotic treatment of streptococcal and staphylococcal endocarditis. *Lancet*, **2**, 815.

British Society of Antimicrobial Chemotherapy (1990) Antibiotic prophylaxis of infective endocarditis. Recommendations from the Endocarditis Working Party. *Lancet*, **1**, 88.

Garrod, L.P., Lambert, H.P. and O'Grady, F. (1981) *Antibiotic and Chemotherapy*, 5th edn. Churchill Livingstone, Edinburgh and London.

Kucers, A. and Bennett, N. McK. (1987) *The Use of Antibiotics*, 4th edn. Heinemann, London.

Lowbury, E.J.L. (1976) Prophylaxis and treatment for infection in burns. *British Journal of Hospital Medicine*, **16**, 566.

Parker, M.T. and Collier, L.H. (1990) *Topley and Wilson's Principles of Bacteriology, Virology and Immunity*, 8th edn. Edward Arnold, London.

Phillips, I. (1979) Antibiotic policies. In *Recent advances in Infection*, (ed. D. Reeves and A.M. Geddes) Churchill Livingstone, Edinburgh and London.

14 *Immunization and specific prophylaxis*

Immunization is important in the control of hospital infection:

1. for the protection of certain members of staff against poliomyelitis, rubella, diphtheria, hepatitis B and certain other infectious diseases which could be contracted from patients;
2. for the protection of patients, when a patient suffering from a communicable disease is accidentally admitted to an open ward;
3. for the protection of patients who, because of their illness or treatment, are particularly susceptible to infection;
4. for the protection against tetanus of patients with open wounds.

For the protection of staff, active immunization with a vaccine or toxoid is the method of choice, and immunity should be established in so far as is practicable before he or she is employed in an area of potential risk (e.g. an infectious disease or paediatric ward). Non-immune patients exposed to certain infections can be given immediate protection against that infection by passive immunization with immunoglobulin, but not by active immunization, which takes time to develop. The importance of both active and passive immunization, prophylactic antibiotics and surgical techniques must be integrated for the prevention of tetanus in hospital.

14.1 Immunization of hospital staff (see also Chapter 15)

14.1.1 GENERAL POLICY

The risks of staff contracting infection vary with the type of hospital, tuberculosis being a special risk in chest wards or hospitals, enteric fever and poliomyelitis in infectious disease units, hepatitis B in renal and liver units and all of these infections in pathology departments. The person in charge of a unit or department must be responsible for ensuring that measures are taken to avoid infection in staff.

It is neither practicable nor desirable to immunize all members of staff against all diseases for which vaccines are available. This is because the risk may not be great (e.g. typhoid fever in the UK), or the vaccine may not be very effective or may have unpleasant side-effects. The risks of side-effects from immunization must be balanced against the potential hazard of spread of the infection from patient to staff in a unit at a particular time, account being taken of the fact that the intestinal infections, in particular, are effectively contained by good hygiene and barrier nursing. Secondly, account must be taken of the effectiveness of specific treatment should infection arise (e.g. antibiotics are effective against typhoid fever, but not against poliomyelitis). Thirdly, the usual rapid turnover of nursing and domestic staff can make it impossible to ensure that well immunized staff are always available: in the average infectious disease unit only the senior nursing staff tend to be permanent. In view of these difficulties, it is impossible to ensure immunity of all staff to meet the chance admission of a patient with unrecognized infectious disease; good hygienic practice is usually a better safeguard for the staff than reliance on an immunity which may not exist. There are, however, circumstances when immunization is useful and necessary; for example, in units dealing with open pulmonary tuberculosis it is important to ensure that all staff have had BCG or are tuberculin-positive.

14.1.2 ACTIVE IMMUNIZATION OF HOSPITAL STAFF

Active immunity results from naturally acquired disease or from immunization. It usually takes at least 10–14 days for active immunity to develop, and it may take longer, depending on the vaccine; immunity develops much more rapidly with some vaccines. Immunity may be good and highly protective (e.g. diphtheria) or rather poor in the face of a large infective dose of bacteria (e.g. cholera).

Smallpox vaccination In 1980 the WHO formally declared the world free from smallpox – the very successful conclusion to its smallpox eradication programme. There is thus no medical reason whatsoever to vaccinate anybody against smallpox.

The vaccinia virus is now being used as a carrier for certain other vaccine antigens. Laboratory staff working with the virus should be vaccinated, but preferably only those requiring re-vaccination should be used in these studies. If primary vaccination is essential, the member of staff should be fully informed of the risks (e.g. a severe local reaction) and be prepared to accept them.

BCG and tuberculosis All hospital staff employed either continuously or intermittently in high risk areas (defined below) must have their resistance to infection tested by the tuberculin reaction (Mantoux or

Heaf test) before being employed in such areas. However, as tuberculosis is likely to be present in many general hospitals, it may be advisable to include all staff in contact with patients in addition to those working in high risk areas. If tuberculin negative, they must be given BCG vaccine and await tuberculin conversion before taking up duties. If having had a successful BCG vaccination, the individual is tuberculin tested a year or more later and is found to be negative he/she should be referred to a chest physician for an opinion. BCG should not be re-administered without such an opinion, for this can produce a severe reaction (chronic ulceration at the site, etc).

High risk areas are:

1. wards, clinics, and isolation units where patients with open (i.e. transmissible) tuberculosis are commonly seen;
2. laboratories where processing of specimens for isolation and culture of the tubercle bacillus takes place;
3. postmortem rooms.

Staff of other departments, such as radiographers and physiotherapists, who visit patients in the tuberculosis wards, should be similarly screened and immunized if tuberculin negative. Screening of staff should be the responsibility of the Occupational Health physician who will keep the necessary records.

Immunization does not exclude the necessity for methods of surveillance or for instruction of staff about potential hazards and how to avoid them, including details of when to seek medical advice, and regular chest x-ray if indicated.

Poliomyelitis Although most young adults in the UK will have been immunized against poliomyelitis, it is desirable to maintain immunity by revaccination, as the disease in the adult is often of the paralytic type and because there exists no specific treatment. Immunization with the Sabin, living attenuated vaccine is easily administered, is safe, has minimal side-effects, and is effective. It should be offered to all hospital staff. It is given by mouth, and three doses must be given at intervals of 4–8 weeks. Although the vaccine contains strains of the three serotypes of poliomyelitis virus, only one of these generally infects the recipient at a time to produce immunity to that serotype. Thus to confer immunity to all types, three doses are required. It is incorrect to assume that two doses will necessarily confer some degree of immunity to all strains. Booster doses can be offered every five years or more often if thought necessary. It is recommended that persons over about 30 years of age who have never previously had poliomyelitis immunization should be given their primary immunity with the formalin-killed or Salk type vaccine. This is because occasionally, primary immunization with the Sabin vaccine (containing live attenuated virus) can in older people give rise to mild paralytic disease, although the risk of this is small.

Diphtheria Most adults born in this country after 1941 will have residual immunity to diphtheria as a result of childhood immunization. Although the vaccine is effective in preventing disease, its administration to adults is not without occasional unpleasant reactions such as painful brawny induration of the arm. Diphtheria vaccine is therefore not recommended routinely even for staff of infectious disease units. Permanent staff should, however, be Schick-tested to determine their immune status; vaccination of the susceptible should be advised. If vaccination is necessary, adults should always be given a low dose vaccine.

If diphtheria is diagnosed in a patient in hospital he/she should be transferred immediately to an infectious diseases unit. Staff in close contact should be given a five-day course of oral erythromycin and placed under surveillance for seven days after contact. Following the course of antibiotic, nose and throat swabs should be taken to detect any possible carriers.

Typhoid and paratyphoid (enteric) fevers It is not essential to immunize staff routinely against typhoid fever, even in infectious diseases units. These diseases are not very communicable, are adequately contained by efficient nursing and hygienic techniques and are treatable with antibiotics.

In hospitals with infectious disease units, engineers and plumbers who may have to clear drains and sewers, and also bacteriology laboratory staff are at slight risk. Staff in these categories working in infectious diseases hospitals but not in general hospitals should be offered immunization. Typhoid (monovalent) vaccine BP has replaced TAB, which also contained the killed bacteria of paratyphoid fevers and was of unproven efficacy.

Rubella (German measles) The Joint Committee on Vaccination and Immunization of the Department of Health has recommended that routine rubella vaccination should be offered to children of both sexes along with measles and mumps vaccine (MMR) at the age of 15 months and also to girls between their eleventh and fourteenth birthdays (DoH 1990). Women of child-bearing age who are exposed to special hazards of rubella (e.g. those in hospitals caring for children or working in maternity units) should have serological testing for susceptibility to rubella; those who are found susceptible (seronegative) and who are not pregnant should be offered rubella vaccination; those who are susceptible and pregnant should be employed in other units. Because of the theoretical possibility (not proven) that rubella vaccine might damage the fetus, pregnancy must be excluded at the time of vaccination and should be avoided for eight weeks thereafter.

Influenza When epidemics of influenza are predicted, those responsible for the health of hospital staff often find themselves under pressure to have the staff vaccinated against this infection. However, the vaccines at present available offer such poor immunity that we are reluctant to advise their routine (yearly) use. When a new strain of virus appears and an epidemic is expected, it is worthwhile vaccinating hospital staff if a vaccine which offers even a modest degree of protection is available. When there are vaccines with greater potency and wider protective powers, these recommendations may be amended.

Measles There is no need to offer active immunization to staff in hospitals, except possibly for those working in paediatric, isolation or infectious diseases wards. Passive immunization is available if required.

Other diseases Active immunization against tetanus should be given to all staff and maintained by booster doses. Hepatitis B vaccine should be offered to certain staff (see Chapter 10).

14.1.3 PASSIVE IMMUNIZATION OF STAFF

Passive immunization is conferred by the injection of human normal immunoglobulin (gamma-globulin), hyperimmune human specific immunoglobulin (e.g. hepatitis B immunoglobulin) or specific immunoglobulins from animal sources (usually horse) e.g. diphtheria antitoxin. The purpose is to confer immediate but short-term immunity to certain diseases. In this situation antibodies are not made by the person immunized (hence the term passive), but are provided from other human or animal sources. Pooled human normal immunoglobulin therapy is effective against measles (adult dose 750 mg), and probably also against poliomyelitis (adult dose 1500 mg). It will also give some protection for about four months against hepatitis A but not against B. However, a specific hyperimmune gamma-globulin has been developed for protection against hepatitis B (see Chapter 10). Convalescent serum may be used for protection against chickenpox; serum from patients with herpes zoster (shingles) can be used for this purpose. Human normal immunoglobulin is not generally indicated for adult contacts of measles, rubella, mumps or chickenpox (see notes below).

14.1.4 DOCUMENTATION

When immunization of staff is mandatory a record must be kept in the hospital; it is desirable that records of other immunizations should also be held in the occupational health department of the hospital (Chapter 15 and Appendix 15.1).

14.2 Immunization of patients

There are few circumstances in which immunization of patients against infectious disease is indicated. When applicable, passive immunisation which is immediately effective should be used. Passive immunity conferred by human immunoglobulin or antitoxin of animal origin is applicable to the following diseases in the circumstances mentioned. For protection against tetanus, see 14.3.

Measles When a case of measles is inadvertently admitted or develops in a paediatric ward, human normal immunoglobulin should be given to patients on immunosuppressive drugs or to those with debilitating diseases, or in whom the clinician considers that it is clinically indicated, e.g. cystic fibrosis, primary tuberculosis, hypogamma-globinaemia and after splenectomy. Children who have not had measles or been vaccinated against it and have been given passive immunization, should be given active immunization at a later date. Immunoglobulin 250 mg, given within 7–10 days of contact will probably modify an attack of measles. The disease may often be prevented with doses of between 250 and 750 mg depending on age. If active immunization of a compromised patient is desired, the live vaccine may be given together with a small dose of specially assayed immunoglobulin. This dose is rather critical and special ampoules containing 0.5 ml, (4–8 i.u. measles antibody) are available. The dose is 0.4 mg immunoglobulin/lb body weight.

Poliomyelitis If a case of acute poliomyelitis is accidentally admitted to or develops on a ward, all persons who have not been immunized with a vaccine (Sabin or Salk) should be given human normal immunoglobulin. Except for close contacts within a family, live polio vaccine is now a much more effective agent for preventing spread in the community.

Hepatitis A   When this disease is diagnosed in a ward, certain patients (e.g. those with chronic diseases requiring long stay in hospital) can be treated with human normal immunoglobulin, which may be used to help in the control of an outbreak. Patients who are on immunosuppressive drugs or who have had extensive radiotherapy should also be protected. It may be desirable to protect staff who are especially at risk. Doses are 250 mg for a child and 500 mg for an adult, which gives protection for about four months.

It is not generally possible or necessary to offer protection to all patients apart from those in the categories mentioned above, as stocks of immunoglobulin have to be conserved. Hepatitis A can probably be controlled to some extent by good hygiene.

Hepatitis B, C and E   See Chapter 10.

Chickenpox   Although chickenpox is not a serious disease in the otherwise healthy person, it will occasionally be necessary to attempt to prevent (or attenuate) an attack in the newborn or in persons on immunosuppressive therapy, or in leukemia patients on cytotoxic drugs. Human normal immunoglobulin is probably not very effective and rather large doses are recommended, for example, 750 mg for a neonate and up to 8 g in an immunosuppressed adult.

Limited supplies of hyperimmune anti-varicella/zoster immunoglobulin (ZIG) are available for such patients.

ZIG may attenuate an attack of chickenpox, but cannot be relied upon to prevent it. There is no evidence of the efficacy of ZIG in the treatment of chickenpox. In herpes zoster, patients normally possess antibodies to the causative virus, so administration of ZIG is not indicated. As a routine measure patients who are at long-term risk (e.g. transplant patients) and who have no history of chickenpox, should be tested for varicella-zoster antibodies. If they are found to be immune then, if subsequently exposed to chickenpox, ZIG will be unnecessary. (Dose of ZIG for prophylaxis is: 0–5 years 250 mg, adults 1000 mg.)

Gas gangrene   An antitoxin prepared in the horse against the toxins of *Clostridium perfringens* (welchii), *Cl. septicum* and *Cl. oedematiens* is available. There is no evidence that this has any value in prophylaxis against gas gangrene when used in patients with open wounds, but the use of a polyvalent antitoxin containing 10,000 u of *Cl. oedematiens* antitoxin (IV or IM) has been advocated by some authorities for extensive soiled wounds. In established gas gangrene it may have some value (dose 75 000 u or more IV) when used together with the most important measures – wide excision of affected muscle, high dosage of penicillin and hyperbaric oxygen; these are probably of greater value than the antiserum, which carries a risk of allergy, including anaphylaxis (see Tetanus, p. 283).

Rabies If a patient is thought to be at risk from rabies (e.g. after being bitten by an animal while abroad), the nearest Public Health Laboratory will give advice on the current prophylactic procedures (see also Chapter 9).

Mumps Convalescent mumps immunoglobulin may occasionally be available but is in short supply. Human normal immunoglobulin has sometimes been used to modify or prevent an attack of mumps but the efficacy of this measure is doubtful.

Rubella Human normal immunoglobulin is of no value in prevention of rubella in pregnant women exposed to infection.

14.3 Protection against tetanus

The risk of tetanus varies with the type and severity of wound or injury, the place where the patient was when injured (e.g. there is a special risk to agricultural workers), and with the presence or absence of immunity induced by a course of toxoid. It was formerly standard practice to give all patients with open wounds (apart from superficial abrasions or minor cuts) an injection of anti-serum (ATS) derived from immunized horses. This practice can be dangerous, because of the risk of anaphylactic shock or serum sickness from injection of foreign protein, and could also be ineffective, because of the rapid removal of antitoxin from the circulation by antibodies to horse serum. It is, in any case, unnecessary when the patient is known to be actively immune and, where possible, human antitetanus globulin (ATG) should now always be used when passive immunization is required.

14.3.1 ASSESSMENT OF THE STATE OF IMMUNITY TO TETANUS

If a patient does not know whether he or she has received tetanus toxoid in the past, consult the patient's general practitioner; if he/she does not know, the patient must, in most situations, be considered non-immune. Many district health authorities hold a record on immunizations, especially of children, so that it may be possible to discover an individual's immune status by telephoning the appropriate authority.

The procedure is outlined in the chart and notes presented here. Table 14.1: Prophylaxis against tetanus in patients with open wounds is based on that which is in use at the Birmingham Accident Hospital. Essential features are:

1. booster doses of adsorbed toxoid (vaccine) for all patients known to have been actively immunized, unless known to have completed a course or a booster dose of toxoid within the previous year;
2. the use of human antitetanus globulin (ATG) for all patients not known to be actively immune (in the event of a shortage of ATG, use ATS);
3. if ATS is used, additional prophylaxis by antibiotics will be given only to patients who have not had prompt and effective treatment or whose wounds are badly contaminated with soil or faeces, or septic;
4. active immunization with adsorbed toxoid for all patients if there is evidence that they are not actively immune;
5. first dose of adsorbed toxoid at same time as ATG, but injected separately at another site.

In the first edition of this book antibiotic prophylaxis was recommended for less severe wounds, and also for severe wounds if promptly treated and not severely contaminated when ATG was not available. Because of the more reliable supply of ATG and the potential shortcomings of antibiotic prophylaxis (see Lowbury *et al.* 1978), we have revised our recommendations for the use of antibiotic prophylaxis against tetanus.

14.3.2   ACTIVE IMMUNIZATION: USE OF TETANUS TOXOID

The patient is considered actively immune (a) for 12 months after the first two injections of an immunizing course of tetanus toxoid (adsorbed) or of diphtheria-tetanus-pertussis vaccine (DTP started at or after the age of six months); (b) for 10 years after three injections (the full immunizing course) of toxoid or DTP vaccine; (c) for 10 years after a boosting dose of toxoid given to an actively immune individual. Patients with open wounds who by the above criteria are actively immune nevertheless require a boosting dose of toxoid unless they are known to have received a full immunizing course or a boosting dose within the previous year.

Table 14.1 Prophylaxis against tetanus in patients with open wounds (Birmingham Accident Hospital)

Types of wound	Other relevant circumstances	Procedure
1. Superficial wound or abrasion		Cleanse and cover
		No ATG
		Start active immunization if not actively immune
2. Puncture wounds	) (If KNOWN to be) ('actively immune'	Cleanse toilet and cover
		Toxoid (adsorbed) booster*
Deep lacerations	) ( ) ( ) (if NOT KNOWN	
Animal or human bites	) (to be 'actively) (immune') (	Cleanse toilet and cover
		ATG 250 i.u. (or 500 i.u. if 24 h delay)
Wounds with devitalized tissue	))	
	) Admit to hospital) if (a) severe	Antibiotic (except for wounds that have had
Wounds more than 4 h old	) if (b) heavily) contaminated)	prompt and effective treatment, including ATG, and not heavily contaminated
Infected traumatic wounds	)))	or septic)
		Start active immunization

* Not necessary if last dose of toxoid in course of active immunization or last booster dose was given less than one year previously
If ATG is not available, use ATS

Immunizing procedure

1. Active immunity is induced by three subcutaneous injections of 0.5 ml of toxoid (adsorbed), the doses being separated by intervals of one month between doses.
2. A patient so immunized should have a booster dose of 0.5 ml toxoid (adsorbed) when wounded, and at intervals of 10 years. In this way immunity is maintained. If a patient with a wound is known to have had a dose of toxoid (the last dose in a course or a booster) less than one year previously, it is not necessary to give a booster dose at the time of injury.
3. Any patient who is given ATG should be actively immunized, the first dose of tetanus toxoid (adsorbed) being injected into the other arm at the same time as ATG is given.

4. Forms – a card is used to record injections of toxoid during the course of immunization.
5. Outpatients:
   (a) if active immunization has been started, the patient is given a card, and told to take it to his doctor for the second toxoid injection in four weeks;
   (b) if a booster dose of toxoid is given, the date of this is entered on the card and duplicates will be sent to the general practitioner.
6. Inpatients – active immunization will be carried out as far as the length of hospital stay allows. According to the stage reached at the time of discahrge, patients will be given a card suitably inscribed, and the duplicate cards will be sent to the general practitioner and health authority.

14.3.3   PASSIVE IMMUNIZATION AGAINST TETANUS

Use of human antitetanus globulin ATG

ATG ('Humotet', Wellcome) is available for prophylaxis of patients not known to be actively immune; it is safer than ATS and likely to be more effective than ATS or antibiotics. A single dose of 1 ml (250 $l\mu$) i.m. injection can give a protective level of antitoxin for 4 weeks. A dose of 500 $l\mu$ is given if 24 h have elapsed since injury or there is a risk of heavy contamination.

Tests for hypersensitivity to ATG are not required, but ATG should be avoided if patients have had adverse reactions to human gamma globulin; such reactions are very rare.

Use of antitoxin (ATS) derived from immunized animals

INDICATIONS
Tetanus antiserum, horse derived (ATS), is used only when a booster dose of toxoid is inappropriate and ATG is not available. This will be mainly in countries with insufficient finance for routine use of ATG. It should not be given to patients with a history of anaphylaxis or severe immediate hypersensitivity reactions. Such patients requiring antiserum should when possible be given an injection of ovine (sheep) tetanus antiserum if ATG is not available; this can be obtained from special centres.

ASSESSMENT OF HYPERSENSITIVITY STATE BEFORE GIVING ATS
1. Patients should be asked if they or members of their family suffer from asthma, hay fever, or other allergies, if they have previously had serum treatment (e.g. ATS, anti-gas gangrene serum, etc.) and if they have previously had reactions to them.
2. If there is no history of allergy or previous serum administration, give a test dose of 0.2 ml ATS (undiluted), by s.c. injection. If there is no general reaction in 30 minutes, give 1500 u ATS.
3. If there is no history of allergy, but patient has received previous serum injections, give a test dose of 0.2 ml 1/10 ATS; if there is no general reaction in 30 minutes, give a test dose of 0.2 ml undiluted ATS; if no reaction in 30 minutes, give 1500 u ATS.
4. If there is a history of allergy (including serum reaction) give a test dose of 1/1000, then 1/10 and then undiluted ATS before giving the full protective dose (1500 u). Have a syringe with 1/1000 adrenaline ready for use when giving ATS or testing for sensitivity to ATS, in case anaphylaxis occurs.

TREATMENT FOR ANAPHYLACTIC SHOCK
At the first sign of dyspnoea, pallor or collapse, inject 1.0 ml of 1/1000 adrenaline solution IM (not IV) (0.5 ml in children), repeat the injection (0.5 ml) every 20 minutes if recovery is delayed (e.g. systolic BP below 100 mm Hg). Antihistamines may also be injected if urticaria or oedema develops; also hydrocortisone sodium succinate (100 mg IV). (The emergency drug cupboard should contain chlorpheniramine – 'Piriton' – for injection 1–2 ml (10–29 mg IV) or by mouth 4 mg thrice daily.)

Warn patients given ATS of the possibility (5 per cent) of a local or general rash, fever and joint pains, generally 7–12 days after serum injections, though sometimes sooner. These can be treated with oral antihistamine preparations.

14.3.4 USE OF ANTIBIOTICS IN PROPHYLAXIS AGAINST TETANUS

Patients who cannot be adequately protected with toxoid, because they are not actively immune, or for whom ATG is not available, will have to rely for protection on surgical cleansing, ATS and supportive prophylaxis by systemic antibiotics. It is essential that the antibiotic treatment should be started as soon as possible after injury. Patients with badly contaminated wounds and those in whom there has been delay in starting treatment should be given antibiotic prophylaxis together with ATG (or ATS, if ATG is not available).

The antibiotic used should be one which is highly active against *Cl. tetani* (penicillins or erythromycin); it is also desirable to give an antibiotic which is not inactivated by penicillase. Suggested schedules are 7–10 days course of oral erythromycin or flucloxacillin; out-patients may be given the same antibiotics – IM flucloxacillin, followed by oral flucloxacillin for 7–10 days is suggested.

14.4   Storage and disposal of vaccines

14.4.1   POTENCY AND STORAGE OF VACCINES

Vaccines are biological products and have a limited effective life. Conditions of storage must be controlled to maintain the potency of the vaccine for as long as possible. Vaccines are normally given an expiry date by the manufacturer and all staff involved in immunization programmes should take great care to ensure that the product is not out of date. Rotation of stocks to avoid expiry is essential.

The optimum storage temperature for most vaccines is between 4° and 10°C (39°F and 50°F); the manufacturer's instructions must be followed. Vaccines should not be left at room temperature for a long time, particularly in summer, nor should they be allowed to freeze, as they may lose potency. Modern domestic refrigerators are now used to store immunizing preparations and these are sometimes set at a temperature which is too low for the storage of vaccines, e.g. 2°C (35°F). The thermostat should be reset to approximately 6°C (43°F) to prevent loss of potency.

14.4.2   DISPOSAL OF UNWANTED VACCINES AND DOSES

Time expired vaccines containing live organisms, for example BCG, measles, poliomyelitis (oral), rubella and yellow fever, should be inactivated by autoclaving or boiling prior to disposal or pouring down a sink drain. Residues of vaccine remaining after an immunizing session must be discarded.

References and further reading

Department of Health (1990) *Immunisation against Infectious Diseases*. HMSO, London.

Lowbury, E.J.L., Kidson, A., Lilly, H.A. *et al.* (1978) Prophylaxis against tetanus in non-immune patients with wounds: the role of antibiotics and human antitetanus globulin. *Journal of Hygiene (Camb)*, **80**, 267.

Sub-committee of the Joint Tuberculosis Committee of the British Thoracic Society (1990) Control and prevention of tuberculosis in Britain: an updated code of practice. *British Medical Journal*, **300**, 995.

15 *Occupational health services in the control of infection*

Transmission of infection in hospitals, from staff to patients and from patients to staff, is well recognized. Medical care is often available for nursing staff, but the extent of this service varies in different hospitals. Health services for hospital staff should, of course, include attention to all forms of illness, but the prevention of infection is a major reason for promoting these services.

The establishment of an occupational health service for hospital staff is outlined in a report of a Joint Committee of the Department of Health and the Scottish Home and Health Department (DHSS 1968). The Health and Safety at Work Act 1974 (see p. 24) regulates the safety of the work place and applies to hospitals. Stress is laid on local policies for each department, and the head of department is responsible for the formulation of such policies. Guidelines for drawing up local policies were published by Boucher (1979). The report of the Health Services Advisory Committee (1991) is relevant to laboratory and hospital staffs (see also p. 347) and a number of other guidelines on HIV infections are available (see Chapter 10). This chapter deals only with the infective aspects of health care for hospital staff.

15.1 Risks to the staff from patients

Members of hospital staff are exposed to risks of acquiring many kinds of infection (see Chapter 9), but some infections, notably tuberculosis, meningococcal infection, poliomyelitis, HIV and HBV infection, enteric fever, other salmonella infections, and viral gastroenteritis, present special hazards. The risk of acquiring HIV infection is small, but the serious outcome of such an infection has had a major influence on preventative measures. A high incidence of staphylococcal or streptococcal infection among the patients may sometimes lead to outbreaks among nurses and other members of hospital staff. However, most staphylococci causing infections in hospitals as well as Gram-negative bacilli, such as *Ps. aeruginosa* and *Klebsiella* spp., are unlikely to infect staff or be transmitted to their relatives. Epidemics of respiratory virus diseases in the community necessitating admissions of patients to hospital may lead to outbreaks of the disease in hospital. Certain infections, such as herpetic whitlow, occur predominantly in members of hospital staff. Head lice and scabies may occasionally be a hazard to staff, the latter especially in mental subnormality units. *Candida* infections may be a problem in maternity and gynaecological units.

In addition to overt clinical infections carrier states may arise. Acquisition of hospital staphylococci in the external nares and on the hands is not uncommon, particularly in burns units and dermatological wards.

15.2 Risks to patients from staff

The commonest infections transmitted to patients by hospital staff, apart from upper respiratory viral infection, are staphylococcal sepsis, streptococcal sore throat, and infective diarrhoea. *Candida* spp. may be transmitted to neonates by staff with paronychia. Spread of pulmonary tuberculosis from a member of staff is a rare but important hazard. The transmission of HIV or HBV infection to a patient is unlikely, and usually carriers continue in their normal work. However, an HIV or HBV positive surgeon is more likely to infect a patient during an operation than other grades of staff during their routine duties. A difficult decision as to whether to allow the member of staff to continue operating has to be made, and counselling and follow-up is always necessary (see Chapter 10; DoH 1990a). The likelihood of transmission clearly depends on the activities of the infected person; for example a boil on the hand of a surgeon or nurse is a greater risk to a patient than a similar lesion on the hand of a clerk or an engineer.

Symptomless carriers of virulent pathogenic bacteria among members of staff are also a potential hazard of infection to patients. Outbreaks of staphylococcal infection in neonatal departments, or of wound sepsis acquired in the operating theatre, may originate from a nasal or a skin carrier of a virulent strain of *Staph. aureus*. An important source of infection especially in surgical wards may be a member of staff with eczema colonized by an epidemic strain of *Staph. aureus*. Nose or throat carriers of Group A β-haemolytic streptococci have been responsible for outbreaks of puerperal sepsis in maternity wards, particularly if carried by delivery-room staff. Kitchen staff carrying dysentery bacilli or *Salmonella* spp. may also be a hazard, although outbreaks of infection arising initially from staff in hospital kitchens are uncommon.

Salmonella carriers are normally allowed to return to work after the acute symptoms have resolved. However, it is usually suggested that they do not work with food or babies and are instructed in good hygiene. This also applies to catering staff if they are known to be conscientious in their personal hygiene, but carriers of *S. typhi* should be kept off duty. Treatment with a quinolone, e.g. ciprofloxacin, will often eliminate salmonella carriage.

During an outbreak of infection in hospital, epidemiological evidence may point to staff members being involved in the occurrence or spread of infection. In these circumstances, a search for carriers or cases among staff may be necessary. Apart from this situation, routine and regular monitoring of otherwise healthy staff members is not required.

15.2.1   INITIAL SCREENING OF STAFF ON APPOINTMENT

All staff, i.e. medical, nursing, administrative, ancillary (laboratory, and other technicians, physiotherapy, x-ray etc.), domestic, portering and mortuary staff, SSD staff, catering and laundry, should be included in the initial screening and immunization programme. This usually involves the completion of a questionnaire (see p. 250). Enquiry should be made for diarrhoeal diseases, recurrent sepsis, tonsillitis or chronic skin diseases; it is advisable that applicants suffering from certain chronic conditions (e.g. severe eczema) should not be accepted for nursing or other duties that bring them into close contact with patients, because of the likelihood of colonization with antibiotic resistant organisms. For those coming into contact with patients, a tuberculin (e.g. Heaf) test for susceptibility to tuberculosis should also be carried out; BCG vaccination should be offered to tuberculin-negative presons who have not previously received BCG vaccination and shown conversion of the tuberculin test. Conversion of the tuberculin test to a positive reaction should be demonstrated before close contact with tuberculous patients or laboratory specimens which might be considered to be tuberculous is allowed. A chest x-ray should only be taken if indicated in the questionnaire or if there are suggestive symptoms (Subcommittee of the Joint Tuberculosis Committee of the British Thoracic Society 1990). See below, and Chapter 13.
Bacteriological examination of nose, throat and faeces and chest x-ray are not recommended as a routine, but may be indicated in certain special circumstances (see Chapters 2 and 12).

An example of a card which might be used for recording hospital staff immunization is shown in Appendix 15.1.

15.2.2   IMMUNIZATION OF STAFF

The principles involved in selecting immunization procedures are discussed in Chapter 14, also DHSS (1990b). For most general hospitals the following are suggested.

All staff should be offered protection against tuberculosis and poliomyelitis. Non-pregnant susceptible women of child-bearing age should also be offered rubella vaccination. The Health Services Advisory Committee report (1991) suggests that tetanus toxoid should be given to laboratory staff and to engineering staff who service laboratory equipment; it seems reasonable to offer tetanus immunization to all engineering and gardening staff, and other staff who request it.

In general hospitals there is no need for routine immunization against typhoid fever. Rubella vaccination is intended for staff in contact with children, but due to rotation of staff it is usually more practical to offer vaccination to all female members of staff at risk. Rubella antibody-negative women should not work in a maternity unit until they have been immunized. Rubella vaccine should be offered also to non-immune male staff who are likely to come in contact with women in the early antenatal period.

Measles vaccine should be offered to staff in paediatric, infectious diseases or leukaemia wards if they have not already had the disease.

Hepatitis B vaccine should be offered to those in regular contact with infected patients or carriers, for example, staff in isolation wards, liver units, drug addiction units, or involved in regular blood taking, for example phlebotomists and all surgeons, junior doctors and nurses.

15.2.3 CONTINUING SURVEILLANCE AND ADVICE

In addition to initial screening, the occupational health service or practitioner and nurse responsible for staff health should be concerned with:

1. training of staff of all grades in personal hygiene;
2. immunization and vaccination of existing staff at the required time interval (DOH 1990b);
3. organization of special precautions for staff particularly at risk of infection, for example regular questionnaires for staff working with tuberculous patients or laboratory specimens and chest x-rays if clinically indicated;
4. examination of staff returning to work after absence due to diarrhoea or sepsis, to ensure that the infection has cleared and to give advice to carriers;
5. arranging tests and possibly treatment for staff with sepsis of hospital origin or who are carriers of pathogens which may be harmful to patients;
6. keeping accurate records of infections in the staff;
7. keeping records of injuries, arranging for prophylaxis following needle-stick injuries and counselling of staff at risk of infection (e.g. HIV, HBV, cytomegalovirus etc.);

8. determining staff contacts of infectious disease, checking immunity and follow-up if necessary;
9. surveys of potential infective and toxic hazards to staff in hospital.

The responsibilities described are concerned mainly with risks of infections and are only a part of the work of the occupational health department. The implementation of the COSHH regulations (see p. 24) is an example. Staff are exposed to potential toxic hazards of disinfectants, especially aldehydes, in addition to risks from microorganisms.

Where an occupational health department exists, a close working relationship must be established between the infection control doctor and nurse and staff of the occupational health department. A member of the occupational health department should be on the control of infection committee.

The infection control and occupational health nurses should work together in tracing contacts of infectious diseases, providing advice and educating staff.

15.2.4 STAFF WITH, OR IN CONTACT WITH, INFECTIOUS DISEASES

The recommended periods of isolation for patients with infectious disease (Chapter 8), are also appropriate periods of time for members of staff with such infections to be kept away from patients in the hospital. Staff who are in contact – at home or in hospital – with infectious disease need not be excluded, but when they are, or have been, in contact with cases of typhoid fever, diphtheria, meningococcal meningitis and other potentially dangerous diseases, the infection control doctor should be consulted for advice. Diphtheria contacts should be given prophylactic erythromycin and kept under surveillance (p. 155). Poliomyelitis and diphtheria contacts should be offered active immunization. Contacts of childhood infections, particularly chicken-pox, should not work where there are high infection risk patients unless they are immune or otherwise protected against the infection to which they have been exposed.

Staff receiving a needle-stick or other sharps injury should report immediately to the occupational health department or inform the duty microbiologist if outside of normal working hours (Chapter 10 outlines the required action).

Appendix 15.1 Hospital staff immunization record

Name .... Card No. ....

Department .... Date of birth ....

Diagnostic tests

	Tetanus	Polio	BCG	Rubella	Influenza	Hepatitis B	Other
Date Test and result							
Date Amount Batch No.							
Date Amount Batch No.							
Date Amount Batch No.							

References

Boucher, B.J. (1979) Guidance on preparing local rules to help implement the Health and Safety at Work Act etc. *British Medical Journal*, **i**, 599.

Department of Health and Scottish Home and Health Department (1968) *The Care of the Health of Hospital Staff*. HMSO, London.

Department of Health (1990a) *Guidance for Clinical Health Care Workers. Protection against Infection with HIV and Hepatitis B Viruses*. Recommendations of the Expert advisory group on AIDS. HMSO, London.

Department of Health (1990b) *Immunization against Infectious Diseases*. HMSO, London.

Health and Safety at Work Act (1974) HMSO, London.

Health Services Advisory Committee (1991) Safe working and the prevention of infection in clinical laboratories: model rules for staff and visitors. HMSO, London.

Subcommittee of the Joint Tuberculosis Committee of the British Thoracic Society (1990) Control and prevention of tuberculosis in Britain: an updated code of practice. *British Medical Journal*, **300**, 995.

16   *Special wards and departments I*

16.1   Intensive care units

Infection is one of the principal hazards to which patients in intensive care (or intensive therapy) units (ICU or, more usually, ITU) are exposed (Wenzel *et al.* 1983). A patient requiring intensive care may be defined as one who requires support of a vital function until the disease process is arrested or ameliorated; such patients are likely to have poor resistance to infection, sometimes due to immunosuppressive or steroid therapy, or due to depression of the immunological response often seen in these patients with multiple organ failure. In addition to being more susceptible, they are exposed in the intensive care unit to greater hazards of contamination and cross-infection than most patients in ordinary wards. This is due to the fact that they receive much more nursing attention and handling, and various forms of instrumentation – in particular tracheostomy, mechanical ventilation, aspiration of bronchial secretions, catheterization of the urinary tract, treatment of open wounds and central venous catheterization. Special difficulties arise through emergencies (e.g. respiratory obstruction requiring immediate clearing of the patient's airway) and the sudden excessive pressure of work which occurs when several patients are admitted at the same time; in such circumstances it may be difficult or impossible to observe all the recommendations of asepsis. Even so, cross-infection is in many cases probably due to thoughtlessness or staff shortages. Intensive therapy requires what is sometimes considered to be an inordinate number of trained nursing staff, but if such a complement is not available, nurses inevitably have to move rapidly between patients without having time even to wash their hands. The amount of technical assistance and the number of cleaners in ITU is much greater than it is in normal wards, but these are essential if nursing skill is to be used effectively and if meticulous cleanliness of equipment is to be maintained.

The microorganisms which cause infection in intensive care units include any of those which are associated with hospital infection, but since the patients are often deficient in resistance to infection, many organisms which have little or no pathogenicity for healthy persons and tissues are potentially important as causes of infection in intensive care patients. The commonest infecting organisms in an ITU are *Staph. aureus*, *E. Coli*, *Ps. aeruginosa*, *Klebsiella* spp., *Proteus* spp., *Acinetobacter* spp., *Enterobacter* spp., and *Bacteroides* spp. Endogenous infection with coliform bacilli and sometimes with *Bacteroides* spp. and other anaerobic non-sporing bacteria is a hazard in patients with abdominal wounds. The reduction of gastric acid by use of H_2 blockers may be followed by colonization of the stomach with Gram-negative bacilli. Aspiration of stomach contents may lead to colonization of the oropharynx and the respiratory tract and possibly to bronchopneumonia. Sucralfate instead of H_2 blockers may reduce the risk of colonization of the stomach and consequently of Gram-negative respiratory tract infection.

Staphylococcal infection may be transmitted by contact or by air, and epidemic strains of MRSA are a particular hazard. Gram-negative bacilli, when not acquired from the patient's own flora of skin, gut or upper respiratory tract, are most likely to be acquired by contact, and from moist vectors such as solutions and medicaments, food, humidifiers of mechanical ventilators, etc. Airborne infection with Gram-negative bacilli is a remote hazard, except from aerosols produced by a contaminated nebulizer, or less commonly from removal of dressings (e.g. of burns) on to which heavily contaminated exudate has dried. Expectoration by patients with tracheostomies or endotracheal tubes may cause heavy local contamination with bronchial mucus, but the air of an intensive care unit has been found usually free from *Ps. aeruginosa*, even when several patients with respiratory and urinary tract pseudomonas infection were in the ward. The suggestion that the expired air of all patients undergoing artificial ventilation in the unit should be filtered or exhausted to the exterior seems unnecessary.

16.1.1   CONTROL OF INFECTION: GENERAL

The general principles of aseptic care and hospital hygiene which are described in Chapters 6 and 7 must be conscientiously applied and with certain additional precautions relating to special procedures of the intensive care unit (Craven and Steger 1989).

16.1.2   DESIGN OF UNIT

Because of the need for quick and unimpaired access of staff to patients, it is usually inappropriate for all the patients to be in single-bed isolation rooms, but one or two isolation rooms are required (e.g. in an 8-bed unit, there could be two 3-bed wards or divisions of a ward, and two isolation rooms). In the 'open' section retractable waterproof curtains between beds may have some value in preventing contamination of adjacent beds with expectorated mucus. There should be adequate space (e.g. 10–12 ft between bed centres) to allow easy access of staff and equipment.

The isolation rooms should be suitable for use either by infected patients (**source isolation**), or by hypersusceptible patients who must be given maximum protection against infection (**protective isolation**), or for combined source and protective isolation – for example, by plenum ventilation into the room and extraction of air, when required, from the room to the outside of the hospital. It is probably desirable that the open section of the Unit should have mechanical ventilation with a turnover of air (e.g. 10 air changes per hour) sufficient to prevent a build-up of bacteria released by persons in the Unit, and to keep air-borne bacteria at a low level. An intensive care unit may, however, be reasonably safe without plenum ventilation, or with a degree of mechanical ventilation to provide maximum comfort.

16.1.3 FURNITURE AND FITTINGS

Floors and walls should be washable. Furniture should be reduced to a minimum. Monitoring equipment should be wall-mounted on a shelf and sealed; suction apparatus and sphygmomanometers should be wall-mounted but detachable.

Sticky mats at the entrance to the Unit have been shown to have no value in reducing infection.

16.1.4 CLEANING OF ENVIRONMENT

As in wards (Chapter 6).

16.1.5 HANDLING OF PATIENTS

A high standard of aseptic care must be used by nurses, doctors, physiotherapists, radiographers, pathology technicians and others in handling intensive care patients. Hands should be washed with an antimicrobial detergent preparation, or preferably disinfected with 70% alcohol rubbed to dryness, which is rapid and effective. Plastic disposable (non-sterile) gloves should be worn for bronchial and oral toilet and as many as possible of the procedures (e.g. oral toilet) should always be done before 'dirty' procedures (e.g. taking rectal temperature).

Protective clothing (gowns or plastic aprons) should be worn when attending to a patient, but this is not necessary if there is no patient contact; all members of staff or visitors should wear a gown or apron used for that patient only. Overshoes, masks and disposable hats are unnecessary. Non-essential visiting should be discouraged, but relatives or close friends of the patient should be allowed. They must have almost unrestricted access to prevent disorientation of the patient, which can cause severe psychological disturbance, one of the major problems for those who survive. Furthermore, there is good evidence that infection is more likely to be acquired from a member of the hospital staff who attends to other patients than from a (healthy) visitor who visits only one patient in the ward.

16.1.6   PROCEDURES

Tracheostomy and endotracheal intubation   The benefits of tracheostomy, by which exudates can be aspirated and mechanical ventilation established, are offset by hazards of infection. Colonization of the oral cavity and trachea, which may sometimes lead to the development of bronchopneumonia, can be caused by various organisms, but predominately Gram-negative bacilli introduced into the respiratory tract at the time of aspiration of exudate or during mechanical ventilation or humidification, or (*Staph. aureus*) from the inspired air. The tracheostomy wound may become infected, and pressure of the tracheostomy tube against the tracheal lining may cause abrasion leading to local wound infection and ulceration. Because of these drawbacks tracheostomy has, to a large extent, been superseded by the long-term use of endotracheal tubes. These also may be a channel of contamination, but they have the advantage of avoiding an operation, with possible infection of the operation wound; there is usually no difficulty in re-intubating patients, and secretions can be aspirated as easily from an endotracheal tube as from a tracheostomy, particularly if a mucolytic agent is used.

The control of infection in patients with a tracheostomy or endotracheal tube is difficult; when any patient in the unit has a multi-resistant Gram-negative infection (of the respiratory tract or of a wound) it is common for the infection to spread to other patients in the unit. Aseptic techniques for aspiration of bronchial secretions should reduce the incidence of infection of patients with tracheostomies and endotracheal tubes. Care is needed in removal of endotracheal tubes and non-sterile plastic gloves should be worn. The most important procedure in reducing the spread of infection is handwashing between patients.

Intravenous catheters   Chapter 7.

Ventilatory equipment   Prevention of infection from this source is very important. Various methods of decontamination are available (Chapter 6). Of importance in the design of all modern lung ventilators is the ability either to isolate the ventilator completely from the patient by bacterial filters, or for the patient's circuit and humidifier to be easily removed for autoclaving, or both.

Urine drainage A fluid balance is required as part of management of patients in the intensive care unit. Drainage bags must be changed or emptied twice daily under aseptic conditions, and the urine collected for 24 hours analysis must not be stored at the bedside (Chapter 7).

16.1.7 EQUIPMENT

All equipment used in intensive care units should be kept meticulously clean and dry. In a study on sources of infection, washing bowls used by patients in an intensive care unit were often found to be contaminated with *Ps. aeruginosa* in residues of moisture; individual bowls, heat-disinfected or at least thoroughly washed and dried after use, are desirable. Shaving brushes should be avoided; electric razors used on one patient and then on another are also potential vectors of infection. An individual shaving kit is desirable (Chapter 6 gives details about disinfection of ventilators, nebulizers, humidifiers and suction equipment). Food mixers are also a potential source of infection. Water in flower vases is frequently contaminated with *Pseudomonas* spp., although this is an unlikely source of infection. Storage of equipment in fluids should be avoided.

16.1.8 ANTIBIOTIC PROPHYLAXIS (Van Saene *et al.* 1989)

Antibiotic prophylaxis should generally be avoided to reduce risks of selecting multi-resistant opportunist organisms. However, selective decontamination of the oropharynx and gastrointestinal tract with antibiotics has been used successfully in several studies, to prevent colonization with aerobic Gram negative bacilli. One such regime includes applications of a paste containing polymyxin B, tobramycin and amphotericin B to the oral pharynx, the introduction of these agents into the stomach with a nasogastric tube and the systemic administration of cefotaxime (Stoutenbeek *et al.* 1984; Ledingham *et al.* 1988). Respiratory infection was significantly reduced by this regime. Other studies have shown similar results, although there is little evidence that mortality is reduced. Further studies over a longer time period are required to determine the specific applications for this routine and to determine whether selective decontamination will also select highly resistant strains.

16.2   Burns and open traumatic wounds

Burns are at first free or virtually free from bacteria, which have been killed by the heat, but soon the layer of dead tissue and exudate becomes heavily colonized by bacteria unless effective measures are taken to keep them out. In small superficial burns and in many deeper and more extensive burns the bacteria cause no apparent ill effects, though this depends on the types of bacteria present and on the patient's resistance. In more extensive burns bacterial infection is the most important cause of illness and death.

Strep. pyogenes, when present, will usually cause the complete failure of skin grafts and delay healing; today it rarely causes invasive infection, though it may cause fever. Of the other bacteria, *Ps. aeruginosa* has proved to be the most important cause of septicaemia and toxaemia; it can also cause the failure of skin grafts, but to a smaller extent than *Strep. pyogenes*. Other Gram-negative bacilli (*Proteus* spp., *Klebsiella* spp., *Serratia*, spp., *Acinetobacter* spp., etc.) and *Staph. aureus* are usually less important pathogens, though they can occasionally cause septicaemia in severely burned patients. Rarer pathogens are *Candida albicans* and other fungi, gas gangrene and tetanus bacilli and Herpes virus.

Ps. aeruginosa and other bacteria are usually acquired from the burns of other patients in the ward, transmitted on hands of nurses, various fomites and by air; air is a less important route, especially for Gram-negative bacilli, but may be important if large dressings are changed in an open ward.

In addition to the burn, the urinary tract, the respiratory tract and intravenous infusion sites are important portals of entry and sites of infection.

Open wounds resemble burns, but there is usually less necrotic tissue in which small numbers of bacteria can multiply. Contaminants acquired at the time of injury, including tetanus and gas gangrene bacilli, are more likely to play a role in infection of open wounds than of burns, but hospital-acquired infection, both exogenous and endogenous, is potentially more important than contamination at the time of injury.

16.2.1   PREVENTION OF INFECTION

The bacterial flora of all burns should be examined on admission and at all changes of dressings for *Strep. pyogenes*, *Ps. aeruginosa* and other common aerobic bacteria. If *Strep. pyogenes* is present, the patient must be treated with systemic erythromycin or flucloxacillin, and grafting operations must be postponed until the organisms are removed from the burn; benzyl or phenoxymethyl penicillin are not suitable for this purpose, because they are likely to be inactivated by penicillinase from other bacteria, especially resistant *Staph. aureus* colonizing the same burn. Prophylaxis against infection of burns can be subdivided into two lines of defence:

The first line of defence (i.e. methods of protecting the patients against microbial contaminants) includes:

1. primary excision and skin grafting (only suitable for relatively small burns of full skin thickness);
2. antisepsis: i.e. application of antibacterial substances to the burn (Lowbury 1976);
3. asepsis.

Antisepsis Local treatment with appropriate antimicrobial agents has been shown in controlled trials to protect burns against colonization by *Ps. aeruginosa, Str. pyogenes, Staph. aureus* and other bacteria, and to reduce the septic consequences of infection, including skin graft failure and mortality. The qualities looked for in such prophylactic agents are effectiveness against all strains of significant burn pathogens, minimal local or systemic toxicity, and failure to select resistant variants in patients under treatment. There is no ideal preparation that fulfils all requirements. Silver sulphadiazine cream has been widely adopted as a standard prophylactic application, but a preponderant flora of sulphonamide-resistant Gram-negative bacilli has been found to emerge in one centre where silver sulphadiazine was in regular use for several years.

When silver sulphadiazine is rejected for such reasons, an alternative prophylactic application is required and can be made available by co-operation of the hospital pharmacy. In patients with extensive burns, silver nitrate compresses (0.5%) have proved highly effective, especially against *Ps. aeruginosa* and *Proteus* spp., but patients having this treatment need supplements of electrolytes by mouth and laboratory control of serum electrolytes to avoid imbalance. The method is not suitable for infants. A further disadvantage is the black staining of all items that come in contact with the silver solution (including walls). Silver sulphadiazine, when acceptable, is more suitable for smaller burns and for children and, though less active against *Ps. aeruginosa* and *Proteus* spp., it is more active against some other Gram-negative bacilli. Alternative preparations which have prophylactic effects similar to those of silver sulphadiazine cream, are creams containing 0.5% silver nitrate with 0.2% chlorhexidine gluconate or 2% phenoxetol, the latter especially effective in controlling *Staph. aureus* infection. For minor burns (especially those treated in outpatient clinics), a tulle gras containing 0.5% chlorhexidine ('Bactigras') has been found appropriate. Burns treated by the exposure method have a physical protective barrier against infection once a dry eschar has formed. This can be anticipated and supplemented by topical chemoprophylaxis with povidone-iodine (7.5%, with 0.75% available iodine), or with aqueous silver nitrate (0.5%) dabbed on three or four times a day for 6–8 days.

Antibiotics should not be used for topical prophylaxis because of the hazards of emergence of resistant organisms and of toxic or allergic effects in the patients (Lowbury 1976). Monitoring of sensitivity of burn flora is an important routine procedure in a burns unit.

Asepsis   Dressing of burns in a ventilated dressing room, barrier nursing, source and protective isolation of patients and good ward hygiene contribute to control of infection (Chapters 7 and 8). The dressing may be carried out in a single isolation room provided the ventilation system and facilities are adequate. For patients with burns in hospital, a dressing technique with two nurses should be carried out if possible in a room with combined source and protective isolation (e.g. plenum ventilation with an exhaust-ventilated air-lock). Exposure treatment, which is clinically desirable for many burns of the trunk and the face, provides some protection by the development of a dry eschar on which bacteria cannot grow (but which may cover a zone of heavy growth and suppuration); exposure treatment is better than moist applications with no antibacterial activity.

The **second line of defence** i.e. methods of preventing invasion of the tissues and bloodstream by bacteria growing on the burn. This includes: **antibiotic therapy, active and passive immunization** and **general supportive measures** (treatment of diabetes, anaemia etc.). Systemic treatment of all *Strep. pyogenes* infections with an appropriate antibiotic (e.g. erythromycin or cloxacillin) protects all patients in the ward by eliminating reservoirs of infection. Severely burned patients who have acquired heavy growths of *Ps. aeruginosa* may be given protection with systemic gentamicin, or another appropriate aminoglycoside, or another anti-pseudomonas agent (e.g. ceftazidime, timentin or a quinolone). A more promising procedure would be the use of a polyvalent *Pseudomonas* vaccine which has been found to give early protection and reduced mortality in patients with severe burns; hyperimmune globulin prepared from immunized human volunteers has also proved valuable. Prophylaxis against tetanus, by use of a 'boosting' dose of toxoid when the patient is known to be actively immune, or by antiserum (human ATG) if there is no evidence of active immunity, should be given to all patients with burns admitted to hospital (Chapter 15).

16.2.2 SPECIAL PROBLEMS OF STERILIZATION AND
DISINFECTION

The principles of sterile supply outlined in Chapter 17 are relevant to
patients with burns. The electric dermatome and the bone saw can be
sterilized by dry heat in a hot air oven at 160°C for one hour. The
outside of electrical equipment, cardiac monitoring equipment, portable
lights, diathermy and x-ray machines, suction apparatus and respiratory
ventilators must be cleaned after use, because of the possibilities of
heavy contamination.

Disinfection of respiratory ventilators and anaesthetic apparatus is
covered in Chapter 6. Water circulating mattresses may be disinfected
with a clear soluble phenolic, and body temperature recorders with 70%
alcohol. Mattress covers may be demaged by repeated application of
phenolic disinfectants or by silver nitrate treatment of patients; Gram-
negative bacilli are then likely to grow in the mattress. Mattresses
should be inspected regularly for damage.

Beds providing air support systems are sometimes used for the management of extensive injuries, including burns, or in patients who are
at special risk of ulcer formation. One type of bed (the 'fluidized bead
bed') has a trough, filled with silica beads and covered with a special
sheet, through which air is pumped. Another type (the 'low air loss
bed') is constructed from a series of inflatable cushions, air being continuously pumped through these, with pneumatic controls to vary the
elevation.

The risk of dispersing bacteria into the environment from these beds,
even when occupied by heavily infected patients, has been shown to
be no greater than that from a standard hospital bed. Normal cleaning
procedures (e.g. with a cloth moistened with a detergent solution) is
generally adequate. If the external surfaces are known to be contaminated, they should be cleansed with a clear soluble phenolic solution,
rinsed and allowed to dry. The air sacs of low-air-loss beds should be
machine-washed at a temperature of 60°C. Advice of the manufacturer
should be sought when internal ducting has become contaminated and
on appropriate agents for disinfection.

Baths are a potential source of Gram-negative infection, particularly
of *Ps. aeruginosa*. Recirculating systems (e.g. jacuzzis etc.) are difficult
to clean and disinfect and should not be used unless adequate disinfection is possible.

16.2.3 HOMOGRAFTS AS VECTORS OF INFECTION

Donor skin cannot be sterilized; pre-operative disinfection of the donor
site destroys most of the transient flora, but a substantial proportion of

the resident flora survives. Homografts are occasionally found to be the source of infection with pathogenic bacteria; HIV can be transmitted in this way from a donor who is a carrier, and it is probable that other viruses (e.g. HBV and cytomegalovirus) can also be transmitted on skin homografts.

As there is as yet no method of sterilizing viable skin grafts or of ensuring that they are virus-free, it is important that they should be applied only when their use is fully justified on clinical and ethical grounds. Prospective donors must be screened for HIV antibodies, but a negative result gives no guarantee of freedom from infection, as antibodies to HIV do not appear until about three months after acquisition of the virus. If non-living homografts are applied, these should be sterilized (e.g. by gamma irradiation), which tends to make the tissue stiffer than living skin. The increased availability of laboratory cultured skin may help to reduce this problem.

16.3 Dermatological wards

Most patients with skin diseases are not physically very 'ill', but their condition often causes them some mental stress. When it is considered necessary to use source isolation procedures, it is important that it should be explained to the patient that, with certain exceptions, the underlying skin condition (e.g. eczema or psoriasis) in itself is not infectious and will not spread to the rest of the family or to visitors. The risk is of the transfer of bacteria capable of causing infection in susceptible patients in hospital (e.g. patients undergoing surgery); healthy people will not become infected from them even when in close contact. This does not apply to certain septic lesions (e.g. impetigo) where there is a definite risk of transfer to healthy subjects.

Patients in dermatological wards often have generalized desquamating lesions which are heavily colonized with *Staph. aureus*. These patients are often heavy dispersers and cross-infection is frequent, but clinical sepsis is rarely caused by these staphylococci. However, such a patient admitted to a surgical ward may be responsible for widespread nasal colonization and wound sepsis. These strains of staphylococci are commonly resistant to two or more antibiotics and MRSA is a particular hazard. Children admitted with clinically apparent staphylococcal infections (e.g. impetigo) not only spread infection, but cause similar septic lesions in other children and sometimes pyogenic lesions in the staff. These strains are often resistant to penicillin only and are initially acquired outside hospital. Some of these infections are caused by β-haemolytic streptococci (often associated with *Staph. aureus*) and may similarly spread to other patients. Cross-infection with Gram-negative bacilli (e.g. *Ps. aeruginosa* and *Proteus* spp.) is also common in dermatological wards and these organisms are usually found in varicose ulcers, but clinical sepsis is unusual.

Candida infection may also occur, although there is little evidence of cross-infection. Patients with dermatophyte infections are not usually admitted to hospital, but the risk of cross-infection exists (e.g. tinea corporis and pedis, which may not be clinically obvious). Transmission of *Tinea capitis* between children occurs readily in schools and could similarly spread in paediatric wards.

The spread of virus infection is not a particular hazard of dermatological wards apart from vaccinia.

16.3.1 CONTROL OF INFECTION

Staphylococcal infection spreads both by contact and by air. Environmental contamination is so heavy that prevention of cross-infection is difficult, but some potentially effective measures are possible, especially the following:

1. children with clinical sepsis must be isolated in single rooms, whether in general or dermatological wards;
2. patients with desquamating lesions must be kept in single rooms, or preferably in an isolation unit, if admitted to general hospital wards;
3. general hospitals should have wards kept solely for dermatological patients;
4. when isolation is required, it must be complete; i.e. patients should not leave the ward to visit other patients.

16.3.2 DRESSING TECHNIQUES

Open lesions (e.g. ulcers) and wounds should be treated as in a general surgical ward, using SSD packs and no-touch technique. A special room should be provided if possible for carrying out surgical techniques (e.g. biopsies). The dressing of patients with non-surgical lesions is rather different, since it is sometimes necessary to apply creams with the hands, but the following points should be observed.

1. Dressing rooms should be immediately adjacent to the bathroom and should have an extractor fan.
2. Couches in dressing rooms should be covered with paper covers which are changed between patients.
3. Dressing materials in contact with broken skin should have been sterilized.

4. Large bags should be provided for disposal of contaminated dressings.
5. Gloves or instruments should be used for carrying out dressing techniques whenever possible; creams and ointments should be applied when possible with a gloved hand. Staff should wash their hands thoroughly with soap or an antiseptic detergent preparation and water after handling each patient.
6. Staff should wear plastic, disposable aprons, which should be discarded at the end of a dressing session.

16.3.3 ADDITIONAL PRECAUTIONS

1. Disposable toilet-seat covers and bath-mats may be of some value; patients should be instructed in their use.
2. Floors should be cleaned with a vacuum-cleaner, never with a broom.
3. Special attention should be paid to the disinfection of baths and wash-bowls after each use. In general, cleaning methods and techniques are similar to those recommended for rooms containing infected patients (Chapter 6).

16.3.4 ANTIBIOTIC TREATMENT

Emergence of resistance is especially likely to occur in patients with skin disease because of the large populations of bacteria on the skin. Antibiotic treatment (especially topical) should be avoided whenever possible and other antimicrobial agents should be used if available or suitable (e.g. silver nitrate, chlorhexidine). Resistance emerges particularly readily to erythromycin, lincomycin (or clindamycin) and fusidic acid, and their use should be severely restricted. Topical preparations of fusidic acid should not be used in hospital. Neomycin and bacitracin are useful topical antibiotics, although resistance of *Staph. aureus* and hypersensitivity to neomycin are common. Gentamicin is a useful systemic antibiotic and should not be used topically in hospital. The combination of neomycin with chlorhexidine in a topical preparation may reduce the likelihood of resistance emerging. When possible, patients receiving treatment with antibiotics on the 'restricted' list (Chapter 12) should be given source isolation. Mupirocin is particularly effective in removing *Staph. aureus* from carriage sites and eczematous lesions. However, resistant strains are now emerging and its use should be restricted preferably to treatment of MRSA carriers. If applied to a skin lesion, its use (and other topical antibiotic agents) should be limited to seven days.

16.3.5   OINTMENTS AND OTHER MEDICAMENTS

Since patients with widespread skin lesions are particularly susceptible to infection and large amounts of topical medicaments are often applied, the application must be free from pathogenic bacteria. Tubes should be used whenever possible for creams and ointments. Jars or bottles should be thoroughly cleaned (or preferably disinfected) and dried before refilling, and occasional bacterial checks should be made on preparations and distilled water in the pharmacy. Topical preparations supplied by manufacturers should also be checked, unless the manufacturer's system of preparation and testing is known to be satisfactory. In the wards, ointments or creams should be supplied for the individual patient and if jars are used the ointment should never be removed with the fingers.

16.4   Ophthalmic departments

16.4.1   PROBLEMS OF INFECTION

The eye is particularly susceptible to infection with Gram-negative bacilli, fungi, adenoviruses and herpes simplex virus, organisms which are often or always resistant to antibiotics sometimes used for prophylaxis. Traumatic wounds and surgical operations increase or determine the risks of severe infection with these organisms.

16.4.2   EXTRA-OCULAR AND ORBITAL SURGERY

Control of infection in extra-ocular and orbital operations present problems which are, in general, similar to those in any other branch of surgery. Many of these operations are performed for cosmetic reasons, so any unsightly scarring due to infection is a serious complication.

There are special considerations when implants are used in the orbit, either on the scleral surface to produce infolding in retinal detachment surgery, or when nucleation implants are used to impart movement to an artificial eye. Any contamination during such operations carries a grave risk of inflammation and possible extrusion of the implant.

16.4.3   INTRA-OCULAR SURGERY

The greatest dangers from contamination occur in intra-ocular operations, and also in patients who have corneal injuries or ulceration. The transparent ocular media have no direct blood circulation and are deficient in antibodies; they are, however, well oxygenated and provide good culture media for exogenous microorganisms (in particular, *Ps. aeruginosa*).

16.4.4 CONTROL OF INFECTION

Pre-operative disinfection of the conjunctiva

1. Present practice is variable and the value of disinfection remains uncertain, but antibiotic drops (e.g. 0.5% chloramphenicol or less commonly 0.3% gentamicin) are usually instilled into the eye pre- and postoperatively. Disinfectants are often not well tolerated, although povidone-iodine 5% has been used and is microbiologically effective. Preoperative microbiological sampling is occasionally carried out, but the value is limited and it may unnecessarily delay the operation.

2. Solutions, eye-drops and ointments; the greatest risks of intra-ocular infection are associated with the use of contaminated fluids due either to inadequate sterilization or to recontamination through inadequate handling or multiple-use-containers. Sterile drops without a preservative should be supplied for pre-operative use and discarded. A fresh supply of multi-dose drops is given postoperatively.

3. Corneal grafts; the cornea is the only tissue from the eye which is transplanted. Donors should be tested for HIV and HBV.

Sterilization of instruments and appliances   While autoclaving provides satisfactory sterilization, some instruments (e.g. cataract knives) may suffer damage to their delicate cutting edge if sterilized in this way. Some authorities accept sterilization by dry heat at 160°C (320°F) for 1 hour, or at lower temperatures for longer periods, as being satisfactory (Ophthalmic Society of the UK 1973). As this method is much slower than autoclaving, a stock of sterile instruments must be held to replace an instrument at short notice, as when an instrument is dropped or otherwise contaminated. Gamma-sterilized disposable knives and autoclaved diamond knives are solving some of these problems. Ethylene oxide has a particular application in the sterilization of cryothermy leads and other heat labile items. As the gas must be allowed to escape for at least 24 hours from the sterilized pack before use of the equipment on patients, this method requires reserve supplies of essential apparatus to cover the 'turnover' of sterilization, especially where transport to another centre adds further delays. Vitrectomy and other aspiration/ infusion apparatus also require sterilization, as the vitreous provides an ideal nidus for colonization by microorganisms.

The adjustment of the operating microscope and other equipment by the surgeon requires special precautions; the provision of dry sterile guards is usually considered satisfactory; most microscopes can now be adjusted by the foot or by other methods not requiring direct handling by the surgeon. The equipment must be kept meticulously clean, as cleaning during the operation is not possible.

16.4.5 SURGICAL TECHNIQUE

During operations instruments are held in such a way that the part which comes in contact with the eye is not touched either primarily or secondarily with the fingers that control them. This is a standard part of the discipline of the surgical team.

Instruments are more effectively controlled when regularly used with an operating microscope, which is also an effective mechanism for excluding foreign material from the operating area. Some surgeons prefer to use the ungloved hand, because of the finer control which they believe they can attain in this way. If it can be assumed that the hands are dry and never touch the operation area or the operating ends of instruments, this may involve little risk; regular and repeated use of an effective detergent antiseptic, such as 4% chlorhexidine detergent ('Hibiscrub') or 0.5% alcoholic chlorhexidine, is a particularly important precaution if gloves are not worn. Risk of infection from the ungloved hand may occur through accidental contact or from dry epidermal scales which are likely to drop from the hands during the course of a long operation. Most surgeons now prefer to accept the slight disadvantage of wearing gloves, when weighed against the disastrous results of a postoperative infection. If the edges of the wound are carefully apposed, the wound is secure and there should be little risk of intraocular contamination from the exterior from about 48 hours after the operation.

16.4.6 WARDS

Dressing packs from the SSD are used; also individual droppers, which are provided by the SSD, and eyedrops sterilized in their final containers, individual to the patient and preferably renewed each day, but these should not be used for more than seven days. Eyedrops may be preserved with benzalkonium chloride (0.01% w/v) or, for short-term use by patients, phenylmercuric nitrate or acetate (0.002% w/v); also chlorhexidine acetate (0.01% w/v), or benzalkonium chloride (0.01% w/v).

16.4.7 OUTPATIENTS

Multiple-use containers are used on patients other than those with external eye disease and are discarded at the end of a clinic session. Multiple-use containers should be discarded after use on a single patient in external eye clinics and in casualty. Epidemics of adenovirus kerato-conjunctivitis have been associated with the use of inadequately decontaminated applanation tonometers (see p. 100).

16.4.8 CONTACT LENSES

Hard lenses are difficult to contaminate and simple hygiene is usually sufficient. However, they may be disinfected with benzalkonium chloride, (0.01% w/v). This method is not suitable for soft lenses. Low water content soft lenses can be satisfactorily disinfected by heating to 80°C for 20 minutes daily. High water content lenses may be damaged by heating and require chemical disinfection. Stabilized hydrogen peroxide 3–6 volumes is commonly used. This should be thoroughly washed off or preferably neutralized. Saline solutions used for storage should be changed daily.

16.5 Ear, nose and throat departments

Patients in ENT departments may be divided into two groups with different problems of hospital-acquired infection. Short-stay patients who are admitted for operations such as tonsillectomy are vulnerable in the postoperative period to endemic hospital organisms, such as staphylococci, but also to β-haemolytic streptococci and other community-type organisms which are brought into hospital by patients. Viruses such as measles and poliomyelitis which are spread by droplet infection are also especially hazardous in the operative period.

Long-stay patients usually are suffering from more severe illness, such as carcinoma of the larynx where the tissues are more susceptible to infection and where, in addition, operative procedures such as tracheostomy provide an alternative route for colonization and ultimately infection by hospital strains of *Ps. aeruginosa* and other Gram-negative bacilli. The mode of spread in these cases is usually by contact; medical apparatus, such as suction tubing or ventilators, may also be important.

Apart from these, many patients with community-acquired infections may be admitted to the wards adding to the hazards. These include patients with tonsillitis, quinsy or acute otitis media (caused by streptococci, pneumococci, haemophilus or staphylococci) and patients with chronic external otitis (often heavily colonized with Gram-negative bacilli, staphylococci, yeasts or fungi).

16.5.1 PREVENTION OF INFECTION

Isolation facilities are essential in ENT departments both to isolate infected cases coming into hospital and to protect those particularly susceptible to infection. Long-stay patients with tracheostomy should ideally be nursed in separate rooms. Patients with streptococcal infections, if admitted at all, must be in a room separate from patients requiring operations. Children admitted for tonsillectomy and found to be pyrexial are best isolated, or, as is common practice, sent home. Patients with chronic ear disease do not generally merit isolation, although the organisms present are often highly resistant to antibiotics and care should be taken to prevent contact spread, particularly by fomites; most of these patients are, however, treated as out-patients. Children and adults should preferably be in separate wards.

Operations on the ear, throat and sinuses require incision through colonized mucous membranes and surface disinfection provides considerable difficulties. Some agents damage the membranes or may lead to fistula formation if they gain access to the middle ear. Patients requiring operation on the middle ear may require intensive out-patient treatment of infection, if present. At the time of operation many surgeons use 1% aqueous cetrimide as a membrane disinfectant, but this agent has poor activity against *Ps. aeruginosa*, and an alternative (e.g. an aqueous solution of iodine or iodophor) should be considered. Care of tracheostomy is dealt with under the section on intensive care units. The hospital hygiene problems associated with ENT wards do not differ from those in other wards. SSDs should be able to supply sterile apparatus for examination of patients and for minor procedures. Nasal and aural specula must be used on one patient only before being treated in SSD or decontaminated on site. Many units without immediate access to SSD may need to decontaminate these small items in the clinic or ward. This may be done by boiling in water for 5–10 minutes or by 5 minutes immersion in 70% alcohol solution. Sterilization in a small autoclave is preferable. In each case the specula should be allowed to dry and be stored covered in the dry state. Tracheostomy tubes, suction catheters and similar apparatus must be supplied sterile either from SSD or in commercial presterilized packs. Most laryngoscopes are capable of withstanding autoclave temperatures and should be so treated. Fibreoptic bronchoscopes are usually disinfected with glutaraldehyde (Chapter 6). The light carrier components must be removed and may be sterilized.

Operating microscopes present some difficulties; wiping with 70% ethyl alcohol is probably the most effective method of disinfection.

Particular risks to and from personnel in the department are similar to those in other wards, but emphasis should be placed on two infections.

Streptococcal disease is especially hazardous in ENT departments, so staff with sore throats should be excluded. **Tuberculous laryngitis** can lead to dissemination of many tubercle bacilli into the air, so that a tuberculin test and routine checks by the occupational health department are mandatory for nurses and doctors working in the unit; tuberculin negative staff must not be employed (Chapter 13).

16.6 The community

16.6.1 PROBLEMS IN THE COMMUNITY

Although this book is mainly concerned with infection in hospital, improved collaboration between medical and nursing staff working in hospital and the home is necessary. Patients are discharged earlier than in former times and a continuity of care at a high standard is important. This applies particularly to hygienic and aseptic techniques. More community nursing staff with better facilities are required if high standards are to be maintained.

Hospital nursing procedures are based on the known availability of equipment, linen, sterile supplies, lotions and antibiotics (all at no direct cost to the patients), which are delivered to the ward or unit. The environment is controlled by the hospital authorities. The community nurse has such supplies and equipment as can be carried in the nursing bag or in her car, or which the patient can buy or loan. As a guest in the home, she has limited control over the environment, and laundry and refuse must be dealt with in the home by patients or their relatives.

Changing patterns of hospital care have influenced domiciliary practice; e.g. early discharge of postoperative patients (possibly with infected wounds or urine, or developing an infection shortly after leaving hospital), more minor surgery carried out by general practitioners, early discharge of mothers who are sometimes carriers of HBV, HIV, or *Salmonella typhi*, or babies carrying hospital-acquired organisms; use of disposable sharps and single-use packs (often bought on prescription, not supplied by an SSD); disposal of used dressings from discharging wounds in the absence of coal-burning fires; disposal of colostomy bags and their contents. Special laundry and refuse collection services are sometimes, but not always, available and may be expensive. Equipment supplied on loan may be difficult to disinfect adequately (e.g. commodes with fabric-covered seats). In addition, family practitioners will have their own views on methods of treatment, both in the home and in health centres or group practices. Both community nurses and family practitioners are often more aware than their colleagues in hospital of the cost to the patient of procedures or treatments which they may recommend.

However, the patient at home has certain advantages over the patient in hospital. He is isolated and 'barrier-nursed' in his own home; care is given by a limited number of trained nurses who tend to use the same methods.

The structure of the community nursing service is such that it is difficult to lay down procedures which can be universally applied. It is, therefore, important for community nurses to be able to apply principles of hygiene and asepsis wherever the patient may be, even in an isolated farm supplied with well water, or an inner city slum with no water supply to the house.

The use of equipment which cannot be readily dried and is used repeatedly should be avoided; this will include cotton hand towels, dish cloths for wiping surfaces, and soap dishes. Paper towels should be used to dry hands, or alternatively a freshly laundered towel. Paper towels should be used to clean and dry work surfaces. Soap should be stored dry. Failing this, washing-up liquid containing a preservative can be used. In either case, running water must be used, not static water in a washing bowl. Provided the hands are physically clean, an alcoholic hand disinfectant containing an emollient rubbed on to the skin until it is dry is effective and should be particularly useful in domiciliary practice. The addition of an emollient is necessary to prevent chapped hands in winter. Alcoholic wipes can also be useful for disinfecting hands and surfaces.

Sterile packs should ideally be supplied by a SSD. Although this is not always possible, SSD managers may be able to supply special packs to meet specific nursing requirements.

Disposable gloves are convenient for carrying out dressing techniques; plastic bags, subsequently inverted and sealed, are useful for removing dressings. Dressing packs containing these items are available.

Although not desirable, disposable insulin syringes may be re-used on the same patient for a limited period (e.g. one week) without increasing the risk of infection, and injections may be given without disinfecting the skin with alcohol. However, the skin must be kept clean. All needles should be discarded into an approved container (BMA 1990).

Disinfectants are seldom required for inanimate surfaces in the home. Washing with soap or detergent and water and thorough drying will usually be adequate, even when a sterile pack is to be opened on the surface. Freshly drawn mains tap water, i.e. collected in a clean, dry container after allowing the water to run for 30 seconds, may be used for wound cleaning, catheter toilet, and inflating catheter balloons. Where possible, however, sterile water or saline should be used for aseptic procedures. Sachets containing antiseptics (e.g. 'Savlodil') for cleaning dirty wounds are convenient.

Notes on the use of disinfectants are given in Chapter 5. Metal instruments, generally scissors or forceps, may need to be disinfected in the home (Hoffman *et al.* 1988; BMA 1989). Although boiling is effective in killing *Staph. aureus* and other non-sporing bacteria and most viruses, instruments should preferably be supplied in sterilized packs. Scissors not used for aseptic procedures should be washed, dried and then wiped thoroughly with an alcohol-impregnated swab. A disposable plastic cover may be used for thermometers or, alternatively, the thermometer can be disinfected by wiping with an alcohol impregnated swab. Inexpensive portable autoclaves are now available, and are used in most health centres. Diaphragms and rings used in family planning clinics can usually be boiled for 5–10 minutes after thorough washing (complete immersion is important), immersed in 70% alcohol for 10 minutes or hypochlorite or other chlorine-releasing solution (1000 ppm av.Cl_2) for 30 minutes. Disposable items are preferred.

A disposable plastic apron should be worn to protect the nurse's uniform. The apron should be longer than those normally used in hospitals, because working heights tend to be lower in the home (e.g. divan beds, armchairs). Often the nurse can work comfortably only when kneeling on the floor; it is then the area immediately above knee height which is likely to be contaminated rather than the waist area. The apron should be discarded immediately, or left in the home, with the outer surface marked so that any organisms surviving on the apron will not be transferred to the uniform of the next nurse to use it.

The early discharge of mothers who are carriers of *Salmonella typhi*, HBV or HIV presents particular problems for community midwives. Salmonella carriers should be careful with their personal hygiene, especially with hand-washing before food preparation and after using the toilet. Simple isolation methods, such as hand-washing and wearing of aprons, are described in Chapter 8, and are equally applicable in the home. A patient infected or colonized with MRSA is not a risk to relatives, but the nurse should be careful to avoid transmitting it to other patients she may subsequently attend. Advice on treatment of carriers may be obtained from the hospital infection control nurse.

If an outbreak of gastroenteritis occurs, hand-washing under running water is again the most important measure. Toilet seats, chamber pots etc. should be washed frequently with a reliable disinfectant, but disinfectants are unnecessary as a routine in the home. Many disinfectants sold to the public are mainly of use as a deodorant, and should not be required if cleaning is satisfactory. Linen from patients with hepatitis or intestinal infection can usually be laundered in the home at the highest temperature the material will withstand, provided care is taken in handling the linen. Cotton or cotton/polyester fabrics should be ironed when dry, using the heat of the iron to destroy any surviving pathogens. Nylon fabrics should be thoroughly dried, preferably out of doors, and stored dry for 48 hours before re-use. Disposal of clinical waste can be a problem. The risk of spread of infection from dressings, incontinence pads and disposable napkins is small. These items can be sealed in a plastic bag and safely discarded with domestic waste, but this may be unacceptable to waste handlers. Arrangements may sometimes be necessary to collect clinical waste for incineration, but this can be expensive. Community nurses should not be expected to carry clinical waste in their cars.

Outbreaks of boils or other superficial sepsis in a family may be caused by strains of *Staph. aureus* brought home from a hospital. Patients should be treated with antibacterial nose creams and antiseptic baths (see Chapter 8). It may be necessary to sample and treat all members of the family (Leigh 1979). Bed linen and underclothes should be laundered at as high a temperature as possible soon after treatment has commenced, and this should be repeated after completion of treatment.

Antibiotic policies are not commonly used in domiciliary practice, but should be introduced. Care is particularly required in the use of topical agents, e.g. gentamicin, mupirocin, fusidic acid, which should not be used except in very special circumstances in hospital. Varicose ulcers and pressure sores are particularly likely to be colonized with antibiotic-resistant *Staph. aureus* and Gram-negative bacilli. If it is thought necessary to use a topical antibiotic, the length of treatment should be no more than 7–10 days. The widespread use of expensive oral agents such as ciprofloxacin will encourage the emergence of resistant strains and restrict the use of a valuable agent for severe infections.

Care is necessary in collection of specimens (Chapter 8) and transport to the laboratory should be as rapid as possible. Urine specimens kept at room temperature for more than three hours may be useless due to growth of contaminants; haemolytic streptococci may die on dry swabs, and sputa are also rapidly overgrown with contaminating Gram-negative bacilli or yeasts.

Further guidance on aseptic and hygienic methods can be obtained from the infection control nurse or infection control doctor at the nearest district general hospital.

16.6.2 DISINFECTION OF LOANED EQUIPMENT

A variety of equipment is available on loan, including hospital beds. Contamination during the period of loan appears to present few practical difficulties.

Generally a deodorant/disinfectant is used, since unpleasant smells are the worst problem.

Decontamination should be done in the home before returning equipment to the central stores. Careful washing, using a detergent such as washing-up liquid, followed by thorough drying is usually adequate, even when the patient was infected. If water cannot be used, 70% alcohol or methylated spirits is effective.

Fabric-covered commodes are widely used and are difficult to disinfect adequately. If the fabric is soiled though not contaminated with known pathogens, a carpet cleaning solution, used in accordance with the manufacturer's instructions, may be effective in improving the appearance of the fabric. If it is contaminated with pathogens, then it should be replaced by the central stores.

Some warning of specific infection risks (e.g. enteric infections) should be given so that equipment can be collected and decontaminated by the hospital. Whenever possible, equipment supplied for home use should be as easy to decontaminate as that used in the hospital.

An area within the central stores of the hospital should be set aside for decontamination of loaned equipment. Adequate sinks and drainage should be available. A member of staff should be properly trained in equipment decontamination techniques.

16.7   Paediatric departments

16.7.1   SPECIAL PROBLEMS OF INFECTION

Many children are admitted to hospital with (or incubating) community-acquired infections. Some of these infections, such as respiratory virus infections, severe gastroenteritis and infected skin lesions, are difficult to keep under control and may spread rapidly. Children are also more susceptible to community-acquired diseases than adults since many have not developed immunity to the common infectious fevers. Most children's wards also contain a few patients who are particularly susceptible, for example those with blood disorders or receiving steroids. The increase in use of invasive techniques has been associated with more infections, including the emergence of the coagulase-negative staphylococcus as a potential pathogen. Patient discipline is understandably rather lax in children's departments and care must be taken to avoid the escape of children from isolation cubicles and misplaced generosity in sharing of toys, dummies, etc.

The organisms which may be involved in cross-infection are many, including viruses such as respiratory syncytial virus (RSV), measles virus, gastroenteritis viruses such as rotavirus, bacteria such as

Group A streptococci, enteropathogenic *E. coli, Campylobacter* spp., fungi such as *Candida albicans*, dermatophytes affecting the scalp, and even skin or intestinal parasites (e.g. cryptosporidium). *Ps. aeruginosa* and *Staph. aureus* are likely to infect children suffering from cystic fibrosis. Outbreaks of tuberculosis occasionally occur in paediatric wards and require special care. Chapter 8 (on isolation and barrier nursing) is particularly relevant to paediatric departments, and procedures are suggested for management of children admitted with community-acquired infections.

16.7.2 PREVENTION OF INFECTION (see also section 16.1 on Maternity departments)

The numbers of nursing staff and the quality of their training are major factors in controlling the spread of infection. It is helpful for senior nursing staff to have some experience of practices in a communicable disease ward.

Isolation facilities are needed for between one in five to one in ten of the patients in the unit, depending on the type of patients admitted. Ideally a separate block for isolation is desirable. Because of the risks of gastroenteritis, no more than four infants should be in any one room and they should preferably be in cubicles with one or two cots only. Adequate washing facilities must be available in each cubicle and each cubicle should have its own weighing machine. Older children should not be in wards with adults. Each ward should have a play room and a separate examination room. There should be beds available to allow some parents to sleep in the hospital. Screening the faeces of all children admitted to paediatric wards for the presence of *Salmonella* spp. has been found useful by some microbiologists, though it is generally not considered practicable or worthwhile.

Outbreaks of rotavirus and RSV infection are particularly common in paediatric wards (see also Chapter 9). Handwashing is important in control of these infections. Rotavirus infection is associated with heavy environmental contamination and the large numbers may be difficult to remove from the hands. The use of gloves is recommended when handling excreta or contaminated materials. An alcoholic hand rub following handwashing is also effective. Prevention of RSV spread to staff is important, and in addition to handwashing staff should be advised to avoid touching the nose and eyes. The use of goggles that cover nose and eyes of staff has been associated with a reduction in infection in the US, although the acceptability of this device remains uncertain.

The increase in IV site infections, often caused by coagulase-negative staphylococci, is mainly associated with central venous catheterization and parenteral feeding. Efficient skin disinfection and care of the site are important requirements (Chapter 7).

There is evidence that frequent and prolonged visiting by parents to their own children does not have any effect on infection rates. It is useful, however, to have a written policy for parents, included in the hospital information booklet, stating that 'parents should consult the ward sister if they have any infection, however trivial, so as to protect other children within the unit whose resistance to infection is poor'. Similar provisos apply to visiting by siblings, but it is advisable to bar children with minor respiratory infections since these may be prodromal signs of measles. Parents should notify staff if a visitor develops a transmissible infection within seven days of visiting, or a patient within the week of discharge. This enables susceptible contacts to be traced. Gowns or plastic aprons should be worn by parents nursing children with gastroenteritis, and handwashing facilities must be available to them, together with instructions on how to avoid acquiring the infection. Visiting of children with dangerous infections, such as diphtheria, poliomyelitis and (for the first 48 hours) meningococcal meningitis, should be restricted to parents and preferably those who are immune, when this is possible.

Visitors should avoid contact with other children.

For preparation of feeds see page 323; for treatment of incubators, suction equipment, thermometers and other equipment, see Chapter 6. Crockery and cutlery need be only domestically clean, but washing in a machine at 70–80°C (158–176°F) is preferred and essential on isolation wards.

16.7.3   TOILET ARRANGEMENTS

Because of the common occurrence of intestinal infections in children, special precautions are necessary for toilet areas and bedpan handling. The toilet areas require a high standard of domestic cleanliness, especially the toilet seat, which should be washed at least daily and more frequently if this is necessary. Spraying the toilet seat and cistern handle with 70% alcohol or cleaning with a clear soluble phenolic (and rinsing) after each patient is useful during outbreaks of gastroenteritis, but attention to handwashing and use of paper towels is of greater importance. A steam or hot water supply capable of destroying vegetative forms of bacteria should be fitted to bedpan washers (Chapter 6).

16.7.4   LAUNDRY

Napkins are sealed in plastic or alginate bags for transport and the bags may be labelled with the words 'used napkins', depending on the laundry policy.

16.7.5   PERSONNEL

Communicable diseases may be acquired by staff from patients if they are not immune and may in turn be passed on to patients and visitors. One of the most important of these is rubella. Staff of both sexes should be screened for immunity to rubella and be immunized if non-immune, because of the number of pregnant women who visit children in hospital. The acquisition of salmonella and shigella by nursing staff can have disastrous effects and most outbreaks of infection in hospital due to these organisms have been associated with the infection in the nursing staff. Herpes simplex infection in attendants may produce a variety of lesions and may cause severe infections in children. Staff with herpetic lesions should not handle babies.

16.7.6   SURVEILLANCE SYSTEMS

A list of patients with infection admitted to the ward or acquired in the ward is useful in the investigation of spread of infection. The infections which are most usefully recorded are those due to salmonella, shigella and enteropathogenic *E. coli*, staphylococcal and streptococcal infections and non-bacterial acute enteritis (as indicated in laboratory reports), and the common infectious diseases.

16.8   Maternity departments

As in paediatric departments, screening of staff, of both sexes, for immunity to rubella is recommended, with immunization of non-immune individuals.

16.8.1   RISKS OF INFECTION

In the maternity department there are three types of patients in whom there are special risks of infection. The antenatal patient is at particular risk only if the fetal membranes have ruptured, allowing access of organisms to the fetus and liquor amnii. The postnatal patient has a large endometrial surface with thrombosed blood vessels which is vulnerable to invasion by many organisms. Wound infection may follow a caesarean section. Thirdly there are problems of the neonate who has very little natural immunity to infection, having come from a sterile environment, and is now meeting bacteria for the first time. Premature or damaged babies are particularly vulnerable to infection. The increased survival of low birth-weight babies has been associated with additional problems of infection.

Almost any organism may give rise to dangerous disease in maternity departments, even those, such as coliforms, enterococci, group B streptococci, coagulase-negative staphylococci or bacteroides, which are often of low pathogenicity; *Staph. aureus* and *Cl. perfringens* are particularly dangerous. The infant may be infected by organisms derived from the mother either *in utero* (rubella, syphilis, tuberculosis, HBV, HIV, cytomegalovirus, toxoplasma, VZ virus, listeria) or during delivery (gonococcal ophthalmia, chlamydial eye infections, salmonellosis) and may be highly infectious. Mothers known to be HBV or HIV carriers may, from time to time, be admitted for delivery. For them special precautions are required (Chapter 10).

Colonization of the child with bacteria begins shortly after birth. The intestinal tract and often the throat are colonized by antibiotic-sensitive coliforms which may be rapidly replaced by resistant strains if the baby is treated with antibiotics. In susceptible infants, these may cause respiratory tract infection, meningitis and septicaemia. Within a few days of delivery, *Staph. aureus* may be found particularly in the flexures and on moist areas of skin (axillae, groin and napkin area) and on the umbilical stump. *Staphylococcus aureus* is found in the throat or nose of many newborn infants after a few days. The carriage of these organisms is usually inconsequential but may be associated with minor skin pustules or eye infections. Severe forms of skin infection, such as bullous impetigo or staphylococcal 'scalded skin syndrome' (epidermolysis bullosa) sometimes occur when strains of staphylococcus, which produce exfoliatin, spread within the hospital. Invasive disease, including septicaemia, osteomyelitis and pneumonia, sometimes occur. Breast abscess may occur in the mother, sometimes weeks after she has been discharged. *Candida albicans* is also common, causing oral and skin infection, and can produce serious disease in weaker babies.

The infant must be guarded, as far as possible, from acquiring a heavy load of pathogenic organisms, for in addition to the risk that it will develop an infection it will in its turn disseminate these organisms into the environment. Poor standards of hygiene may be followed by heavy contamination; good hygiene lowers the risk. Infants are apt to get sticky eyes within a few days of birth; a variety of organisms may be isolated from these and it seems likely that conjunctivitis is often of chemical origin, caused by the antiseptics used during labour. Gonococci, chlamydia, Group B streptococci, staphylococci, coliforms and other organisms should be excluded. Napkin rash is due to the action of bacteria (chiefly coliforms) which produce ammonia and other substances which damage the wet skin.

Spread of infection after delivery is mainly by contact, usually on attendants' hands, with some additional spread of Gram-negative bacilli by way of apparatus or disinfectants, and, less commonly, of staphylococci in the air.

16.8.2 PREVENTION OF SPREAD

Isolation facilities are necessary for both mothers and babies. Maternal diseases requiring isolation include puerperal sepsis, which may be due to a Group A β-haemolytic streptococcus, gastrointestinal infections, breast abscesses, and staphylococcal skin sepsis. Infected neonates should also be placed in isolation as soon as an infection is suspected. It may be necessary to separate infants from their mothers if the latter are infected, particularly in cases of maternal typhoid or shigella infections. Infant nurseries should be small and preferably contain not more than four beds and should be equipped with handwashing basins. Overcrowding and staff shortages may be associated with cross-infection in the nursery. Cross-infection may also be reduced by rooming-in, i.e. keeping the baby in the mother's room. If there are insufficient numbers of small rooms, cohort nursing is a particularly useful routine measure for prevention of infection or for ending an outbreak; babies born over a period of 24 to 48 hours are kept in one nursery; when all these babies are discharged from hospital the room is cleaned if necessary and another batch of babies admitted. A nursery should be designed to allow cohort nursing in the event of an outbreak.

Babies born with gastroenteritis should be isolated immediately. If an infection is severe, or more than two cases occur, the ward should be closed to further admissions. The other infants should be screened and all carriers kept in one nursery. If possible, separate nurses should attend babies in the infected and non-infected nurseries. Nurses preparing feeds should not handle infected babies or their contacts.

As the main method of spread of infection is by way of attendants' hands, these require special care. Hands should be washed after any procedure involving handling of a baby or its immediate environment. Washing with soap and water is usually adequate, but an antiseptic preparation should be used for handwashing by staff in premature baby units and in outbreaks of infection; povidone-iodine, or chlorhexidine-detergent preparations are equally suitable, but use of an alcoholic handrub (see Chapter 6) is equally effective and more convenient. In overcrowded nurseries and during outbreaks of staphylococcal infection, dusting the axillae, groin and umbilicus with hexachlorophane powder until discharge from hospital, but for no longer than seven days, is a safe and effective method of reducing staphylococcal colonization. Chlorhexidine bathing is also effective and may be introduced during outbreaks of infection (p. 174). Baths should be thoroughly cleaned and disinfected between patients (Chapter 6). Masks are unnecessary in nurseries. Gowns or aprons should be worn and changed regularly, but not necessarily after attending each baby. Separate gowns or aprons should be worn for handling babies in special care units, but are not necessary if the baby is not removed from the incubator. Specific procedures requiring standardization are napkin changing and disposal, bottle feeding, tube feeding and bathing. Napkins should be disposed of into a bucket lined with a plastic bag which is sealed when full. Alginate or hot water-soluble bags may also be used. Disposable napkins should be considered during outbreaks of infections. Separate sterile catheters should be used for each tube feed and discarded after use. If not disposable, catheters should be processed in the SSD and autoclaved. If it is necessary to leave the tube *in situ* for feeding (e.g. nasal catheters), its use should be limited to essential times only.

Although the administration of antibiotics may be necessary as soon as infection of a neonate is suspected, the widespread use of chemoprophylaxis is not recommended. The use of antibiotics selects resistant strains of bacteria, including *Klebsiella* and *Enterobacter* spp, *Ps. aeruginosa* and *Serratia marcescens*. The prevalence of resistant bacteria (e.g. gentamicin-resistant organisms in nurseries) should be determined from time to time as a guide to the choice of antibiotics for treating undiagnosed infections arising in the unit.

The sterile services department (SSD) can provide much of the equipment needed in maternity departments. Delivery packs, episiotomy sets, dressings and sterile sanitary pads are routine supplies in most hospitals. In addition, as far as possible the SSD should sterilize equipment for preparing special feeds on the wards, and the containers and teats and tube feeding equipment for neonates. Cleaning and disinfection of incubators and suction equipment is also best carried out in the SSD if conveniently near. If incubators must be processed in the maternity department, space must be set aside for this purpose and procedures similar to those used in SSD (Chapter 6) followed.

Disinfection of teats and bottles on wards should be regarded as second best to presterilized feeds or SSD processing. Milk kitchens and infant feeds are discussed below.

The risks of infection spreading from workers in the unit to the patients are similar to those in other wards, but two special infections, herpes (facial lesions or herpetic whitlow of the fingers) and candida paronychia, are readily spread to neonates; attendants with these lesions should be excluded while infected.

Colonization of the genital tract with group B streptococci occurs in up to 40% of pregnant females. Many are carriers early in pregnancy whilst others only become colonized immediately preterm, making screening logistically difficult. Antibiotics make little difference to the spontaneous loss of the carrier state. Not all babies become colonized from their mother and less than 1% of these develop overt infection. For these reasons we do not recommend routine screening. Group B streptococcal infection must be borne in mind in any sick neonate, particularly the low birth-weight or premature, and in those with respiratory distress.

Some maternity units require nose and throat swabs from new members of staff before starting work, to exclude carriers of pathogenic staphylococci and streptococci, but most units have abandoned these procedures without ill-effect. Other routine screening systems have been suggested, including that of mothers for carriage of *Salmonella* or *Shigella* spp. before admission to the unit. These suggestions followed the occurrence of several outbreaks of gastroenteritis in maternity departments, but are impractical as a routine procedure. *Salmonella* spp. may not be detected even if present; the organisms may be acquired after the faeces have been examined and some infected patients are unbooked. Furthermore, most laboratories could either not offer such a service without reducing their more essential services, or if they did, the examination would be of poor quality and without significant value. However, if there is reason to suspect a patient of having a gastrointestinal infection or of being a *Salmonella* or *Shigella* carrier, her faeces must be examined and she must immediately be isolated. After delivery of a patient with enteric fever, careful follow-up of other patients in the unit is necessary.

Surveillance of infections is particularly important in neonatal wards, so that immediate action may be taken to prevent extension of an outbreak.

16.8.3 MANAGEMENT OF DELIVERY OF MOTHERS WHO ARE CARRIERS OF HBV OR HIV

The recommended precautions are described in Chapter 10.

16.9 Preparation of infant feeds and use of milk kitchens

Milk is an excellent growth medium for most pathogenic or potentially pathogenic bacteria and contamination of feeds is a particular hazard in neonatal nurseries. Although there is little published evidence that contaminated feeds have caused outbreaks of infection, it seems likely that such outbreaks have occurred more commonly than reported. Many organisms, sometimes in large numbers, have been isolated from feeds, for example *Salmonella* spp., enteropathogenic and other strains of *E. coli*, Group A and other Groups of β-haemolytic streptococci,

Candida albicans, Proteus spp., *Klebsiella* and *Pseudomonas* spp., *Staph. aureus* and many other organisms.

Contamination of feed can occur due to faulty disinfection of bottles, teats, dispensing and mixing equipment. Milk, water or other additives may be contaminated prior to use. Recontamination or additional contamination can occur at any time during the preparation process or when feeding the baby. This may be from the air, from the hands of preparation room or ward staff or from the mother.

Usually the initial contamination of the feed is low, and the main hazard is storage at room temperature for a sufficient time to allow organisms to grow. An additional hazard is warming the feed in a contaminated sink or container immediately before administration.

All feeds must be free from intestinal pathogens. The greatest hazard is from these organisms, but other bacteria (e.g. *Proteus* and *Klebsiella* spp.), may cause infection if abundant.

The hazard of a major outbreak is much increased if one milk kitchen supplies feeds for all babies in a large unit.

16.9.1   PREFERRED METHODS

Commercially supplied pre-sterilized or, if locally produced, terminally sterilized or heat-disinfected feeds should be used in all of the larger maternity units (e.g. over 50 beds with a single milk kitchen). The choice of methods must be made on the basis of effectiveness, economy, availability of staff and space.

Where possible, one of these methods should be introduced into all maternity units. When feeds are sterilized or disinfected by heat, controls to ensure exposure of the feed for the required time at the correct temperature are necessary. Charts showing this information should be regularly inspected by the head of the department. Disinfection by heat, including pasteurization in a specially designed machine, is satisfactory if the processes are adequate; in these instances bacteriological tests should also be made at intervals (e.g. monthly). Commercially prepared presterilized feeds should be bacteriologically safe, provided their control and testing process is satisfactory. Bottles and caps should be inspected before use for obvious damage, and if any doubt exists the bottle should be discarded. Commercially supplied presterilized feeds with the teat already attached to the bottle and adequately protected from contamination are preferable. Single-use tears packed separately are almost as satisfactory, if put on (preferably by the mother) immediately before giving the feed. If teats are used repeatedly, they should be thoroughly cleaned and autoclaved after each use.

16.9.2   OTHER METHODS

Chemical disinfection of bottles and teats (by hypochlorite) is reliable if correctly performed, but more difficult to control than those methods already described and more susceptible to individual staff errors. The hypochlorite method of disinfection is suitable for use in small units and at home. The hazard of infection in large, well controlled units using chemical methods is not very great if dispensing equipment involving taps which can be easily taken apart and autoclaved are used, and if disinfection is well supervised. Bottles and teats should be thoroughly cleaned before disinfection or sterilization by any method, but particularly prior to chemical disinfection. The disinfectant solution should be made up to the correct strength (hypochlorite – 125 ppm available chlorine). All equipment should be completely immersed, with removal of air bubbles, and should be left for at least the recommended time. Autoclaving of bottles and teats is preferable to chemical disinfection because of the greater reliability of the process. Boiling, correctly performed, should also be more reliable than a chemical method, but the boiling of bottles and teats in an open container is difficult to control and is not recommended.

16.9.3   PAEDIATRIC FEEDS

The recommendations are similar to those for maternity units. Commercially prepared feeds are often not suitable, since a number of babies may require special feeds. Arrangements for terminal sterilization, or autoclaving of bottles and teats, are still necessary in these units.

16.9.4   MILK KITCHEN AND STAFF (Burnett *et al.* 1989)

For hospitals where commercially prepared presterilized feeds are used a clean store-room is all that is required. In small units a kitchen which is used only for preparation of feeds is required. In all milk kitchens, washing up of used bottles, teats and other equipment should be carried out in a room separate from that used for preparing feeds. A hand-washing basin should be available immediately adjacent to the milk kitchen. Staff should be trained in techniques of feed preparation, and in personal hygiene. The training should include methods of preventing contamination, for example thorough cleaning of equipment, and the reduction of airborne and contact transfer by hands to a minimum. The preparation of feeds should, if possible, be carried out by staff not handling babies and supervised by a senior member of the nursing staff. After preparation, feeds (unless sterilized) should be placed in a refrigerator (4°C; 39°F) preferably within 30 and not more than 60 min.

Non-sterile feeds should be discarded after 24 hours. Supplements should be added to the feed immediately before use.

Newborn infants will usually accept a feed at room temperature and, if possible, warming before use should be avoided. If the feed is warmed, a special container should be used and kept for this purpose only. The container should be filled with boiled water, or with fresh water and boiled for five minutes. The bottle with intact teat cover should be placed in the container at body temperature, and the water level should be well below the neck of the bottle. After use the container should be immediately emptied, cleaned and dried.

16.9.5 HUMAN EXPRESSED BREAST MILK

Human milk contains antimicrobial factors which are believed to provide some protection to premature infants against infection. These factors may be heat-labile, although the inactivating effect of pasteurization on the antimicrobial factors at relatively low temperatures such as 63–65°C (145–149°F) remains to some extent uncertain. Inadequately collected or stored milk may be heavily contaminated with potential pathogens such as *Klebsiella* spp., *Ps. aeruginosa* and *Staph. aureus*. Unless microbiological tests are made on all samples, apart from milk from the mother fed to her own baby, pasteurization is required.

To ensure milk of an acceptable microbiological standard, careful attention must be paid to hygienic methods of collection. These high standards are more easily attained in hospital than in the home. Potential donors should be free of infection including HBV and HIV, not excreting drugs in the milk, and able to produce sufficient milk to make collection worthwhile. They should be trained in aseptic practices and supplied with suitable equipment for disinfection. The home conditions should be hygienically acceptable. In addition, several samples should be tested microbiologically before the donor is accepted. Instructions on collection and storage should be clear and precise, and should include hand-washing, care of the breast, and methods of cleaning, disinfection and storage of the pump. Whenever possible, sterilized equipment should be supplied. The first 5–10 ml of milk should be discarded and the remainder transferred to a sterile bottle which is labelled with the time of collection, storage time and temperature. It must be placed in a refrigerator as soon as possible at 4°C (39°F) and the temperature during transport should not be allowed to rise above 10°C (50°F). The time out of the refrigerator should not exceed two hours, and refrigerated transport or insulated containers may be required for transport.

Although samples are collected from HIV negative mothers, pasteurization is still advisable, but excessive heating should be avoided.

Exposure at 65°C (149°F) for 10 minutes is recommended. The process must be carefully controlled and temperatures checked with a thermometer initially and at regular intervals afterwards. A standard volume of milk should be treated, and should be cooled rapidly. As well as temperature checks, microbiological tests should be made on setting up the process and at regular intervals afterwards. Milk should be deep frozen (9–28°C; −18°F) as quickly as possible after collection, and repeated heating and freezing avoided.

16.9.6 MICROBIOLOGICAL STANDARDS

Since the numbers of organisms required to infect the infant – as well as the role of relatively non-pathogenic organisms – remain uncertain, proposed standards are variable. The resistance of the infant to infection is also variable and the possible deleterious effect of pasteurization is uncertain. It is generally agreed that Gram-negative bacilli should be absent, but the acceptable numbers of *Staph. aureus* or of the normal skin flora are controversial. Some authorities accept the presence of normal flora up to 10^8/ml (Carroll *et al.* 1979), but we prefer higher standards and suggest the following:

1. total counts should not be above 10^5 organisms/ml;
2. *Staph. aureus* should preferably be absent and not above 10^2/ml;
3. no Enterobacteriaceae, pseudomonas, other Gram-negative bacilli or groupable streptococci should be present.

Although there is little evidence of infection occurring from milk containing much larger numbers of normal flora or *Staph. aureus*, it seems illogical to have lower standards than would be acceptable for milk feeds for normal infants. It is obviously safer to pasteurize all breast milk before use. An exception would be freshly expressed milk which is given to the woman's own infant.

References and further reading

British Medical Association (1989) *A Code of Practice for Sterilization of Instruments and Control of Cross-infection.* BMA, London.

British Medical Association (1990) *A Code of Practice for the Safe Use and Disposal of Sharps.* BMA, London.

Burnett, I.A., Wardley, B.L. and Magee, J.T. (1989) The milk kitchen Sheffield Children's Hospital before and after a review. *Journal of Hospital Infection*, **13**, 179.

Carroll, L., Osman, M., Davies, D.P. and McNeish, A.S. (1976) Bacteriological criteria for feeding raw milk to babies on neonatal units. *Lancet*, **ii**, 732.

Craven, D.E. and Steger, K.A. (1989) Nosocomial pneumonia in the intubated patient. In Nosocomial infections: new issues and strategies for prevention. (Eds D.J. Weber and W.A. Rutala) *Infectious Disease Clinics of North America*. W.B. Saunders, Philadelphia, London.

Department of Health and Social Security (1975) *Preservation of Sterility in Ophthalmic Preparations in Hospitals*. Health Service Circular HSC(75)122. HMSO, London.

Hoffman, P.N., Cooke, E.M., Larkin, D.P., *et al.* (1988) Control of infection in general practice: a survey and recommendations. *British Medical Journal*, **297**, 34.

Ledingham, I., McAlcock, S.R., Eastaway, A.T., *et al.* (1988) Triple regime of selective decontamination of the digestive tract, systemic cefotaxime and microbiological surveillance for prevention of acquired infection in intensive care. *Lancet*, **i**, 785.

Leigh, D.A. (1979) Treatment of familial staphylococcal infection. *Journal of Antimicrobial Chemotherapy*, **5**, 497.

Lowbury, E.J.L. (1976) Prophylaxis and treatment for infection of burns. *British Journal of Hospital Medicine*, **16**, 566.

Lowbury, E.J.L. (1992) Special problems in hospital antisepsis. In *Principles and Practice of Disinfection, Preservation and Sterilization*, 2nd ed. (Eds A.D. Russell, W.B. Hugo and G.A.J. Ayliffe) Blackwell Scientific Publications, Oxford.

Ophthalmic Society of the United Kingdom (1973) The sterilization of surgical instruments. *Transactions of the Ophthalmic Society of the UK*, **92**, 539.

Stoutenbeek, C.P., van Saene, H.K.F., Miranda, D.R. *et al.* (1984) The effect of selective decontamination of the digestive tract on colonization and infection rate in multiple trauma patients. *Intensive Care Medicine*, **10**, 185.

van Saene, H.K.F., Stoutenbeek, L.P. and McA Ledingham, I. (1989) Update in intensive care and emergency medicine/infection control by selective decontamination. Springer–Verlag, Berlin, Heidelberg.

Wenzel, R.P., Thompson, R.L., Landry, S.M. *et al.* (1983) Hospital acquired infections in intensive care unit patients: an overview with emphasis on epidemics. *Infection Control*, **4**, 371.

17 Special wards and departments II

17.1 Neurosurgery departments

The meninges are particularly susceptible to infection, and clinical infection may be caused, through contamination occurring at operation or during a lumbar or ventricular puncture, by Gram-negative bacilli of low pathogenicity, as well as by the usual organisms causing wound infection. Infections caused by these opportunistic organisms, e.g. *Ps. aeruginosa*, *Serratia marcescens* and flavobacteria, have occurred because of inadequate sterilization or maintenance of sterility of instruments or water applied topically. Organisms normally present on the skin (e.g. coagulase-negative staphylococci) which are usually of low pathogenicity may also cause low grade infections, particularly in association with Spitz-Holter valves. Infections may be transmitted on the hands of staff from infected patients or following the use of contaminated nailbrushes, hand-creams, soaps or detergents. Inadequate disinfection of the patient's skin pre-operatively, or use of contaminated shaving equipment, may also be followed by infection. As regards other types of infection, neurosurgical units have the same problems as other departments, and some neurosurgical patients are in hospital for long periods. They may have indwelling catheters, and tracheostomy or endotracheal intubation is sometimes necessary. Patients with ear infection may be admitted to the unit. Unconscious patients are apt to acquire chest infections or bedsores. Although cerebral abscesses are usually endogenous in origin, hospital strains of Gram-negative bacilli and *Staph. aureus* are likely to spread in the ward and be acquired in the nasal and intestinal flora to become a potential source of endogenous infection unless effective control measures are employed.

17.1.1 PREVENTION OF INFECTION

Isolation and barrier-nursing of infected patients, particularly of patients with pseudomonas infection, are important in neurosurgical units. Dressings of wounds exposing the meninges should, if possible, be changed in the operating theatre or, if not, in a plenum-ventilated dressing room; the patient's own single-bedded room, if the facilities are adequate, may be suitable for many of the routine procedures. Special wards are required for intensive care treatment, including patients with tracheostomies (see the section on Intensive care units in Chapter 16). Other procedures, e.g. lumbar puncture and catheterization, may be carried out in non-specialized wards; the relevant precautions are described elsewhere (Chapter 7). Pre-operative shaving should be carried out on the day of operation, to avoid the possibility that small scratches or excoriations which sometimes occur might become heavily colonized. Shaving either of head hair or of pubic hair for vertebral angiography should be completed before disinfection of scalp or skin. Shaving brushes should not be used; razors should be sterilized or adequately disinfected and individual sterilized gauze swabs should be used for applying shaving cream. If shaving cream is used, it should contain an antiseptic which prevents the growth of organisms that might cause infection. A povidone-iodine shampoo or chlorhexidine detergent may also be used before shaving. Subsequent skin preparation in the operating theatre is carried out with 0.5% alcoholic chlorhexidine. Equipment for aseptic procedures should be autoclaved, and SSD packs supplied whenever possible, e.g. for lumbar puncture, catheterization, wound dressing and tracheostomy toilet. Particular care is required to avoid contamination of lotions. If aspiration of an effusion from a craniotomy wound is required, insert the needle through intact skin and not through the suture line. Organisms may enter the bloodstream from monitoring equipment and set up an infection at the operation site. This equipment should be regularly disinfected or sterilized, preferably by heat.

17.2 Urological units

Urinary tract infection is the commonest type of acquired infection in hospitals. Many patients already have urinary infection when they enter the unit, but instrumentation and operations on the urinary tract can lead to infection, either by introducing organisms into a previously uninfected tract or by replacing the existing organisms with hospital strains which are more resistant to antibiotic therapy (Slade and Gillespie 1985).

Although some patients acquire urinary tract infections without having had instrumentation, most infections follow catheterization, cystoscopy, drainage or more extensive operative procedures. In particular, the indwelling catheter can be hazardous and, if precautions are not taken to prevent contamination, the incidence of bladder infections in patients on continuous drainage approaches 100% after a few days.

17.2.1 ROUTES OF CONTAMINATION AND CROSS INFECTION

The entry of bacteria into the bladder may occur either through the lumen of the catheter or between the catheter and the wall of the urethra. Both routes are important and every effort is needed to close both.

The organisms most likely to be found in urological patients with urinary tract infection vary. If there has not been any manipulation of the urinary tract the organisms are usually *E. coli* or *Proteus mirabilis* sensitive to many common antibiotics, such as sulphonamides, ampicillin and nitrofurantoin. In hospital-acquired infections *Klebsiella* spp., indole-positive *Proteus* spp., *Ps. aeruginosa* and *Strep. faecalis* are commoner. Less frequent are *Acinetobacter* spp. and *Providencia* spp. These organisms are usually resistant to many antibiotics and may prove difficult to eradicate. They are likely to spread to other patients. The emergence of strains resistant to gentamicin and the newer agents such as the third generation cephalosporins and the isoquinolones is particularly worrying as they limit the available treatment in a unit. These organisms are commonly associated with indwelling catheterization and the mode of spread is thought to be mainly on the hands. The management of catheterized patients is discussed in Chapter 7, p. 129. However, some attention should be given to the environment, for example disinfection of bedpans and urinals by heat (not a tank of disinfectant), correct drying and stacking of washbowls, disinfection by heat or use of disposable containers for emptying urine bags and urine testing equipment, and adequate disinfection of baths etc.

Urine from patients with renal tuberculosis should be disposed of with care. The bottle used for collecting the urine must be disinfected and the patient should have his own urine bottle. Collection of specimens for laboratory examination should be made directly into a sterile universal container. The use of the urine bottle as an intermediary container has often given false positive results, because of failure to decontaminate the bottle between patients.

Although routine microbiological monitoring of the environment is not recommended, periodic surveys of the microbial flora in the environment serve a useful educational function and may bring to light defects in cleaning. Single room isolation is not usually recommended for Gram-negative infections, but this may be advisable to eradicate a highly resistant strain from a unit. Restriction of certain antibiotics may be desirable.

17.3   Out-patients and casualty departments

Since many of the patients who attend out-patient departments have recently been in hospital wards, their wounds and other lesions may be infected with antibiotic-resistant Gram-negative bacilli and *Staph. aureus* which they acquired in hospital. Patients with skin diseases may have been treated with a variety of antibiotics and are also likely to be carrying antibiotic-resistant strains. Most patients with infections are either carrying or infected with antibiotic-sensitive strains, which are usually less transmissible than hospital organisms; the risk of cross-infection with Gram-negative bacilli and *Staph. aureus* in out-patient or casualty departments is less than in wards but, owing to the large number of patients attending out-patient departments, there is a high risk of spread of community-acquired infections, e.g. measles, influenza etc. The consequences may be severe if a case of undiagnosed Lassa fever is brought into the department.

Many patients are also particularly susceptible to infection (e.g. those with immunodeficiency diseases) and they may come into close contact with infected patients. The range of surgical procedures carried out in out-patient theatres is increasing, and clean operations may alternate with incisions of abscesses. Diagnostic procedures, such as endoscopy, are also now more frequently done in out-patient departments.

17.3.1   PREVENTION OF INFECTION

Surgical procedures should, when possible, be carried out in a mechanically ventilated operating theatre; aseptic and cleaning techniques should correspond to those used in the main operating theatres (Chapter 10). These recommendations are particularly applicable to the types of operation which previously required admission to hospital for several days, though the wearing of masks and caps is not essential for incision of abscesses. The risk of airborne spread of infection after drainage of abscesses to patients subsequently undergoing operations in the same operating room is not great, especially if the theatre is mechanically ventilated, but precautions against contact spread, for example adequate cleaning of operating tables, are necessary. The general principles of prevention of infection are similar to those which apply in other areas in the hospital and a few reliable techniques will reduce the risk to a minimum. Accident departments may be associated with considerable blood spillage from injured persons. Wearing of gloves and a plastic apron for handling wounds is advised. Facilities for minor surgery and for dressing wounds should be adequate, with rooms for laying-up of trolleys and disposal of contaminated dressings and linen.

Sufficient hand-washing basins and disposable paper towels should be provided for the staff. Hand-washing by the staff between handling patients and before and after procedures is one of the most important measures. Wearing of a gown or plastic apron when handling infected patients and covering of couches with paper or a cleanable plastic material when examining potentially infected patients are also useful measures. Linen should be changed after use on an infected patient, and at least daily. Gowns for patients to wear during examination should preferably be disposable, but owing to expense and since the risk of transfer of infection is usually not great, it may be necessary to use gowns for a whole morning or afternoon session. A separate gown should be provided for patients with infections or with a skin disease in which heavy skin colonization by potential pathogens is likely. Some segregation of patients is also advisable; in particular, hypersusceptible patients should not be mixed with those who are likely to be infected (e.g. chronic bronchitics with leukaemics, or dermatological with surgical cases). A separate clinic for patients with varicose ulcers may also be advisable.

Facilities should be provided for examination of patients with communicable disease. A room, which can be fumigated, is required for isolation of cases of suspected viral haemorrhagic fever and other dangerous or highly transmissible infections; and a routine for management of these cases must be available (Chapter 9). Plentiful supplies of specula and other instruments, either disposable or provided by the SSD, should be available in the departments. If not available, such equipment should be sterilized in a small autoclave. Disinfection by chemicals or by boiling should be avoided if possible; although disinfection by immersion of a clean instrument in 70% alcohol, with or without 0.5% chlorhexidine, or by boiling in water for five minutes, is effective (against vegetative organisms and most viruses), it should rarely be necessary to do without proper sterilization. Inexpensive autoclaves are now available. Instruments and needles should be stored in a dry state and not in chemical disinfectants. They should be disinfected by heat immediately before use, or, if possible, sterilized in the SSD and supplied in packs. A routine for disinfection of endoscopes and other instruments which are heat-labile and of emergency equipment should be known and always followed in the department (Chapter 7). The use of 2% glutaraldehyde should be avoided if possible except for disinfection of endoscopes. If used, adequate safety precautions are required (p. 96).

17.4   Radiology and radiotherapy departments

17.4.1   RADIOGRAPHY

Patients are brought to this department from all parts of the hospital and from the community. Patients coming from different wards may be responsible for spread of infection between wards. The radiographers also visit patients in the wards and may transmit infection on their hands or clothing or on equipment. The principles of control are similar to those which apply in other areas of the hospital. The staff should be informed of any patient with communicable disease sent to their department, or if an x-ray is required on such a patient in the ward. In the ward, the radiographers should follow the recommended barrier-nursing routine, paying particular attention to hand-washing and gowning techniques. Similar procedures may be necessary if the patient is brought to their department, and it may be necessary to cover the x-ray table with disposable paper, or to disinfect it after use. X-ray equipment is not an important source of infection, and routine cleaning with a detergent and allowing it to dry will usually be sufficient. Cleaning the equipment between patients is not necessary, except when a patient is known to be infected. Disinfection by wiping over with 70% alcohol is quick and fairly effective and it may be necessary after x-raying an infected patient, or on taking the equipment into the operating theatre; wiping with other disinfectant solutions is rarely necessary. For cleaning of the environment, see Chapter 7.

Many procedures involving aseptic techniques are now carried out in the x-ray department, and facilities should be adequate, including a hand-washing basin. The room used for such procedures should be well ventilated and unnecessary equipment should be excluded; it should, if possible, be reserved for procedures involving aseptic techniques. As few people as possible should be in the room during the procedure, particularly if a catheter remains *in situ*. Good surgical techniques are as necessary for these procedures as they are in operating theatres. Instruments and dressings should be supplied by the SSD. The use of patients' gowns is described in the section on Out-patient departments.

17.4.2   RADIOTHERAPY

Patients treated in this department may be particularly susceptible to infection, for example, immunosuppressed patients, or those with low natural immunity; if in wards, these patients should be nursed in single-bed cubicles with full protective isolation precautions (see Chapter 8). Special skills are often necessary in nursing these patients, and suitably trained staff should be available. Other patients (e.g. those with fungating carcinoma or with thrush) may be sources of infection. Isolation of these patients and techniques to prevent contact infection, such as hand-washing and wearing of plastic gowns, are necessary. The protection of examination couches and provision of patients' gowns are discussed above (see Section on Out-patients and casualty). Equipment used is often difficult to sterilize or disinfect. Whenever possible it should be autoclaved and supplied in packs by the SSD. If the equipment is heat-labile, ethylene oxide or low-temperature steam and formaldehyde is preferred to chemical solutions.

Immersion in 2% glutaraldehyde or preferably 70% alcohol (with or without 0.5% chlorhexidine for 5–10 minutes) will be appropriate for most other purposes, but great care is necessary in rinsing (or drying, with alcohol alone) if the equipment is likely to contact mucous membranes or the conjunctiva. If possible, the use of glutaraldehyde should be avoided owing to toxicity, but if used the precautions should meet safety requirements. For rapid disinfection of surfaces of larger items of equipment, wiping with 70% alcohol is satisfactory and preferable to aqueous disinfectants.

It is essential that x-ray staff are trained in aseptic techniques and control of infection, and that the system for warning the radiological department of infection hazards is effective. This applies particularly to patients with or at high risk of blood-borne infection to ensure appropriate precautions are taken.

17.5 Physiotherapy departments

Physiotherapists treat many ill or infected patients and move from one patient to another and from ward to ward. Infected wounds are exposed during certain treatments. Patients are handled and the opportunities for contact transfer of infection are high. Patients attend the physiotherapy department from all parts of the hospital and from outside. Infection from patients with wounds or skin lesions may readily be transferred on couches, equipment, other fomites and on the hands of the staff. Treatment with wax or water baths and in hydrotherapy units may aid the spread of infection. Fungal infection of the feet may be spread in the gymnasium, particularly if patients exercise with bare feet or wear communal shoes.

17.5.2 PREVENTION OF INFECTION

The physiotherapy department should be informed of patients known to have a communicable disease or hospital infection which could spread to other patients. Meticulous care in hand-washing before and after handling any patient, and wearing a plastic apron when treating an infected patient, are important. This applies both to wards and to the physiotherapy department. Infected wounds should be effectively sealed whenever possible with an impermeable dressing during treatment and contaminated dressings should only be handled with forceps or plastic gloves. The department should have adequate facilities for dressing wounds and lesions, a comprehensive SSD supply and an effective disposal system for contaminated linen and dressings. Recommended aseptic dressing techniques should be used. Other facilities are described in the sections on wards and out-patients, but, in particular, treatment couches should be covered with paper or cleaned after each infected patient. Bedding should be changed after use by an infected patient and at least daily. Physiotherapists should also be aware of 'blood and body fluid' precautions and techniques for source and protective isolation.

The skin of the hands of patients undergoing paraffin wax treatment should be inspected, and any patients with an infected lesion should not be treated until healed; if this is not possible they should wear polythene gloves. Patients should wash their hands before and after treatment and used wax should be heated to disinfect before being returned to the wax bath.

17.6   The hydrotherapy unit

17.6.1   THE HYDROTHERAPY POOL

A variety of infections have been attributed to hydrotherapy and recreational pools. These include skin infections and otitis externa caused by *Ps. aeruginosa*, and more recently legionella infection. Dermatophyte infections of the feet are acquired from the area surrounding the pool. Good hygienic standards are required, particularly the pools used by hospital patients. A senior physiotherapist trained in hydrotherapy and pool management should be in charge and responsible for daily maintenance. A daily log should be kept of cleanliness, bathing load, pH and chlorine concentration and temperature. The physiotherapist should collaborate with the engineer and microbiologist to ensure correct conditions are maintained (Penny 1991; PHLS 1990). If any health problems occur they should be reported immediately to the infection control doctor or occupational health physician. Clean footwear should be worn in the pool area.

The following are some of the important measures required.

1. Patients should be adequately prepared, e.g. emptying of bladder,

ensuring safe bladder drainage, and bowel evacuation of incontinent patients before entering the pool.

2. Patients' feet and skin should be inspected for infected lesions.
3. Patients should take showers before entering the water and after leaving it.
4. Everyone entering the water must step through a footbath containing a hypochlorite or an iodophor solution. Use of a mycostatic powder after bathing might have some value.
5. Patients should keep the same swimsuit for the duration of their course of teatment, and the suit should be laundered after each attendance.
6. The water is continually circulating and is treated daily for adequacy of chlorination. Residual chlorine levels should be maintained at 1.5–3.00 mg/1 (ppm). Periodically, bacteriological tests should be made on the water.
7. Contamination of poolside with urine or faeces should be cleaned immediately with a solution containing 1000 ppm of free chlorine. 'Shock' chlorination of the pool (2–5 fold higher than normal levels) may be required after heavy faecal pollution.
8. Floors should be washed down each evening with pool water, and at least weekly with a solution containing 200 mg/l available chlorine.

17.6.2 THE GYMNASIUM

1. All patients should be inspected for skin infections, especially of the feet (e.g. athlete's foot).
2. Patients should be issued with a pair of shorts which are kept by them for the course of treatment and sent to the hospital laundry upon completion of treatment.
3. Staff should wear special training shoes which are kept only for the gymnasium.
4. Patients should wear preferably their own or disinfected gym shoes when entering the gymnasium.
5. The gymnasium, patient toilet and changing room floors should be cleaned each evening.
6. Equipment should be washed at regular intervals.
7. Patients should be encouraged to take a shower after their classes and be supplied with towels.

17.6.3 TRAINING

Physiotherapists should be trained in aseptic methods and control of infection.

17.7   Pharmaceutical department

The pharmaceutical department issues medicinal products, disinfectants and other related preparations to wards and departments and sometimes to other hospitals; it has an important responsibility for preventing hospital infection caused by the use of contaminated supplies of these products. The department also has an important role in monitoring and implementing antibiotic and disinfectant policies in collaboration with the infection control team.

Medicinal products for injection into blood or for instillation into tissues or viscera which are normally sterile must be provided sterile. Though sterility is not essential for preparations which are ingested or applied to surfaces which have a normal microbial flora (skin, mouth, vagina), pathogens must be excluded and large numbers of any microorganisms must be avoided in these products. Contamination may occur due to inadequate sterilization of preparations required sterile, or to the subsequent acquisition of microorganisms by sterilized or aseptically prepared medicaments through inadequate storage or handling. Safeguards to prevent contamination by either of these channels are necessary. Aqueous solutions, which may allow bacterial growth during storage, present a special hazard. Unlike human tissues, pharmaceutical preparations cannot protect themselves against small numbers of bacteria, so the degree of environmental cleanliness in areas where aseptic dispensing is carried out must be very high. Areas where fluids are being prepared for sterilization do not demand such a high standard of environment as those used for aseptic preparation of medicaments which are not to be sterilized. Nevertheless, strict measures are currently in force as an insurance policy against unforeseen hazards.

17.7.1   STERILE PHARMACEUTICAL PRODUCTS

Sterile medicinal products and pharmaceutical preparations are produced in pharmaceutical departments having specialized facilities as described in the Guide to Good Pharmaceutical Manufacturing Practice (1977) (known as GMP). The manufacture of medicinal products is controlled by the application of the Medicines Act 1968 to Health Authorities (DHSS 1975), and manufacturing activities are inspected by the Medicines Inspectorate and approved by the Medicines Division, Department of Health.

Products to be terminally sterilized are prepared under standard 'clean room' environmental conditions to Class 2 specifications of BS 5295 (BSI 1976) Parts 1–3, other sterile airflow work stations provide Class 1 environmental conditions. These are solutions to be sterilized by filtration, admixtures of sterile solutions, and radiopharmaceuticals.

The standards suggested for preparing products for terminal steriliz-ation, although required in industry, are rather excessive and not related to risks of infection. A clean room with natural ventilation and good hygienic methods by staff should be adequate.

Pharmaceutical production now has quality control built into its procedures, so that the quality, safety and efficacy of the manufactured product is assured. Final product analysis and testing of samples for sterility completes the quality control procedure before the product is released for use in the hospital. Sterility testing of samples must not, however, be regarded as providing guarantees of sterility – nothing short of tests on the whole batch could provide that. It can, of course, provide evidence of gross or moderate contamination; but since bacteria can grow rapidly from very small numbers in many solutions, the value of sample testing, though cumulative, is uncertain, and the main emphasis in producing sterile pharmaceuticals must rely on other cri-teria.

Sterile production units concentrate on the non-commercially avail-able sterile preparations required to treat patients in hospital; e.g. sterile topical solutions, antiseptic solutions, solutions for irrigation and injec-tions.

Further details of the requirements to produce sterile pharmaceuticals are set out in the GMP (1977) where guidelines are given for personnel and training, documentation, work flow systems, changing rooms, preparation and filling rooms, sterilizing, and product quarantine area. Equipment should be designed, located, and maintained to suit the processes and products for which it is to be used; for example autoclaves should have planned operational and maintenance programmes as rec-ommended by the DHSS (1980).

Sterile pharmaceuticals are also prepared as a dispensing service for named patients. This specialized service is available for injections, creams, powders, and sterile medicinal products required for the treat-ment of patients without undue delay.

A back-up service of drug information is provided by the pharmaceut-ical department. Whenever possible, pharmaceutical preparations are supplied in unit-dose packs, to minimize bacterial contamination of the preparations; for example, eyedrops may be supplied in single-dose applicator packs, tablets in unit-dose strip packs, injections in single-dose glass containers, and oral mixtures in small volume containers for use by a single patient. As pharmaceuticals are good media for bacterial growth, opened containers should be exposed for a minimal period of time. As a rough guide, injections should be administered at once and any residue discarded, oral mixtures may be kept for up to 10–14 days after opening, whilst tablets can be kept for a longer time, if properly stored for an indefinite period, or until the activity of the drug diminishes or alters. A practicable storage time of 28 days for tablets has been suggested.

17.7.2   WORK OF THE PHARMACEUTICAL DEPARTMENT

The work in pharmaceutical departments is segregated into a number of specialized areas. Sterile products are manufactured in controlled production areas; those terminally sterilized by heating in an autoclave are prepared in Clean Rooms. Thermolabile preparations are produced in Aseptic Rooms which have a very high standard of cleanliness. The prepacking of tablets takes place in rooms provided with dust extraction facilities to minimize contamination. Oral mixtures and ointments are prepared in manufacturing areas maintained to the requisite standards laid down in the GMP (1977).

It is of greatest importance that an efficient workflow pattern should obtain in manufacturing areas so that every product is subjected to the full quality assurance procedures before it is released from quarantine for administration to patients.

The work flow in the pharmacy should not permit 'dirty' returned containers from wards intermingling with 'clean' supplies to be issued to the wards. Re-use of containers is an economical part of the pharmaceutical service and such containers must be thoroughly washed and dried prior to recycling. Containers which are damaged or cannot be satisfactorily cleaned and disinfected or sterilized are destroyed. Staff are provided with the appropriate clean clothes, suitable for the purpose, which are worn only in specific areas in the pharmacy department, and the staff must observe a high standard of personal hygiene.

17.7.3   STORAGE AND HANDLING

Pharmaceutical products require special conditions of storage and handling. Directions as to storage (e.g. in a refrigerator or protected from light) should be noted and adhered to. Ampoules and vials should be kept in their outer containers or wrappings to protect them, as far as possible, from external contamination.

Parenteral solutions
1. **Ampoules** The contents of the opened ampoule must be withdrawn into a syringe immediately, and any surplus discarded. Ampoules of solution for intrathecal injections should be sterilized by autoclaving inside a sealed container. Some solutions are not thermostable and these will not withstand this process, so before subjecting injections to this procedure the Pharmacist's advice must be sought.

2. **Multidose vials** The cap or diaphragm must be swabbed with an antiseptic solution that acts rapidly, such as ethyl alcohol (70%) or a spirit-impregnated swab (available in sachets) of the type commonly used for preparing the skin before injection.

   On no account should an injectable solution be transferred to a gallipot before it is drawn into a syringe. This increases the risk of contamination and also introduces the more dangerous risk of administering the wrong injection.

   Contents of multidose containers do not keep indefinitely and must be inspected routinely for opalescence before use; such containers must not be held over for subsequent use after a clinic.

3. **Rubber-capped vials of dry powder for preparing injections** The cap should be swabbed with an antiseptic solution, e.g. ethyl alcohol (70%) or a spirit-impregnated swab, before injecting the vehicle into the vial. Most of these are intended for single doses, but some may be used for several doses provided that the solution is stable enough to retain its potency and that it is used within 24 hours of being reconstituted. The pharmacist will give advice on particular preparations.

4. **Intravenous infusion solutions and emulsions (see also Chapter 7)** Solutions for infusion are supplied in glass bottles with rubber plugs or more usually in PVC bags. The rubber plug or diaphragm must be swabbed with, for example, ethyl alcohol (70%) or one of the spirit-impregnated swabs available in sachets before the cannula is introduced or drug solutions are injected into the container.

Topical preparations
This ideal situation can only be approached as closely as facilities will permit. Many chlorhexidine or chlorhexidine/cetrimide ('Savlon') solutions are available in sterilized sachets (e.g. 'Savlodil' or 'Hibidil') for immediate use or for dilution immediately before use. Alternatively, antiseptic solutions may be issued in clean and disinfected bottles with preservatives if required, e.g. isopropanol 7% w/v. Such solutions need to be diluted as appropriate.

Bladder irrigation solutions
These should be isotonic and pyrogen free. Commercially available solutions, usually in one or three litre plastic containers, are now mainly used, although solutions may be prepared in a hospital pharmacy if facilities are available.

Irrigation solutions for the eye, wounds, and body cavities
These are sterile solutions diluted ready for use, and they should be used on one occasion only.

17.8   Sterile services departments (SSD)

The function of the SSD is to supply a range of sterilized or disinfected items to theatres, wards and other health care establishments. The manager, advised by the infection control doctor or microbiologist, is responsible for monitoring all decontamination processes and for ensuring that all protocols for the handling and processing of equipment meet the required standards. Records must be kept of tests of efficacy of sterilizers and of all sterilization cycles. These records must be related to packs issued to users. The SSD is also responsible for the safe and effective processing of re-usable equipment, preventing any risk of transfer of infection to patients or staff. The responsibility for re-use of expensive 'high risk' single use items such as cardiac catheters is ultimately that of the user, with advice on processing and packaging from the infection control doctor and the SSD manager. This practice, however, is rarely endorsed by employers in developed countries. The SSD must develop good communications with the users, i.e. medical and nursing staff, and should remain a clinical service as well as an efficient distribution and cost-effective processing unit. The manager should be a member of relevant committees (e.g. theatre users and control of infection).

Central supply services were developed in the US and the first purpose-built civilian central sterile supply department (CSSD) in the UK was opened in Belfast in 1958. Since then there have been many developments, including the addition of independent sections or units, such as a theatre sterile supply unit (TSSU) and a hospital sterilization and disinfection unit (HSDU). The latter unit processes large items of medical equipment, such as respiratory ventilators, suction pumps and infant incubators. Periodic maintenance and instrument calibration may be carried out either in the unit or in an adjacent area. This should be done after decontamination and before the items are returned for use.

The present SSDs have rationalized their function and now obtain a large range of sterile procedure packs, dressings and single-use supplementary instruments from commercial sources.

With the introduction of consumer legislation and loss of Crown Immunity, departments should operate good manufacturing practices, which should be in accordance with the guidelines produced by the Institute of Sterile Service Management (1989) and endorsed by the Department of Health. Most of the recommendations in these guidelines are satisfactory, but some are rather excessive in terms of microbiological requirements (Atfield 1991), for example rooms used for packing dressings and instruments etc. which will be subsequently sterilized by heat. These standards may be appropriate for new SSDs but may be unnecessarily expensive to implement, particularly in developing countries. However, packs should be assembled in a room which is as clean and dust free as is reasonably practical.

17.8.1 DESIGN OF DEPARTMENTS AND WORKFLOW

The design features for a SSD are described in DHSS, Hospital Building Note no. 13. The design provides for two distinct flow lines:

1. for routine processing of surgical instruments/utensils, and
2. for medical equipment.

The work-flow should be in one direction only, but where medical equipment requires cleaning and disinfection after processing or maintenance this should be incorporated in the overall plan.

The typical work flow for surgical instruments and utensils is as follows:

1. sorting, washing, heat disinfection and drying;
2. inspection, setting trays and assembling packs;
3. sterilization;
4. transfer to sterile goods store;
5. distribution to wards and other units.

Medical equipment is similarly treated, but may require stripping down to component parts before cleaning, re-assembling and checking after processing.

17.8.2 COLLECTION AND RETURN OF USED EQUIPMENT TO THE SSD

Equipment should be effectively contained so that there is no risk to personnel during transport to the SSD. Single-use items should be correctly disposed of by the user, especially sharps (e.g. needles and blades) and not returned with reprocessable equipment. Delicate items must be well protected. Body fluids in suction bottles or hollow ware should be discarded by the user. The reception area in the SSD should be separate from clean areas and have readily cleanable surfaces.

17.8.3 PROCESSING PROCEDURES FOR USED EQUIPMENT

Sterile services staff (and most other health service staff) have become increasingly concerned with the risk of acquiring HBV and HIV infection despite the extremely low risk. However, staff must assume that there is a possibility of infection from any used item returned to the SSD. Risk can be reduced by wearing gloves and plastic aprons when handling all items, particularly those that are blood-stained, and taking care when handling sharp instruments. Any cuts or damaged skin on the hands should be covered with a waterproof dressing, and the hands thoroughly washed after removal of gloves. All staff handling potentially contaminated instruments or equipment should be immunized against hepatitis B.

Known high risk equipment should be decontaminated as soon as possible after receipt with minimal handling. All returned items that require cleaning should preferably be disinfected by heat at this stage. For high risk items, i.e. those marked 'biohazard', it may be possible for them to be returned to the department in a container that can be placed directly into a washer/disinfector. This is preferable to using chemical disinfectants, such as glutaraldehyde, which is irritant and a potential hazard to staff, and may not kill organisms in the presence of protein. Autoclaving before cleaning will coagulate protein, making it more difficult to remove during subsequent washing. It is always preferable to clean items before disinfection or sterilization. A washer/disinfector is preferable, but cleaning by hand should be a safe procedure if carried out by experienced staff wearing the correct protective clothing. The choice of methods for dealing with contaminated items must be made by the manager in association with the infection control committee. Washer/disinfectors are also of considerable value for processing anaesthetic and respiratory equipment since the items can then be dried and packaged without further treatment.

If equipment has been used on patients diagnosed or suspected of being infected with high risk pathogens, prior notification to the department is required in addition to labelling with a 'biohazard' notice and transporting in an approved container.

17.8.4   TESTING OF WASHER/DISINFECTORS AND STERILIZERS

If washer/disinfectors are to be used for the decontamination of high risk items, agreement should be reached with the infection control doctor on what is an acceptable process. Cleaning efficacy and time/temperature parameters should be checked when commissioning washer disinfectors and at periodic intervals. To ensure adequate disinfection the coolest part of the most difficult load would need to reach a temperature of at least 80°C for one minute (Central Sterilizing Club Working Party No. 1 1986). Rigorous attention should be paid to the method and frequency of testing of sterilizers (HTM (10) 80, Chapter 4).

17.8.5 RETURNING EQUIPMENT FOR SERVICING OR REPAIR

It is a requirement of the DoH that certificates are issued stating that equipment returned for servicing or repair is microbiologically safe. It is, however, not always possible to ensure that the internal surfaces of some items of equipment have been adequately decontaminated. It may also be necessary to return equipment that has not been decontaminated due to failure in use (e.g. an endoscope with a blocked channel). In these circumstances, a note should be attached to the returned equipment indicating safe methods of handling and suitable decontamination methods. All single-use components should be removed and discarded as clinical waste. Non-disposable components should be cleaned and preferably autoclaved (if heat tolerant) or disinfected in a washing machine. If this is not possible, immersion in a disinfectant such as 70% ethanol, a solution of a chlorine-releasing agent (1000 ppm av Cl_2) or 2% glutaraldehyde is acceptable provided it is effective and compatible with the surface (see Chapters 5 and 6 for choice of disinfectants and advantages and disadvantages of these agents).

Following immersion, items should be thoroughly rinsed and dried. If there are difficulties in decontaminating the internal surfaces, all external surfaces should be cleaned before returning an item to the manufacturer. Maintenance staff should be provided with suitable protective clothing, disinfectants and decontamination equipment. They should also be trained in handling and disinfection procedures.

17.9 Wards of psychiatric, geriatric and mentally handicapped patients

Many of these patients are incapable of understanding the principles of personal hygiene or of carrying out normal hygienic procedures; some may be incontinent of faeces or urine or both. In addition, the elderly are particularly susceptible to infection. Effective isolation of these patients in single rooms may be difficult to maintain and can often have adverse psychological effects. Gastrointestinal and skin infections or infestations, pulmonary tuberculosis, influenza, hepatitis A and hepatitis B are likely to spread in these units.

Methods of control are similar in principle to those used in other wards and are described elsewhere in the book, but there are special problems. Surveillance and immediate action are particularly important. New patients should be admitted to a special ward and screened for skin infection and infestation and for pulmonary tuberculosis; faeces should be examined if there is a history of diarrhoea and swabs should be taken from superficial lesions. Food poisoning is a particular hazard in these wards and should be considered in any outbreak of diarrhoea and vomiting. Ward staff should inform the infection control nurse of cases of diarrhoea which are probably of infective origin, particularly if there is more than one case. Patients with diarrhoea should be isolated, and if more than one case of a salmonella or shigella infection occurs in a ward, the faeces of other patients and staff should be examined. However, outbreaks of diarrhoea of viral origin are common and usually self-limiting; isolation of all patients may be impractical. Hygienic measures, particularly hand-washing and disinfection of toilet seats etc. should be reinforced. New patients should not be admitted until the ward is clear of infection (see also p. 179).

Outbreaks of hepatitis A can occur in units for children with mental handicaps. Screening for antibody in patients and staff may be required and the administration of gamma globulin to uninfected patients and new admissions should be considered, in addition to improvements in hygiene. Hepatitis B can also be a problem in units for the mentally handicapped and for drug addiction, and staff should be advised to have vaccination. Particular care is required in psychiatric units with violent or unpredictable patients with known or suspected HBV or HIV infection, particularly in taking blood samples.

Pulmonary tuberculosis is sometimes detected in a patient who has been in the ward for a long period. Patient contacts and staff should have a chest x-ray, which should be repeated after three months. Staff should be checked for previous tuberculin test results and BCG administration by the occupational health department.

Outbreaks of influenza tend to have a high mortality in geriatric wards and vaccination is advised if an epidemic is likely. The administration of a pneumococcal vaccine should also be considered for geriatric patients.

Patients with long term catheterization are likely to have urine infected or colonized with antibiotic-resistant Gram-negative bacilli which could be a cross-infection hazard if transferred to an acute surgical ward. Removal of the catheter and use of incontinence pads should be considered whenever possible. Pressure sores and varicose ulcers may similarly be colonized with antibiotic-resistant organisms. If the lesion is colonized with MRSA, every effort should be made to eliminate it (Chapter 9). Medical notes should be marked appropriately and, if the patient is transferred to another hospital, the infection control department of that hospital should be informed. MRSA are rarely responsible for clinical problems in geriatric wards, but could be if transferred to an acute surgical unit.

Scabies may also spread in these units and, if several cases have occurred, it may be advisable to treat all patients and staff.

Skin infections should be treated promptly, particularly if caused by β haemolytic streptococci of Group A. If there is an outbreak of skin sepsis, all patients and staff should use antiseptic soaps or detergents for all washing and bathing. Staff should maintain as high a standard of hygiene as possible, including washing hands (patients' and their own) before eating, and regular cleaning of toilets and baths. Communal towels and flannels should be avoided. Floor, walls and furniture should be washable. Although carpets may seem desirable in such units, these are difficult to keep clean and maintain and should generally be avoided if contamination from incontinent patients is frequent (p. 83). It is desirable that patients wear clothes that can be disinfected by heat; where psychological considerations require that patients wear their own clothes, it must be recognized that some risk of infection exists.

17.10 Pathology laboratories

Reports of outbreaks of laboratory-acquired infection and the introduction of the Health and Safety at work Act (1974) have been followed by the publication of guidelines from several committees. As new evidence emerges, these guidelines continue to be modified (ACDP 1990a, 1990b; DHSS 1990; Health Services Advisory Committee, 1991a,b).

The ACDP has classified organisms into four hazard and containment categories. Category 1 includes agents unlikely to cause human disease and requires no special precautions. Category 2 (formerly 'Howie' category C) includes most organisms isolated in clinical laboratories and requires good microbiological practice. Category 3 (formerly Howie group B) includes organisms of special hazard to laboratory workers (e.g. *Salmonella typhi*, *Mycobacterium tuberculosis*) and requires special containment facilities. Category 4 (formerly 'Howie' category A) includes organisms that are extremely hazardous to laboratory workers and may cause serious epidemic disease (e.g. Lassa and Marburg viruses), which require particularly stringent containment. It is recognized that Category 3 organisms may be isolated in routine laboratories, and on identification subsequent work on them must be carried out in the appropriate containment category. Modified requirements are also considered to be adequate for handling samples from patients with hepatitis B or HIV antibody or in high risk groups for these infections. These viruses are transferred by contact with blood and not by the airborne route.

The recommendations in these codes and guidelines are extensive and demand much from the laboratory worker and also from those who design or direct laboratories. They comprise all the sensible and feasible precautions which need to be taken in diagnostic clinical (and research) laboratories, although no code of practice can prevent infections due to negligence or poor technique of the laboratory worker. Everyone who works in a pathology department must develop habits of safe and careful technique. However, precautions against laboratory-acquired infection should be reasonable and, whenever possible, based on scientific or clinical evidence. Rituals should be discouraged; for example, ventilated rooms or cabinets cannot be expected to influence the transmission of blood-borne infections such as HBV or HIV or organisms transferred by the faecal-oral route such as *S. typhi*.

17.10.1 SPECIAL RISKS OF INFECTION

There are several ways in which the pathology department may be involved in the spread of infection in hospital. Patients are at risk from infection carried from the laboratory by laboratory staff collecting specimens in wards or outpatients, and may also be infected by procedures carried out by the technician involving transfer of microbes from one patient to another. Laboratory staff are at risk both from patients and from specimens of biological material and cultures examined in the laboratory. This last involvement, i.e. risk to laboratory staff from biological specimens, is in practice the most likely to have serious consequences. Many hazards are well known and precautions are taken to prevent spread, but infections can also arise from unsuspected sources, such as a request form contaminated by faeces and handled by clerical staff, or from serum containing HBV examined in the biochemistry department.

There are many ways in which infections are acquired in pathology departments, for example infected aerosols or sprays generated when pipetting or pouring liquids in the laboratory may be inhaled by workers; HBV or HIV may enter through skin abrasions. Tuberculosis and hepatitis B have been particularly important in hospital and laboratory infections in the UK, but hepatitis B has been acquired less in microbiological than in biochemical and haematological laboratories; in recent years such infections have become less frequent through better training in safe working. There is no evidence that HIV has been transferred to clinical laboratory workers, but in spite of the very low risk of transmission, HIV infection is such a dangerous infection that particular care is necessary. In general, it is usually not a specimen which is already known to be infective that causes trouble but one which is not suspected as being dangerous. Nevertheless, it is not necessary or cost-effective to treat every specimen as though it contained a highly dangerous pathogen. Some areas of the laboratory (e.g. animal houses, tuberculosis laboratories, and hospital mortuaries) are especially hazardous and require special precautions.

17.10.2   PREVENTION OF INFECTION

Methods of collecting specimens to minimize infection risks are described in Chapter 7. Ward staff should ensure that high-risk specimens (hazard Category 3) are transferred in sealed plastic bags labelled 'biohazard'. These samples should be handled with disposable gloves. However, all specimens must be handled with care since the diagnosis of a hazardous infection may not be known until laboratory tests have been completed. Specimens must be received in an area used exclusively for the purpose. The general office can be used if the reception area is separated from the clerical area. Staff handling specimens should be adequately trained. A handwash basin with pedal or elbow taps should be readily available, as well as appropriate materials and disinfectants for cleaning up any spillage and a container for disposal of spillage.

Laboratory staff visiting the wards should be trained in barrier nursing techniques and must follow carefully the instructions for handling infected patients.

17.10.3   TRANSPORT OF SPECIMENS

Attention should be given to the containers used to transport specimens from patient areas to laboratories. The specimen containers should be leakproof, robust and transported in trays or boxes which will hold the specimens upright. Some laboratories seal all specimens in plastic bags with a pocket to keep the forms from contamination. Simple clear rules need to be formulated for staff involved in transporting specimens. The Code of Practice (Health Services Advisory Committee, 1991a) recommends that metal boxes used for transporting specimens should be autoclaved weekly. Staff involved in transport of specimens should be trained to cope with spillage. Specimens from patients at risk for HIV infection, or known to be antibody-positive, should be taken to the laboratory by the doctor or a trained member of staff. The laboratory should always be informed in advance (Chapter 10).

17.10.4   PROCEDURES WITHIN THE LABORATORY

Details of hazards and their avoidance are given in several publications (for example, Collins 1988). In handling specimens, particular attention should be given to centrifuges and other possible sources of infective aerosols. Infected materials (e.g. slides and pipettes) should be discarded into jars containing a phenolic or chlorine-releasing disinfectant which is replaced daily (Chapters 5 and 6). Plastic pipettes should be used whenever possible to reduce hazards of trauma when handling.

The elimination of unnecessary glassware is one of the most important measures to reduce risks of bloodborne infection. Plastic petri dishes involve problems of disposal; they should be made safe before removal from the laboratory, and this is best achieved by autoclaving in a suitable container or in stainless steel buckets. The resultant lumps of polyethylene can be handled by the refuse collectors, but should be kept in sealed plastic bags. Difficulties have arisen when plates have been discarded without treatment and subsequently appear on local refuse sites. Incineration, preferably on site, without prior autoclaving is acceptable provided the waste is effectively contained during transport. Incineration of plastic plates in bulk may lead to an unacceptable smoke pollution and should be discontinued unless a satisfactory incinerator is available. Used glass petri dishes should be autoclaved by trained staff before handling by domestics. Other glass containers, such as bijou bottles containing infective material, should be similarly autoclaved before leaving the laboratory, whether they are going to be reprocessed or disposed of.

Care is needed in selection of the container for autoclaving. Failure to remove air from bags or buckets is likely to cause failure in decontamination. Various designs of containers have been suggested as well as autoclave modifications (PHLS 1981; Oates *et al.*, 1983). Sterilizing temperatures are usually recommended but are rarely required to achieve adequate decontamination, unless the work of the laboratory involves spore-bearing organisms hazardous to workers (e.g. *B. anthracis*, *Clostridium tetani* or *Cl. botulinum*). It is important that temperatures in the coolest part of the load are regularly checked with thermocouples.

17.10.5   IMMUNIZATION OF LABORATORY STAFF

Infections against which immunization should be offered to laboratory staff include tuberculosis, poliomyelitis and tetanus. Female staff should also be offered rubella vaccination, preferably after testing the immune state. None of these procedures is mandatory, except for BCG protection of tuberculin-negative staff, who must be excluded from work with material that contains or is likely to contain tubercle bacilli until conversion has taken place (British Thoracic Society 1990). Other protective measures should be strongly urged on all staff on joining the laboratory (Chapter 15).

The hepatitis B vaccine should be offered to all laboratory staff handling clinical specimens.

17.10.6 TRAINING AND INSTRUCTIONS FOR STAFF

Training of staff in aseptic procedures and in methods of handling infected material is part of the routine education in microbiology departments. In many hospitals the various branches of pathology recruit their own staff and there may be no opportunity for biochemists or technicians to acquire experience in microbiology departments. In these cases, some basic instruction should be given on methods of spread of infection, aseptic procedures and handling of potentially infected biological or toxic materials. The Code of Practice and other relevant documents should be readily available for consultation. The COSHH regulations apply to microorganisms as well as toxic chemicals (p. 24) and each laboratory should produce its own Safety Code which includes the most important rules, for example:

17.10.7 PRECAUTIONS AGAINST LABORATORY INFECTION

Any specimen entering the laboratory may be infectious. Some will certainly contain the agents causing HBV and HIV infection, typhoid, tuberculosis, and other infections. Your safety, your family's safety, and your colleagues' safety depend on observing the following instructions.

General No smoking, no eating, no drinking in the laboratory. Keep your bench clean and tidy.

Wash your hands thoroughly on leaving the laboratory; before taking food or drink, or handling personal possessions; after handling specimens; after changing tubing or dialysers or diluters in the autoanalysers and if you think you have contaminated them: thoroughly wash with soap and water; if contamination with bacterial cultures has occurred and in 'high risk' laboratories, use an antiseptic handwashing method. Thorough application of 70% alcohol after washing is particularly effective.

Handwashing is your most important safeguard Wear gloves when handling high risk specimens (or when cleaning up spillage).

Cuts and abrasions Wash well in running water. Cover with waterproof protective dressing. If you splash your eye with serum or a culture, wash it out with saline or tap water. Report to chief medical laboratory scientific officer or deputy at once. Enter in accident book (needle-stick injuries must be entered and immediately reported).

Spilt specimens: treatment of contaminated area, floor or other surfaces
Swab with plenty of a 2% clear soluble phenolic solution on the areas

of contamination or with a chlorine-releasing agent containing 10 000 ppm av Cl_2 when cleaning up blood or organic materials possibly containing viruses; 1000 ppm is adequate for small amounts of spillage or routine cleaning; rinse well, particularly if metal surface (for which 2% glutaraldehyde is an effective alternative, but precautions against staff exposure to aldehyde vapours are required, e.g. disinfect in a fume cupboard). Thoroughly covering the spillage with a chlorine-releasing or peroxygen powder or granules before removal with paper towels is also effective. Do not use a chlorine-releasing powder or granules for large amounts of spillage, since excessive chlorine may be released. Wear gloves when handling contaminated materials or disinfectants.

Pipettes Avoid mouth suction. Use automatic pipettes, or rubber bulbs, or teats. Discard all Pasteur pipettes and graduated pipettes into enough clear soluble phenolic (2%) or a chlorine-releasing solution – 0.25% (2500 ppm av Cl_2) – to cover them completely.

Other equipment Plastic tubes, pilot tubes and other plastic disposables should be incinerated. Slides should be autoclaved in the discard jars in which they have been placed. Syringes and needles should be discarded into an approved container (Chapter 10).

Centrifuging Use only closed centrifuges, with wind-shields if possible, and preferably with sealed buckets which should be opened only within a protective exhaust cabinet when dangerous pathogens are involved.

Swab out the centrifuge bowl with a clear soluble phenolic or, for virus infections, an aldehyde disinfectant (formalin 10% or glutaraldehyde 2%) weekly with appropriate precautions against staff exposure to toxic vapours. Wear disposable gloves for this. In view of problems of aldehyde toxicity, 70% ethanol may be preferred.

If a breakage occurs, autoclave the bucket and its contents. Swab the bowl as above.

White coats A plentiful supply is necessary. Coats must be changed immediately if contaminated; all coats should be treated as infected linen in the laundry; coats known to be contaminated with particularly hazardous pathogens should be autoclaved in the laboratory autoclave. Fully protective coats should be worn when handling Category 3 pathogens.

Do not wear your laboratory coat to visit the wards.

Do not wear *any* white coat to visit the coffee room or toilet.

17.10.8 INFECTIONS IN CONTAINMENT CATEGORY 3:
LABORATORIES

Since this containment category is required for handling sputum specimens that may contain *M. tuberculosis*, most large laboratories will now
have this facility. The room will contain a cabinet with exhaust ventilation, filtered before discharge usually to the outside. The cabinet
and system should be disinfected with formalin routinely and before
maintenance, and airflows should be regularly checked. Gloves should
be worn for all manipulations and staff must be adequately trained to
avoid a false sense of security when using a cabinet. Careful work on
an open bench may often be safer, particularly if working with viruses
such as HBV or HIV, which do not spread in the air. It is, therefore,
recommended that for the clinical examination of samples containing
HBV or HIV the work may be carried out at a defined work station
which allows sufficient seclusion to avoid inoculation accidents.

A fully protective gown or plastic apron should be worn as well as
disposable gloves for more dangerous manipulations. Staff must be
adequately trained in the use of aseptic measures in addition to provision of this protective clothing, otherwise a false sense of security
may lead to simple errors which would not arise if gloves were not
being worn.

Fungi Cultures of fungi causing communicable systemic infection (e.g.
histoplasma) should be processed in a ventilated cabinet, as recommended for tubercle bacilli.

17.11 Postmortem room and mortuary (see also Health Services
Advisory Committee, 1991c)

The dead body, whether previously infected or not, may be a source
of infection: mortuary and postmortem staff are at risk. As in the ward,
bacteria may spread by air or by contact, but there are special hazards
when a postmortem examination is being made. Contaminated aerosols
or splashes may be released through squeezing sponges, cutting tissues
such as the lung or incising abscesses, and the sawing of bones may
also release small contaminated chips into the air. Cutting or pricking
a finger with a contaminated instrument or ragged bone edge is one of
the commonest modes of infection. Although most organisms in the
dead body are unlikely to infect healthy people with intact skin, there
are some particular hazards. Tubercle bacilli may be spread in large
numbers in aerosols. Salmonella, shigella and other intestinal pathogens may be transmitted from the intestinal tract. Following a break in

the skin of the operator, large numbers of *Staph. aureus* or *Strep. pyogenes* may be introduced, and unless treatment with appropriate antibiotics is given promptly these may cause a severe local infection and sometimes septicaemia; HBV or HIV introduced by a cut or needle-prick is a major potential hazard. The conjunctiva may be infected by splashes or aerosols, and a severe local infection may follow; HBV and HIV may also enter the body by this route (Chapter 10).

17.11.1 PREVENTION OF INFECTION

The risks of infection are not high if adequate precautions are taken. Cleanliness of mortuary, refrigerator, postmortem room and good personal hygiene of members of staff are essential.

The postmortem room should be mechanically ventilated and designed so that cleaning can be readily carried out. Fly-proofing arrangements in the mortuary and postmortem room should be efficient. A shower, with soap and towels supplied, should be available for the postmortem room staff. When performing postmortem examinations, the pathologist and mortuary technicians should completely change their outer clothing and a disposable plastic apron, disposable gloves and rubber boots should be worn. Clean white trousers, vests and jackets should be supplied daily if possible, or at least several times a week, or if contaminated. Visitors to the postmortem room not in close contact with the body should wear a gown and overshoes. A wash-basin with disposable paper towels, soap and an antiseptic hand-washing preparation (povidone-iodine or chlorhexidine detergent, or 70% ethanol) should be available in postmortem rooms.

Staff should wash their hands thoroughly after handling any contaminated surface or material irrespective of whether gloves are worn, and always on leaving the postmortem room. If hands are likely to have become contaminated, they should also be washed before handling case notes or any other clean items.

If the skin or eye is splashed, it should be thoroughly washed. An eyewash bottle containing sterile saline should be available. Any cut or finger-prick should be immediately reported to the pathologist, after thorough washing under running water and application of an antiseptic (e.g. 0.5% alcoholic or aqueous chlorhexidine or 1% iodine in 70% alcohol). All pre-existing cuts or open lesions on the hands should be covered with a waterproof dressing. Open injuries, other than minor ones, should be treated in the casualty department.

Instruments should be routinely cleaned before disinfection since the presence of organic matter may protect the organisms from the disinfectant. Boiling or immersion in 2% 'Stericol' or other phenolics for ten minutes are less satisfactory alternatives to autoclaving, but if properly carried out are safe procedures, a small washer disinfector would be preferable, since washing by hand would be avoided. After treatment with a disinfectant, instruments should be rinsed and dried. Immersion in 2% glutaraldehyde rather than a phenolic is advised after a postmortem on a patient with an HBV or HIV infection. Although autoclaving or treatment in a washer disinfection would be preferable. For disinfection and cleaning instruments and room at autopsies in patients with slow-virus infections see below. The room and other equipment should be thoroughly cleaned after use with a phenolic disinfectant (e.g. 2% 'Stericol'), or with a chlorine-releasing agent (1000 ppm av Cl_2) if HBV, HIV infection or poliomyelitis was diagnosed in the patient before death. If chlorine-releasing agents are used on metal surfaces, they should be immediately rinsed to avoid corrosion.

Linen should be sent in a sealed bag and treated as 'infected' by the laundry. Dressings, waste materials and body tissues should be sealed in plastic bags and treated as clinical waste and preferably incinerated on site.

Special precautions should be taken with certain infections. In post-mortem examination of patients with untreated pulmonary tuberculosis, filter type masks should be worn by operators. Postmortems on patients with known or suspected HBV or HIV infection should be avoided unless absolutely essential (for general precautions, see Chapter 10). Special care is necessary to avoid cuts and needle-pricks.

Viruses causing spongeiform encephalopathy (Creutzfeldt-Jakob disease) and other slow virus infections are relatively resistant to heat and are resistant to most chemical disinfectants, especially aldehydes. The environment should be disinfected with a strong chlorine-releasing solution (containing 0.25% available chlorine); blood should be mopped up with a solution containing 1% (10 000 ppm) av Cl_2 or following the application of a chlorine-releasing powder. If the skin is contaminated, wash thoroughly with soap and water and apply 1N sodium hydroxide for 10 minutes. Instruments should be autoclaved at 134°C for 18 minutes (e.g. six three-minute cycles). (See also p. 101.) Immersion in 1N sodium hydroxide is a possible alternative if autoclaving is not possible.

Formaldehyde used for the preservation of tissues is an effective antimicrobial agent, but thorough penetration should be ensured before handling, particularly if lesions are caused by potentially dangerous infections, such as tuberculosis, typhoid or hepatitis. It is ineffective against 'slow' viruses.

It is most important that the mortuary staff should be informed about the bodies of patients who have died or were suffering from a communicable disease. These should be enclosed in a plastic bag and a warning label could usefully be attached to them in the ward. Training of mortuary staff in prevention of infection is also necessary.

Immunization should be offered as for laboratory staff.

References and further reading

Advisory Committee on Dangerous Pathogens (1990a) HIV – The Causative Agent of AIDS and Related Conditions, 2nd revision of guidelines. HMSO, London.

Advisory Committee on Dangerous Pathogens (1990b) Categorization of Pathogens According to Hazard and Categories of Containment, 2nd edn. HMSO, London.

Atfield, R.D. (1991) Hospital hygiene – a continuing assessment: a microbiological view of sterile services production. Journal of Hospital Infection, 18 (Supplement A), 524.

British Standards Institution (1976) Environmental Cleanliness in Enclosed Spaces. BS 5295: Parts 1, 2 & 3. BSI, London.

British Thoracic Society (1990) Subcommittee of the Joint Tuberculosis Committee of the British Thoracic Society. Control and prevention of tuberculosis in Britain: an updated code of practice. British Medical Journal, 300, 995.

Central Sterilizing Club (1986) Working Party Report No. 1. Washer/disinfection Machines. Obtainable from the Hospital Infection Research Laboratory.

Collins, C.H. (1988) Laboratory Acquired Infections. Butterworths, London, Boston.

Department of Health and Social Security (1975) Application of Medicines Act to Health Authorities. Health Circular HSC (1S) 128. HMSO, London.

Department of Health and Social Security (1980) Hospital technical memorandum (HTM No. 10) Pressure steam sterilizers. HMSO, London.

Department of Health and Social Security (1990) Recommendations of the Expert Advisory Group on AIDS. Guidance for Clinical Health Care Workers. Protection against infection with HIV and hepatitis viruses. HMSO, London.

Guide to Good Pharmaceutical Practice (1977) HMSO, London.

Health Services Advisory Committee (1991a and b) Safe working and the prevention of infection in clinical laboratories – model rules for staff and visitors. HMSO, London.

Health Services Advisory Committee (1991c) Safe working and the prevention of infection in the mortuary and post-mortem room. HMSO, London.

Hospital Building Note No. 13. (1961) Hospital Sterilization and Disinfection Unit. London, HMSO (Revised edition 1992).

Institute of Sterile Services Management (1989) Guide to Good Manufacturing Practice for National Health Sterile Services Departments. ISSM, UK.

Institute of Sterile Services Management (1990) Teaching and Training Manual for Sterile Services Personnel. ISSM, UK.

Oates, K., Deverill, C.E.A., Phelps, M. and Collins, B.J. (1983) Development of a laboratory autoclave system. Journal of Hospital Infection, 4, 181–90.

Penny, P.T. (1991) Hydrotherapy pools of the future – the avoidance of health problems. Journal of Hospital Infection, 18 (Supplement A) 535.

Public Health Laboratory Services (1990) Report: Hygiene for Hydrotherapy Pools. PHLS, London.

Public Health Laboratory Services Subcommittee (1981) Specifications for laboratory autoclaves. Journal of Hospital Infection, 2, 377.

Slade, N. and Gillespie, W.A. (1985) The Urinary Tract and the Catheter: Infection and Other Problems. John Wiley, Chichester and New York.

18   *The special problems of renal units*

The general considerations regarding hospital infections apply to dialysis and transplant units, but the particular nature of the work there poses special, although not unique, cross infection hazards, which may sometimes be a threat to staff as well as to patients.

The special infection hazards of renal units may be summarized as:

1. impaired immune responsiveness of uraemic subjects or of patients immunosuppressed to prevent graft rejection;
2. use of extracorporeal circulation of blood or repeated access to the peritoneal cavity;
3. the need for blood transfusion in many circumstances;
4. the transplantation of organs, often from cadaveric donors.

These factors have come under particular scrutiny with regard to the transmission of blood-borne or tissue-borne viruses, in particular HBV and HIV.

18.1   Prevention and control of hepatitis and other tissue or blood-borne virus infections (ACDP 1990; Hospital Infection Society 1990)

Viral hepatitis is considered in some detail in Chapter 10, but the disease has been a particular problem in renal units and requires further comment in this context. Hepatitis in renal units has nearly always been due to HBV, though outbreaks of hepatitis C infection have been reported with increasing frequency. Spread of infection with HIV has not been reported in a renal unit, but similar precautions are required for 'at risk' or antibody positive patients as for hepatitis B.

Patients suffering from chronic renal failure and other conditions associated with immunological insufficiency (including those receiving immunosuppressive therapy) are often not made ill when infected with the HBV virus, but become carriers of the virus. Healthy carriers in the general population usually carry virus in comparatively low titre in their blood, but patients with chronic renal failure, or those on immunosuppressive therapy, often carry the virus in very high titre. Infection has, in the past, entered dialysis units by transfusion of blood from a carrier or through the introduction of an unsuspected patient carrier to the unit's treatment programme; the virus has then been spread from patient to patient by shared dialysis equipment.

Infection may be spread to staff by patient's blood entering a scratch or via the conjunctiva, or by a needle stick accident. All blood donations in the United Kingdom are nowadays tested for HBV, but no test can be guaranteed to exclude all infected donations.

In the absence of sensible precautions, hepatitis can become a major problem in renal units. In 1977, 23.5% of patients receiving hospital dialysis in Europe were infected (EDTA 1978); 671 members of staff were infected, with eight deaths. The efficacy of sound preventative measures against hepatitis B is confirmed by the UK experience since 1972, very few patients becoming hepatitis positive after starting treatment and infection in staff becoming a rarity. The main procedures adopted in the UK have been based on the report of the Rosenheim Committee (DHSS 1972).

Organ donors have been recorded as a source of infection with HBV and HBC and there is evidence of transmission of cytomegalovirus, HIV and even of rabies by organ or tissue grafting. Clearly careful screening and exact diagnosis of donors, both living and cadaveric, is important. Of the virus infections other than hepatitis, it would seem that only HIV is likely to pose a hazard to individuals other than graft recipients. HIV positive patients may present for dialysis therapy, or in inner city areas with a large population of intravenous drug abusers, patients on regular dialysis may become infected. Present evidence suggests that precautions taken to prevent the spread of HBV will be more than adequate to prevent cross-infection with HIV.

18.1.1   GENERAL MEASURES FOR PREVENTION AND CONTROL OF HBV AND HIV INFECTION (see also Chapter 10)

1. **To prevent virus infection entering units**
   (a) Screen patients with appropriate counselling before admission for the HBV antigen and HIV antibody and thereafter at regular intervals while they are in-patients. Patients found to be positive will need to be treated in a separate dialysis facility. Routine screening and segregation of HIV positive patients remains controversial.
   (b) Give only blood transfusions screened for HBV, HBC and HIV; use only screened organ donors. The introduction of erythropoietin has greatly reduced transfusion requirements of dialysis patients. The improved success of renal transplantation has been outweighed with the possible exception of donor specific transfusion by improved immunosuppressive regimes and organ

matching by reducing the risks of sensitization to transplant organs. Blood transfusion in dialysis units is now largely confined to emergencies and should be kept to a minimum.

(c) Consider the use of home haemodialysis or continuous ambulatory peritoneal dialysis (CAPD) to reduce contact between patients.

(d) Minimize transfer between dialysis units. In recent years there has been a temptation to relax this practice because long term dialysis imposes considerable restrictions on holiday and business travel for patients and their families. Holiday centres for dialysis patients have been developed, but it is important that the risks are appreciated and that there is full liaison between units to minimize risk of transmission of HBV and HIV.

(e) Immunization against HBV should be considered (see below and Chapter 10).

2. **To protect patients against transfer of virus within the unit**
Use disposable dialysers. If re-use is practised, great care should be taken to identify the patient's dialyser. Re-use is not recommended if a patient is HB$_s$Ag or HIV antibody positive.

Use separate dialysate proportionating and monitoring units for each patient, or for a restricted group of patients whenever possible. Pressure monitors connected directly to blood lines should be isolated from direct contact with blood by disposable gauge isolators. Transfer of HBV has been directly attributed to contamination of pressure monitors in past outbreaks.

Segregate new 'acute' dialysis patients from those having 'chronic' dialysis.

Secretions and peritoneal dialysis effluent, may contain virus; for disposal see the section on Standard isolation in Chapter 8.

Screen staff for HB$_s$Ag and abnormal liver function before they start to work in the unit, and every six months thereafter.

Staff who get hepatitis B or become antigen-positive must not return to work in a dialysis unit until three successive blood samples have proved negative for HB$_s$Ag.

3. **To enhance host-resistance of staff and patients**
Effective and safe vaccination against hepatitis B is now available, and it is recommended that all staff in direct contact with dialysis patients, their laboratory specimens or environment, should receive a full course of hepatitis B vaccine and their antibody response subsequently checked.

The active immunization of uraemic patients is more controversial because only 60% of uraemic patients respond to currently available hepatitis vaccines with a satisfactory antibody response, although a better response may be obtained if patients are inoculated early in the course of renal failure. For antibody negative staff who may be accidentally contaminated with infected blood, normal pooled human gamma globulin has no prophylactic value but specific gamma globulin prepared from plasma selected for its content of antibody to hepatitis B is available in limited supply, and gives good, but not infallible, protection against clinical hepatitis: 500 mg should be injected as soon as possible, preferably within 24 hours but at least within seven days, into any person put at risk by accidental injection or splashing of infected blood into mouth, eyes or open skin lesions. A second dose should be injected one month later (Chapter 10).

18.1.2   OTHER MEASURES

Responsibility for safety   A member of the medical staff of the renal unit should be designated Safety Officer. Any accident or untoward happenings, illness etc., must be reported to this person. The Safety Officer will also be responsible for ensuring that agreed safety precautions are observed and that newly appointed staff are trained to work safely. Ultimate responsibility is with the consultant in charge of the unit.

Instruction to Staff   New members must be instructed and trained in methods of work to minimize hazards of infection. The importance of neat and tidy working should be emphasized.

Smoking, eating and drinking   These must be forbidden to staff in the unit.

Overcrowding   Overcrowding in the unit must be avoided.

Protective dressings   Staff must wear waterproof dressings over cuts and abrasions. Those with extensive untreated cuts or epithelial deficiency (e.g. eczema) should not work in renal units.

Protective clothing   Surgical or disposable gloves must be worn on all occasions when taking blood, and when handling shunts or dialysis apparatus. The use of surgical gowns and disposable long plastic aprons is recommended when there is a risk that much blood may be shed, as for instance in setting up dialysis or declotting a cannula. Goggles are recommended in these situations if the patient is a known HBV or HIV carrier. *Change of clothing, gowns, etc* – Gowns or uniforms must be changed if they become splashed with blood.

Specimen collection   When taking blood with a syringe the specimen container should be filled from the syringe with the needle still attached (Chapter 10). Great care should be taken to avoid frothing. The syringe and attached needle should then be disposed of, placing them in an approved container. Needles not attached to syringes (e.g. those of drip sets) should be similarly discarded. Accidental cuts or pricks by sharp instruments are an important hazard and are the principal route of infection for staff. Sharp instruments must be disposed of with care.

Spills (see Chapter 7)   Any spilt blood from a patient must be mopped up and a wide area disinfected around the spill. A strong hypochlorite solution or chlorine releasing powder is the best disinfectant to use. If used on metals, rinsing must be thorough. Some newer agents (e.g. peroxygen compounds) may be less corrosive to certain metals.The 'mopping-up' material should be sealed in a plastic bag for subsequent incineration.

Decontamination of instruments   (Chapter 6).

Hazard to others   Staff must ensure that contaminated material is not transferred to other departments (e.g. to pharmacy or SSD) before it has been disinfected, and that it is appropriately contained and labelled.

Accidents   There must be a routine to prevent accidents, and to deal with, report and record any that do occur.

1. Cuts, pricks – if a finger or hand is accidently pricked the venous return should be occluded and the injury made to bleed if possible, and thoroughly washed. The area should be treated with tincture of iodine or other alcoholic preparation. If the patient is HBV positive and the member of staff is antibody negative when injured, human specific immunoglobulin should be offered; its administration should not be delayed if the person at risk cannot be tested for HBV antigen immediately (see Chapter 10).
2. Splashes in eyes – if contamination of the conjunctiva occurs the eye should be immediately washed out with saline or tap water and anti HBV gammaglobulin offered as above.

Action when a patient is found to be HBV antigen or HIV antibody positive
1. Isolate HBV or HIV positive patients (see p. 358).
2. discharge HBV or HIV positive patients as soon as possible to home dialysis or, if possible, to a special unit for positive patients.
3. Use disposable dialysers and do not re-use.

4. Incinerate or disinfect articles contaminated with blood or other secretions (e.g. menstrual discharge).
5. Linen should be transported to the laundry in sealed alginate bags contained in an outer bag as appropriate for infected linen (Chapter 12).
6. Clean and disinfect baths, toilet areas etc., possibly contaminated by HBV or HIV positive patients.
7. Limit laboratory investigations as far as possible.

Staff in high risk areas   Specially trained staff should be selected for these duties.

Consultation   There should be regular consultation and collaboration between staff of the renal unit, the microbiology department and the infection control team.

Blood and blood products   These should be screened to exclude any found to be HBV antigen or HIV antibody positive.

18.2   Prevention and control of bacterial infection

18.2.1   GENERAL PREVENTATIVE MEASURES: THE ENVIRONMENT

The general measures designed to protect patients and staff from cross-infection are described elsewhere: these include meticulous attention to all aspects of general hygiene. Unless this is done, gross contamination of the environment can occur, with attendant high risk of vascular or peritoneal access site infection.

In particular, extensive use of pre-sterilized disposable dressing packs, syringes and instruments, strict control and safe disposal of linen, and cleaning (and disinfection if necessary) of bed, furniture and floors after use of a cubicle should be routine practice.

18.2.2   GENERAL PREVENTATIVE MEASURES: THE PATIENT

The patient's general cleanliness must be carefully assessed, and tactful guidance in these matters by the ward sister is invaluable. In patients with external cannulae or peritoneal catheters bathing may present difficulties, in that keeping the access site dry is of paramount importance in the prevention of infection. Methods must be improvised to achieve this, depending upon the access site and presence of external cannulae and materials available.

Carrier sites On acceptance of a patient for long term dialysis, all carrier sites – nose, throat, axilla and groin – are swabbed. Where multi-resistant *Staph. aureus*, especially MRSA are found, appropriate measures are taken to eradicate them by topical application of ointments or creams, e.g. 'Naseptin' or mupirocin, to the nasal mucosa, and repeated use of 4% chlorhexidine detergent solution, or an iodophor or alcoholic chlorhexidine for the disinfection of the skin (Chapter 9). There is evidence that intermittent applications of mupirocin to the nose reduces the incidence of staphylococcal bacteraemia (Boelart *et al.* 1989). Swabs should be taken after such measures to ascertain their effectiveness.

This swabbing is repeated at intervals as indicated by previous findings or repeated infections.

Care of blood access sites Access to the circulation is most commonly obtained by needle puncture of veins draining a subcutaneous arteriovenous fistula. This has largely replaced the external silastic-teflon arteriovenous shunt which poses special bacteriological hazards. Use is being made of prosthetic devices to create subcutaneous arteriovenous fistulae including grafts of bovine carotid artery and polytetrafluoroethylene (TFE) ('Gortex' or 'Impra') in patients with veins unsatisfactory for fistula formation. For short term dialysis (up to six weeks or more) or for plasmapheresis or haemofiltration, increasing use is being made of percutaneous cannulation of the subclavian or femoral veins using a Seldinger technique with or without subsequent subcutaneous tunnelling. More permanent cannulation of large veins with subcutaneous tunnelling is possible with newer devices such as the 'pericanth' for patients in whom satisfactory fistulae cannot be created.

18.2.3 SUBCUTANEOUS ARTERIOVENOUS FISTULAE

The subcutaneous fistula has a great advantage over the external shunt in that there is no open wound once postoperative healing has occurred. The technique for management is as follows.

1. A wide area of the arm is cleaned with 0.5% chlorhexidine in 70% ethyl alcohol. It is essential that this preliminary skin preparation should be very thorough, in order to avoid introduction of bacteria directly into the bloodstream.
2. Local anaesthesia is usually necessary in view of the wide bore of the needle to be inserted. Lignocaine (2%) in 2 ml ampoules is recommended for this purpose.
3. It is desirable to avoid inserting the needle through the identical point of insertion made during the preceding dialysis where a small infected clot or scab may have formed.

4. The fistula needle is strapped into position after reinsertion into the fistula sites, but no dressing is necessary.
5. Haemorrhage after withdrawal of the needle can occur and severe blood loss can be troublesome if adequate steps are not taken. To prevent this, a protamine-soaked or other haemostatic swab is placed over the site and held in place firmly for 10 minutes. This is replaced by a sterile gauze square, and firmly bandaged for two hours.

18.2.4 EXTERNAL ARTERIOVENOUS SHUNTS AND VENOUS CANNULAE

The basic bacteriological problem presented by the external access device can be simply stated: it is how to avoid infection in a permanently open wound containing a foreign body. This obviously presents considerable difficulties. However, prevention of infection at the access site is of major importance if suppuration is to be avoided. This may lead to destruction and abandonment of an important site when the number of sites is strictly limited and to the risk of septic emboli and fatal septicaemia. The organisms concerned are most commonly coagulase-positive and coagulase-negative staphylococci, but Gram-negative bacilli, such as *Ps. aeruginosa*, may also be involved. The major pathogen in this context, however, is the staphylococcus, and 80% of strains of *Staph. aureus* isolated in one series, were derived from the patient's own carrier sites, the remainder being cross-infection acquired from other patients.

In view of these considerations, the care of the access site must be seen to begin in the wider context of general hygiene and ward cleanliness, and the measures used to control cross-infection in the general hospital ward situation should be applied even more rigorously to the renal unit.

Routine care of access site   the main object is to prevent introduction of pathogens. This is achieved by observance of strict aseptic principles in the dressing and handling of the access site, by an occlusive dressing, and by keeping the site dry at all times as far as possible.

Dressing technique   Standard aseptic practice must be used throughout. A dressing pack made up especially for shunt toilet by the SSD is desirable. A pack containing two dressings and one waterproof towel, two gallipots, gauze squares and swab-mounted cotton-wool 'buds' has been found suitable for this purpose.

The operator scrubs up, using an approved hand preparation, e.g. 4% chlorhexidine or povidone-iodine with detergent, or 5 ml of 0.5% chlorhexidine in 70% ethanol with 1% glycerol, rubbed into the skin till dry (the most effective method for single use). A sterile gown and gloves are worn. If the site of cannulation appears clean it is sufficient to gently cleanse the area with 4% chlorhexidine detergent solution or with povidone-iodine detergent. If there is crusting or congealed blood at the site of entry this should be gently cleaned with chlorhexidine or povidone-iodine detergent using cotton-wool buds, and then dried.

Finally, it is disinfected with 10% solution of povidone-iodine in 70% ethanol, or 0.5% chlorhexidine in 70% alcohol.

The shunt ends are now separated, or the cannula cap removed, and the lines attached to the dialyser and dialysis commenced. The access site is covered with a loose sterile gauze square during dialysis.

At the end of dialysis the ends are disconnected from the machine and attached to each other once more. The area is again cleaned with a 4% chlorhexidine detergent solution or with povidone-iodine detergent, dried and then treated with an application of an alcoholic chlorhexidine or povidone-iodine solution. A dry sterile gauze is placed over the access site; occlusive dressings such as 'Opsite' are often used for sub-clavian cannulae.

It must be emphasized that techniques will vary with local practice and we are not at present able to present evidence that the method outlined gives appreciably better long-term results in sepsis control than any other. It is possible that excessive use of local skin disinfectants may, in some patients, devitalise tissue and later render it more liable to infection. Similarly, there may be a tendency to damage tissues by poking too vigorously with a cotton wool bud around the site, so that unmounted cotton wool swabs may be preferred.

18.2.5   TRAINING FOR HOME DIALYSIS

While it is important that home dialysis patients be trained to be self-sufficient, it is valuable in most circumstances for the spouse, relative or friend who may help the patient, to be fully instructed in both the principles and practice of access site care, bearing in mind that both they and the patient find the technique completely foreign and the aseptic precautions without apparent reason. Experience suggests that teaching is best done by example. At the same time, the dangers of autogenous infection must be stressed to encourage the highest standards of personal hygiene.

18.2.6   INFECTION IN ACCESS SITE

When there is clinical evidence of infection at the site, a swab is taken for bacteriological examination, and swabs of nose, throat, axilla and groin are taken also.

If the clinical condition warrants antibiotic therapy pending the bacteriological report, antistaphylococcal drugs (e.g. flucloxacillin or an initial dose of vancomycin) are started. Treatment is reviewed and altered if necessary on receipt of the bacteriological report. If possible, avoid antibiotics that may accumulate to toxic levels in renal failure (Chapter 13).

Treatment is continued until there is bacteriological evidence of clearance. Carrier sites are treated as outlined above if found to carry pathogens.

The maintenance of an infection-free access depends upon rigorous attention to basic aseptic principles, keeping the site dry, prevention of colonization of carrier sites by pathogens, and on a high level of personal and environment hygiene.

18.3   Cleaning and sterilization of dialysis equipment

Although much attention has been focused upon the hepatitis risk, the greatest hazard to patients in dialysis units is bacterial infection. Techniques must take into account both factors.

The general measures required to avoid the introduction of hepatitis or HIV infection have been discussed in the first section of this chapter. This section will deal with routine cleaning and sterilizing of dialysis equipment.

In general, proportionating machines should be used for a designated small group of patients rather than at random, to confine the area of potential spread of infection. Re-used dialysers should be clearly labelled and each dialyser restricted to the treatment of one individual.

Adequate and safe containers must be provided for the disposal of needles and cannulae.

18.3.1   ROUTINE MEASURES

The dialyser   Disposable dialysers (coils, flat plate and hollow fibre) will normally be disposed of by incineration without dismantling.

It is the practice of some dialysis units to re-use these disposable items to reduce unit cost, and because they function well for several dialyses and reduce the incidence of 'first-use' reactions. The cost of these units has been reduced in recent years and single-use is usually possible. When re-use is contemplated, the dialyser (with or without the blood lines) is thoroughly washed through to remove all traces of blood. Until recently 2% formalin has been the most effective sterilizing agent for dialyser re-use. Formalin is cheap and does not destroy the dialysing membrane but it is unpleasant to use, is potentially toxic and sensitizes a proportion of patients and renal unit personnel. When formalin is used there must be adequate ventilation in the room to meet safety requirements. For re-use the dialyser is filled with 2% formalin and stored until shortly before the individual's next dialysis. Sterilants for re-use need to kill spore-forming bacteria and viruses. Hypochlorites tend to damage the membranes. Sterilants now replacing formalin for re-use include agents releasing chlorine dioxide. These should be used according to the manufacturer's recommendations.

During dismantling and washing, staff should wear plastic aprons and gloves.

Proportionating machines The dialysing fluid used for haemodialysis does not need to be sterile, but heavy bacterial growth leads to the dangers of contamination and changes the chemical composition of the solution, and there is evidence that bacterial products including endotoxins may cross the membrane.

There is now a wide choice of machines on the market. These employ one of three methods of sterilization and disinfection:

1. chemical disinfection, usually with formalin;
2. heat disinfection by hot water circulation at temperatures of 80–90°C; or
3. in a few models, autoclaving of the dialysate circuit.

Whichever method is used, careful physical cleaning is required, particularly for units using chemical or hot water disinfection. For hot water systems a periodic thorough cleaning of the flow systems is recommended, followed by disinfection with a solution of a chlorine-releasing agent or by a period of recirculation with water for four hours at 80°C.

Particular care is required to ensure the cleanliness of those parts of the circuit which, in some machines, are not included in the sterilizing or disinfecting pathway.

Pressure gauges Particular danger attaches to 'blind' connections to pressure monitors which permit bacterial growth and subsequent contamination of the circuit, or, in the case of the venous pressure monitors, direct contamination by blood. The use of gauge isolators is essential, except with machines fitted with pressure transducers which can easily be cleaned.

Contaminated gauges must be cleaned and sterilized with ethylene oxide. Otherwise they should be replaced.

18.4   Peritoneal dialysis

18.4.1   ACUTE AND INTERMITTENT DIALYSIS

Peritoneal dialysis may be used for the treatment of acute renal failure, usually via a semi-rigid catheter inserted percutaneously into the abdomen followed by fairly rapid (e.g. hourly) exchanges of dialysis fluid, often with automated control of inflow and outflow using a suitable design of peritoneal dialysis machine. Such a procedure can also be applied intermittently to patients with chronic renal failure using a more permanent form of peritoneal access.

Sterile pyrogen-free solutions and sterile cannulae and tubing are required for this procedure. Bottles of dialysate should be inspected for evidence of bacterial or fungal contamination. Abdominal drainage should be through a closed system.

Adequate skin preparation and stringent aseptic techniques, as previously described, are required for insertion of the peritoneal cannula. A suture should be placed around the catheter and tied so that the latter cannot be pushed freely in and out by the staff attendant and the site should be covered by a simple gauze dressing.

Dialysis bottle tops should be adequately swabbed with alcoholic chlorhexidine or povidone-iodine solution before inserting needles.

Manual methods often include the use of a water bath or sink for warming the bottles of dialysate before use. This water is likely to become contaminated with Gram-negative bacilli, including *Pseudomonas* spp. The water should be changed frequently.

Automated systems for peritoneal dialysis usually include adequate instructions for sterilization.

Parts of the system likely to be in contact with dialysate must either be pre-sterilized disposable items, or be autoclaved.

Routine addition of prophylactic antibiotics to peritoneal dialysis fluid is not recommended. It is desirable to send samples to the laboratory every 24 hours for culture.

Peritoneal dialysis for chronic renal failure requires the use of a permanent indwelling silicone rubber peritoneal catheter. Such a catheter is plugged between use except when continuous dialysis is practised. The insertion and care of these catheters closely resembles the care of external arteriovenous shunts or cannulae. Whenever connections or disconnections are made, rigorous aseptic or no-touch techniques must be used. Peritonitis remains a common and serious complication of chronic peritoneal dialysis.

18.4.2 CONTINUOUS AMBULATORY PERITONEAL DIALYSIS (CAPD)

The technique of continuous ambulatory peritoneal dialysis (CAPD) utilizes plastic bags of dialysate which are changed by the patient several times daily. Patients must be taught to avoid contaminating the connections during these changes. Several types of connecting systems for CAPD are in use and the manufacturer's instructions for each pattern should be followed. Various methods are available to reduce contamination of the line, for example flushing with hypochlorites and use of disinfectant-impregnated cuffs (*Lancet* 1991; Ludlam, 1991) as well as systems using UV light and local heat application. Spraying with 70% ethanol is also effective. Systems are available which can be safely operated by blind patients. A type of connection is recommended which, while secure between bag changes, is easily undone by the patient with little risk of touching the parts coming in contact with dialysate. The catheter connection is usually changed periodically by the staff of the 'parent unit' using full aseptic precautions.

The major hazard of peritoneal dialysis is, of course, peritonitis. Infection in CAPD is most commonly by skin organisms, particularly *Staph. epidermidis*. There is no doubt that meticulous attention to detail, including catheter care and avoidance of wetting the exit site, greatly reduces the incidence of infection. Peritonitis, often indicated by cloudy dialysis effluent and abdominal pain, requires antibiotic therapy – often added to the peritoneal dialysis fluid. Whilst awaiting positive cultures a broad spectrum antibiotic regime, including drugs active against *Staph. epidermidis* is usually instituted. Gram-negative and particularly fungal infections usually require temporary removal of the peritoneal catheter.

18.5 Disinfection of equipment and materials (see also Chapter 7)

Equipment and materials should be autoclaved or heat-treated whenever possible. Chemical disinfection is less reliable. A strong chlorine-releasing agent yielding 1% (10 000 ppm) available chlorine should be used for removal of spilt blood and containers for discarded specimens of blood. A weaker solution containing 0.1% (1000 ppm) available chlorine should be used for routine environmental cleaning in a dialysis unit, or in rooms occupied by patients with hepatitis. Chlorine-releasing solutions may be corrosive to metals and fabrics, but some chlorine-releasing powders or newer agents, such as peroxygen compounds, are less so and may be preferred for use on equipment (section 18.3 above). Glutaraldehyde (2%) is less corrosive, but it may cause skin sensitization on repeated use, and its use should be avoided if possible. Iodophors are relatively non-corrosive and active against a wide range of bacteria. Their activity against enteroviruses is uncertain and at present chlorine-releasing agents are preferred if possible where a virucidal action is required in dialysis units.

18.6   Renal transplant units

The special problems associated with renal transplantation arise because of the effects of immunosuppressive agents used to prevent graft rejection. Many of the opportunistic infections in transplanted patients are due to organisms already carried by the patients, including the more common bacteria, *M. tuberculosis*, fungi, *Pneumocystis carinii*, Herpes simplex virus and cytomegalovirus. The latter infection may sometimes be transmitted in the actual graft. It is unwise to use organs from grossly infected donors and a routine culture should be taken from the donor fat and perfusate at the time of grafting. Donors should be screened for hepatitis B antigen and HIV antibodies.

Isolation practice varies between different units, but strict protective isolation with barrier nursing and positive pressure ventilation is not often used now because, with less intensive immunosuppression, it is felt that the possible benefits of strict isolation are outweighed by the difficulties of ensuring adequate patient care in this environment. Nevertheless, cross infection can be a major problem and isolation in cubicles is desirable during the first two weeks, or when steroid dosage is increased for rejection episodes. Staff should take every precaution to avoid transmitting infections from themselves or other patients, as described elsewhere in the book.

References

Advisory Committee on Dangerous Pathogens (1990) *HIV – the Causative Agent of AIDS and Related Conditions*, 2nd revision of guidelines. HMSO, London.

Boelart, J., De Smedt, R.A., De Baere, Y.A. *et al.* (1989) The influence of calcium mupirocin nasal ointment on the incidence of *Staphylococcus aureus* infections in haemodialysis patients. *Nephrology, Dialysis & Transplantation*, **4**, 278.

Department of Health and Social Security (1972) *Rosenheim Advisory Group: Hepatitis and the Treatment of Chronic Renal Failure*. HMSO, London.

EDTA (1978) *Proceedings of the European Dialysis and Transplant Association*, **15**, 66.

Hospital Infection Society (1990) Acquired Immunodeficiency Syndrome. Recommendations of a Working Party. *Journal of Hospital Infection*, **15**, 7.

Lancet. (1991) Editorial: Prevention of peritonitis in CAPD. **1**, 22.

Ludlam, H.A. (1991) Infectious consequences of continuous ambulatory peritoneal dialysis. *Journal of Hospital Infection*, **18** (Supplement A), 341.

Bibliography

Altemeier, W.A., Burke, J.F., Pruitt, B.A. and Sandusky, W.R. (ed. committee) (1984) *Manual on Control of Infection in Surgical Patients.* Lippincott, Philadelphia.

Ayliffe, G.A.J., Coates, D. and Hoffman, P.N. (1984) *Chemical Disinfection in Hospitals.* PHLS, London.

Ayliffe, G.A.J., Collins, B.J. and Taylor, L.J. (1990) *Hospital-Acquired Infection. Principles and Prevention.* John Wright, London.

Bartlett, C.L.R., Macrae, A.D. and Macfarlane, J.D. (1986) *Legionella Infections.* Edward Arnold, London.

Benenson, A.S. (1985) *Control of Communicable Disease in Man,* 14th edn. American Public Health Association, New York.

Bennett, J.V. and Brachman, P.S. (1986) *Hospital Infections,* 2nd edn. Little Brown, Boston.

Block, S.S. (1983) *Disinfection, Sterilization and Preservation,* 3rd edn. Lea & Febiger, Philadelphia.

Caddow, P. (1989) *Applied Microbiology.* Scutari Press, London.

Castle, M. and Ajemiam, E. (1987) *Hospital Infection Control: Principles and Practice,* 2nd edn. John Wiley, Chichester, New York.

Christie, A.B. (1987) *Infectious Diseases, Epidemiology and Clinical Practice,* 4th edn. Churchill Livingstone, Edinburgh.

Collins, C.H. (1988) *Laboratory-Acquired Infections.* Butterworths, London and Boston.

Crow, S. (1989) *Asepsis, the Right Touch.* Everett Co., Louisiana.

Daschner, F. (1986) *Forum Hygienicum. Hygiene in Praxis und Klinik.* (Handbook on Control of hospital infection, text in German). MMV Medizin Verlag, München.

Gardner, J.F. and Peel, M.M. (1991) *Introduction to Sterilization and Disinfection and Infection Control.* Churchill Livingstone, Edinburgh.

Haley, R.H. (1986) *Managing Hospital Control for Cost-effectiveness.* American Hospital Publishing, Chicago.

Hobbs, B.C. and Roberts, D. (1987) *Food Poisoning and Food Hygiene,* 5th edn. Edward Arnold, London.

Johnston, I.D.A. and Hunter, A.R. (1984) *The Design and Utilization of Operating Theatres.* Edward Arnold, London.

Mandell, G.L., Douglas, R.G. and Bennett, J.E. (1989) *Principles and Practice of Infectious Diseases.* Churchill Livingstone, Edinburgh.

Maurer, I.M. (1985) *Hospital Hygiene,* 3rd edn. Edward Arnold, London.

Parker, M.T. and Collier, L.H. (1990) *Topley and Wilson's Principles of Bacteriology, Virology and Immunity,* 8th edn. Edward Arnold, London.

Russell, A.D., Hugo, W.B., and Ayliffe, G.A.J. (Editors) (1992) *Principles and Practice of Disinfection, Preservation and Sterilization.* Blackwell Scientific Publications, Oxford.

Shanson, D.C. (1989) *Microbiology in Clinical Practice*, 2nd edn. John Wright, Bristol.

Sim, J.W. and Jeffries, D.J. (1990) *AIDS and Surgery*. Blackwell Scientific Publications, Oxford.

Slade, N. and Gillespie, W.A. (1985) *The Urinary Tract and the Catheter: Infection and Other Problems*. John Wiley, Chichester, New York.

Weber, W.C. and Rutala, W.A. (1989) Nosocomial infections: New issues and strategies for prevention. *Infectious Disease Clinics of America*, **3**(4), W.B. Saunders, Philadelphia.

Wenzel, R.P. (1987) *Prevention and Control of Nosocomial Infections*. Williams & Wilkins, Baltimore.

Williams, R.E.O., Blowers, R., Garrod, L.P. and Shooter, R.A. (1966) *Hospital Infection: Causes and Prevention*, 2nd edn. Lloyd-Luke, London.

Willis, A.T. (1977) *Anaerobic Bacteriology: Clinical and Laboratory Practice*, 3rd edn. Butterworth, London and Boston.

Worsley, M.A., Ward, K.A., Parker, L., Ayliffe, G.A.J., and Sedgwick, J.A. (1990) *Infection Control: Guidelines for Nursing Care*. ICNA, Great Britain.

Index